Gynecologic Imaging

Editor

KATHERINE E. MATUREN

MAGNETIC RESONANCE IMAGING
CLINICS OF NORTH AMERICA

www.mri.theclinics.com

Consulting Editors
SURESH K. MUKHERJI
LYNNE S. STEINBACH

August 2017 • Volume 25 • Number 3

ELSEVIER

1600 John F. Kennedy Boulevard • Suite 1800 • Philadelphia, Pennsylvania, 19103-2899

http://www.mri.theclinics.com

MRI CLINICS OF NORTH AMERICA Volume 25, Number 3
August 2017 ISSN 1064-9689, ISBN 13: 978-0-323-53241-9

Editor: John Vassallo (j.vassallo@elsevier.com)
Developmental Editor: Meredith Madeira

Magnetic Resonance Imaging Clinics of North America (ISSN 1064-9689) is published quarterly by Elsevier Inc., 360 Park Avenue South, New York, NY 10010-1710. Months of issue are February, May, August, and November. Business and Editorial Offices: 1600 John F. Kennedy Blvd., Ste. 1800, Philadelphia, PA 19103-2899. Customer Service Office: 3251 Riverport Lane, Maryland Heights, MO 63043. Periodicals postage paid at New York, NY and additional mailing offices. Subscription prices are $380.00 per year (domestic individuals), $661.00 per year (domestic institutions), $100.00 per year (domestic students/residents), $420.00 per year (Canadian individuals), $861.00 per year (Canadian institutions), $545.00 per year (international individuals), $861.00 per year (international institutions), and $275.00 per year (international and Canadian students/residents). International air speed delivery is included in all *Clinics* subscription prices. All prices are subject to change without notice. **POSTMASTER:** Send address changes to *Magnetic Resonance Imaging Clinics*, Elsevier Health Sciences Division, Subscription Customer Service, 3251 Riverport Lane, Maryland Heights, MO 63043. Customer Service (orders, claims, online, change of address): Elsevier Health Sciences Division, Subscription **Customer Service, 3251 Riverport Lane, Maryland Heights, MO 63043. Tel:1-800-654-2452 (U.S. and Canada); 314-447-8871 (outside U.S. and Canada). Fax: 314-447-8029. E-mail: journalscustomerservice-usa@elsevier.com (for print support); journalsonlinesupport-usa@elsevier.com (for online support).**

Reprints. For copies of 100 or more of articles in this publication, please contact the Commercial Reprints Department, Elsevier Inc., 360 Park Avenue South, New York, NY 10010-1710. Tel.: 212-633-3874; Fax: 212-633-3820; E-mail: reprints@elsevier.com.

Magnetic Resonance Imaging Clinics of North America is covered in the *RSNA Index of Imaging Literature, MEDLINE/PubMed (Index Medicus),* and *EMBASE/Excerpta Medica*.

Contributors

CONSULTING EDITORS

SURESH K. MUKHERJI, MD, MBA, FACR
Department of Radiology, Michigan State University, East Lansing, Michigan

LYNNE S. STEINBACH, MD, FACR
Professor of Radiology and Orthopaedic Surgery, Department of Radiology and Biomedical Imaging, University of California, San Francisco, San Francisco, California

EDITOR

KATHERINE E. MATUREN, MD, MS
Associate Professor, Departments of Radiology and Obstetrics and Gynecology, Abdominal Radiology Fellowship Director, University of Michigan Health System, University of Michigan, Ann Arbor, Michigan

AUTHORS

MONICA D. AGARWAL, MD
Abdominal Imaging Section, Department of Radiology, Beth Israel Deaconess Medical Center, Boston, Massachusetts

BETHANY ANDERSON, MD
Department of Radiation Oncology, University of Wisconsin Hospital and Clinics, Madison, Wisconsin

LISA BARROILHET, MD
Department of Obstetrics and Gynecology, University of Wisconsin Hospital and Clinics, Madison, Wisconsin

SPENCER C. BEHR, MD
Assistant Professor, Department of Radiology and Biomedical Imaging, University of California, San Francisco, San Francisco, California

JAMES BOYUM, MD
Department of Radiology, Mayo Clinic, Rochester, Minnesota

JOCELYN S. CHAPMAN, MD
Assistant Professor, Department of Obstetrics, Gynecology and Reproductive Services, University of California, San Francisco, San Francisco, California

LEE-MAY CHEN, MD
Professor, Department of Obstetrics, Gynecology and Reproductive Services, University of California, San Francisco, San Francisco, California

SUZANNE T. CHONG, MD, MS
Emergency Radiology Division, Department of Radiology, University of Michigan Health System, Ann Arbor, Michigan

PIERRE EMMANUEL COLOMBO, MD, PhD
Department of Surgery, Montpellier Cancer institute, Montpellier, France

DANIA DAYE, MD, PhD
Resident, Department of Radiology, Massachusetts General Hospital, Harvard Medical School, Boston, Massachusetts

ALBERTO DIAZ DE LEON, MD
Assistant Professor, Division of Abdominal Imaging MRI, Department of Radiology, University of Texas Southwestern Medical Center, Dallas, Texas

MANJIRI DIGHE, MD
Section Chief, Director of Ultrasound, Professor, Radiology, UWMC, University of Washington, Seattle, Washington

SHINYA FUJII, MD, PhD
Department of Radiology, Tottori University, Tottori, Japan

MARTA E. HEILBRUN, MD
Department of Radiology and Imaging Sciences, University of Utah, Salt Lake City, Utah

THOMAS A. HOPE, MD
Assistant Professor, Department of Radiology and Biomedical Imaging, University of California, San Francisco, Department of Radiology, San Francisco Veterans Affairs Hospital, San Francisco, California

SHRUTI JOLLY, MD
Department of Radiation Oncology, University of Michigan Health System, Ann Arbor, Michigan

AYA KAMAYA, MD
Associate Professor, Department of Radiology, Stanford University Medical Center, Stanford University, Stanford, California

ZAHRA KASSAM, MD, FRCPC
Assistant Professor, Diagnostic Radiology and Oncology, Department of Medical Imaging, Western University, Associate Scientist, Lawson Health Research Institute, St. Joseph's Health Care, London, Ontario, Canada

GAURAV KHATRI, MD
Assistant Professor, Division of Body MRI, Department of Radiology, University of Texas Southwestern Medical Center, Dallas, Texas

URSULA S. KNOEPP, MD
Emergency Radiology Division, Department of Radiology, University of Michigan Health System, Ann Arbor, Michigan

YULIA LAKHMAN, MD
Department of Radiology, Memorial Sloan Kettering Cancer Center, New York, New York

SUSANNA I. LEE, MD, PhD
Associate Professor of Radiology, Department of Radiology, Massachusetts General Hospital, Harvard Medical School, Boston, Massachusetts

MARK E. LOCKHART, MD, MPH
Chief, Abdominal Imaging, Professor, Department of Radiology, University of Alabama at Birmingham, Birmingham, Alabama

WILLIAM R. MASCH, MD
Assistant Professor, Department of Radiology, University of Michigan Health System, Ann Arbor, Michigan

KATHERINE E. MATUREN, MD, MS
Associate Professor, Departments of Radiology and Obstetrics and Gynecology, Abdominal Radiology Fellowship Director, University of Michigan Health System, University of Michigan, Ann Arbor, Michigan

MICHAEL B. MAZZA, MD
Emergency Radiology Division, Department of Radiology, University of Michigan Health System, Ann Arbor, Michigan

CHRISTINE O. MENIAS, MD
Professor, Department of Radiology, Mayo Clinic in Arizona, Scottsdale, Arizona

JENNIFER NI MHUIRCHEARTAIGH, MBBCh
Abdominal Imaging Section, Department of Radiology, Beth Israel Deaconess Medical Center, Boston, Massachusetts

AIDA MOENI, MD
Department of Radiology and Imaging Sciences, University of Utah, Salt Lake City, Utah

KOENRAAD J. MORTELE, MD
Abdominal Imaging Section, Department of Radiology, Beth Israel Deaconess Medical Center, Boston, Massachusetts

STEPHANIE NOUGARET, MD, PhD
IRCM, Montpellier Cancer Research institute, Department of Radiology, Montpellier Cancer institute, INSERM, U1194, University of Montpellier, Montpellier, France

MICHAEL A. OHLIGER, MD, PhD
Assistant Professor, Department of Radiology and Biomedical Imaging, University of California, San Francisco, Department of Radiology, Zuckerberg San Francisco General Hospital, San Francisco, California

JEFFREY D. OLPIN, MD
Department of Radiology and Imaging Sciences, University of Utah, Salt Lake City, Utah

KRUPA PATEL-LIPPMANN, MD
Department of Radiology and Radiological Sciences, Vanderbilt University, Nashville, Tennessee

IVA PETKOVSKA, MD
Assistant Professor of Radiology, Weill Cornell Medical Center, Staff Radiologist, Department of Radiology, Memorial Sloan Kettering Cancer Center, New York, New York; Assistant Professor, Department of Medical Imaging, University of Arizona, Tucson, Arizona

LIINA PODER, MD
Professor, Department of Radiology and Biomedical Imaging, University of California, San Francisco, San Francisco, California

CAROLINE REINHOLD, MD, MSc
Department of Radiology, McGill University, Montreal, Quebec, Canada

ELENA L. RESNICK, MD
Abdominal Imaging Section, Department of Radiology, Beth Israel Deaconess Medical Center, Boston, Massachusetts

JESSICA B. ROBBINS, MD
Department of Radiology, University of Wisconsin Hospital and Clinics, University of Wisconsin School of Medicine and Public Health, Madison, Wisconsin

ELIZABETH A. SADOWSKI, MD
Departments of Radiology and Obstetrics and Gynecology, University of Wisconsin Hospital and Clinics, Departments of Radiology and Obstetrics and Gynecology, University of Wisconsin School of Medicine and Public Health, Madison, Wisconsin

EVIS SALA, MD, PhD
Department of Radiology, Memorial Sloan Kettering Cancer Center, New York, New York

ANDREW P. SCIALLIS, MD
Assistant Professor, Department of Pathology, University of Michigan, Ann Arbor, Michigan

ANUP S. SHETTY, MD
Assistant Professor of Radiology, Mallinckrodt of Institute Radiology, Washington University School of Medicine, St Louis, Missouri

ERICA B. STEIN, MD
Assistant Professor, Department of Radiology, University of Michigan, Ann Arbor, Michigan; Department of Radiology, University of Pittsburgh Medical Center, Pittsburgh, Pennsylvania

ANGELA M. TRINH, MD
Staff Radiologist, Sutter Medical Foundation, Sacramento, California

HEBERT ALBERTO VARGAS, MD
Department of Radiology, Memorial Sloan Kettering Cancer Center, New York, New York

CAROLYN L. WANG, MD
Assistant Professor of Radiology, University of Washington, Seattle, Washington

ASHISH P. WASNIK, MD
Assistant Professor, Abdominal Imaging Division, Department of Radiology, University of Michigan Health System, University of Michigan, Ann Arbor, Michigan

RODERICK J. WILLMORE, MD
Department of Radiology and Imaging Sciences, University of Utah, Salt Lake City, Utah

Contents

Foreword xv

Suresh K. Mukherji

Preface: Be an Advocate for Women's Health: Get a Pelvic MRI xvii

Katherine E. Maturen

MR Imaging of the Female Perineum: Clitoris, Labia, and Introitus 435

Monica D. Agarwal, Elena L. Resnick, Jennifer Ni Mhuircheartaigh, and Koenraad J. Mortele

The female perineum has a complex anatomy and can be involved by a wide range of pathologies. In this article, we specifically focus on the clitoris, labia, and introitus. We discuss the normal anatomy of these structures, the MR imaging techniques to optimize their evaluation, and several common and uncommon entities that may affect them, including benign and malignant tumors, as well as infectious and inflammatory, vascular, iatrogenic, and developmental entities.

MR Imaging of the Pelvic Floor 457

Gaurav Khatri, Alberto Diaz de Leon, and Mark E. Lockhart

Pelvic floor dysfunction is a term used to describe a broad set of conditions including pelvic organ prolapse, urinary or fecal incontinence, defecatory dysfunction, and chronic pelvic pain that frequently affects multiple compartments of the pelvic floor. Imaging is important, because physical examination may not be adequate as the only means of evaluating pelvic floor disorders. This article reviews pertinent pelvic floor anatomy as well as the technique for performing, interpreting, and reporting abnormalities seen on MR defecography examinations in the anterior, middle, and posterior compartments.

MR Imaging of Vulvar and Vaginal Cancer 481

Anup S. Shetty and Christine O. Menias

Vulvar and vaginal cancer are uncommon gynecologic malignancies, most frequently diagnosed clinically. MR imaging is a powerful tool for local staging of these tumors and to detect posttreatment complications and recurrent disease. This review presents anatomic delineation of the female pelvis, pathology and staging of vulvar and vaginal cancer, MR imaging techniques of the pelvis, MR features of vulvar and vaginal cancer, and the differential diagnosis of potential mimickers.

MR Imaging of Pelvic Emergencies in Women 503

Ursula S. Knoepp, Michael B. Mazza, Suzanne T. Chong, and Ashish P. Wasnik

MR imaging is a useful adjunct imaging modality for evaluating women presenting with acute lower abdominal/pelvic pain who have negative or inconclusive sonographic findings. In pregnant women, although obstetric complications are of prime concern, gastrointestinal pathologies also warrant careful attention, and MR imaging is often useful in refining the diagnosis. In nonpregnant women, gynecologic pathologies and gastrointestinal pathologies are of major concern, and may necessitate evaluation with MR imaging. Knowledge of imaging features in the appropriate

clinical setting helps in early and accurate diagnosis, enabling timely management for better clinical outcomes.

MR Imaging for Incidental Adnexal Mass Characterization 521

William R. Masch, Dania Daye, and Susanna I. Lee

Incidentally detected adnexal masses are common, and the overwhelming majority of them are benign. As many of these adnexal masses are considered indeterminate at CT or US, a large number of benign oophorectomies occur. Of the malignant adnexal masses, high-grade primary ovarian neoplasms with fast doubling times and early dissemination are the most common. Due to their aggressive behavior, diagnosis of malignancy by interval growth on surveillance imaging represents an undesirable option. Immediate MR characterization allows for a decreased rate of benign oophorectomies and expedited triage of patients to definitive treatment when malignancy is suspected.

MR Imaging–Pathologic Correlation in Ovarian Cancer 545

Erica B. Stein, Ashish P. Wasnik, Andrew P. Sciallis, Aya Kamaya, and Katherine E. Maturen

There are many ovarian cancer subtypes, giving rise to a range of appearances at gross pathology and magnetic resonance (MR) imaging. Certain fundamental concepts at MR, arising from underlying tissue characteristics, can provide guidance to radiologists in suggesting a diagnosis. The ability of multiparametric MR to risk stratify ovarian masses can contribute substantially to clinical decision making and patient management.

MR Imaging of Müllerian Fusion Anomalies 563

Jeffrey D. Olpin, Aida Moeni, Roderick J. Willmore, and Marta E. Heilbrun

Müllerian duct anomalies, also called congenital uterine anomalies, are developmental structural disorders of the female genital tract. These anomalies are clinically relevant in patients with a history of infertility and pregnancy-related complications. The American Society for Reproductive Medicine classification system is the most well known, although newer systems, such as from the European Society of Human Reproduction and Embryology/European Society for Gynaecological Endoscopy, are becoming more widely accepted. MR imaging remains the optimal imaging modality due to its superior multiplanar capability and spatial resolution. This review article describes the typical MR appearance of congenital uterine anomalies.

Benign Gynecologic Conditions of the Uterus 577

Zahra Kassam, Iva Petkovska, Carolyn L. Wang, Angela M. Trinh, and Aya Kamaya

In this article, the authors review the anatomy, pathophysiology, MR imaging features, and diagnostic criteria for benign uterine conditions, including adenomyosis, uterine leiomyomas, retained products of conception, and uterine arteriovenous malformations. Pearls, pitfalls, and variants are discussed for each entity as well as important imaging features that can affect management decisions.

MR Imaging of Abnormal Placentation 601

Manjiri Dighe

Morbidly adherent placenta (MAP) encompasses a spectrum of conditions characterized by abnormal adherence of the placenta to the implantation site. Classification

of MAP is based on the degree of trophoblastic invasion through myometrium and uterine serosa and includes accrete, when the villi are attached to the myometrium but do not invade the muscle; increta, when the placenta invades partially through the myometrium; and percreta, when it invades up to and beyond the uterine serosa. Knowledge of the common findings of MAP on MR imaging is important to be able to provide an accurate diagnosis.

From Staging to Prognostication: Achievements and Challenges of MR Imaging in the Assessment of Endometrial Cancer **611**

Stephanie Nougaret, Yulia Lakhman, Hebert Alberto Vargas, Pierre Emmanuel Colombo, Shinya Fujii, Caroline Reinhold, and Evis Sala

Endometrial cancer is the most common gynecologic malignancy in the United States, with recent increasing incidence mostly owing to obesity. Preoperative MR imaging is essential to stratify patients according to their risk of recurrence and to guide surgical management. In the combination of T2-weighted imaging, diffusion-weighted imaging, and dynamic contrast enhancement, MR imaging provides a "one-stop shop" approach for patient-specific accurate staging including the evaluation of the depth of myometrial invasion, cervical stromal invasion, extrauterine extension, and lymph node status.

MR Imaging of Cervical Cancer **635**

Krupa Patel-Lippmann, Jessica B. Robbins, Lisa Barroilhet, Bethany Anderson, Elizabeth A. Sadowski, and James Boyum

Cervical cancer is a significant cause of morbidity and mortality worldwide despite advances in screening and prevention. Although cervical cancer remains clinically staged, the 2009 International Federation of Gynecology and Obstetrics committee has encouraged the use of advanced imaging modalities, including MR imaging, where available, to increase the accuracy of staging, guide treatment, and detect recurrence. Understanding the multiple roles of advanced imaging in the evaluation of cervical cancer will help radiologists provide an accurate and useful report to the referring clinicians.

MR Imaging in Gynecologic Brachytherapy **651**

Jessica B. Robbins, Elizabeth A. Sadowski, Shruti Jolly, and Katherine E. Maturen

Magnetic resonance–based image-guided adaptive brachytherapy is gaining popularity in the United States in the setting of gynecologic malignancies. This technique improves local control, increases overall survival, and minimizes toxicity to the adjacent organs at risk. The purpose of this article is to familiarize radiologists with image-guided adaptive brachytherapy by describing its history, detailing MR imaging techniques, describing treatment considerations, and reviewing image interpretation.

PET/MR Imaging in Gynecologic Oncology **667**

Michael A. Ohliger, Thomas A. Hope, Jocelyn S. Chapman, Lee-may Chen, Spencer C. Behr, and Liina Poder

MR imaging and PET using 2-Deoxy-2-[^{18}F]fluoroglucose (FDG) are both useful in the evaluation of gynecologic malignancies. MR imaging is superior for local staging of disease whereas fludeoxyglucose FDG PET is superior for detecting distant

metastases. Integrated PET/MR imaging scanners have great promise for gynecologic malignancies by combining the advantages of each modality into a single scan. This article reviews the technology behind PET/MR imaging acquisitions and technical challenges relevant to imaging the pelvis. A dedicated PET/MR imaging protocol; the roles of PET and MR imaging in cervical, endometrial, and ovarian cancers; and future directions for PET/MR imaging are discussed.

MAGNETIC RESONANCE IMAGING CLINICS OF NORTH AMERICA

FORTHCOMING ISSUES

November 2017
Update on Imaging Contrast Agents
Carlos A. Zamora and Mauricio Castillo, *Editors*

February 2018
Update in Head and Neck Imaging
Girish M. Fatterpekar, *Editor*

May 2018
Breast Cancer
Jessica W.T. Leung, *Editor*

RECENT ISSUES

May 2017
Hybrid PET/MR Imaging
Weili Lin, Sheng-Che Hung, Yueh Z. Lee, and Terence Z. Wong, *Editors*

February 2017
MR Imaging of the Foot and Ankle
Mary G. Hochman, *Editor*

November 2016
Imaging of Brain Tumors
Rivka R. Colen, *Editor*

ISSUE OF RELATED INTEREST

Radiologic Clinics, May 2017 (Vol. 55, No. 3)
Breast Imaging
Sarah M. Friedewald, *Editor*
Available at: www.radiologic.theclinics.com

PROGRAM OBJECTIVE

The goal of *Magnetic Resonance Imaging Clinics of North America* is to keep practicing physicians up to date with current clinical practice by providing timely articles reviewing the state of the art in patient care.

TARGET AUDIENCE

All practicing physicians and healthcare professionals who provide patient care utilizing findings from Magnetic Resonance Imaging.

LEARNING OBJECTIVES

Upon completion of this activity, participants will be able to:

1. Review imaging techniques of the pelvic floor.
2. Discuss innovations in imaging of gynecologic oncology.
3. Recognize updates in MR/PET imaging for gynecologic abnormalities.

ACCREDITATION

The Elsevier Office of Continuing Medical Education (EOCME) is accredited by the Accreditation Council for Continuing Medical Education (ACCME) to provide continuing medical education for physicians.

The EOCME designates this enduring material for a maximum of 15 *AMA PRA Category 1 Credit*(s)™. Physicians should claim only the credit commensurate with the extent of their participation in the activity.

All other health care professionals requesting continuing education credit for this enduring material will be issued a certificate of participation.

DISCLOSURE OF CONFLICTS OF INTEREST

The EOCME assesses conflict of interest with its instructors, faculty, planners, and other individuals who are in a position to control the content of CME activities. All relevant conflicts of interest that are identified are thoroughly vetted by EOCME for fair balance, scientific objectivity, and patient care recommendations. EOCME is committed to providing its learners with CME activities that promote improvements or quality in healthcare and not a specific proprietary business or a commercial interest.

The planning committee, staff, authors and editors listed below have identified no financial relationships or relationships to products or devices they or their spouse/life partner have with commercial interest related to the content of this CME activity:

Monica D. Agarwal, MD; Hebert Alberto Vargas, MD; Bethany Anderson, MD; Lisa Barroilhet, MD; James Boyum, MD; Jocelyn S. Chapman, MD; Lee-may Chen, MD; Suzanne T. Chong, MD, MS; Dania Daye, MD, PhD; Alberto Diaz de Leon, MD; Pierre Emmanuel Colombo, MD, PhD; Anjali Fortna; Shinya Fujii, MD, PhD; Marta E. Heilbrun, MD; Shruti Jolly, MD; Aya Kamaya, MD; Zahra Kassam, MD, FRCPC; Gaurav Khatri, MD; Ursula S. Knoepp, MD; Yulia Lakhman, MD; Susanna I. Lee, MD, PhD; William R. Masch, MD; Katherine E. Maturen, MD, MS; Michael B Mazza, MD; Christine O. Menias, MD; Aida Moeni, MD; Koenraad J. Mortele, MD; Suresh K. Mukherji, MD, MBA, FACR; Jennifer Ni Mhuircheartaigh, MBBCh; Stephanie Nougaret, MD, PhD; Michael A. Ohliger, MD, PhD; Jeffrey D. Olpin, MD; Krupa Patel-Lippmann, MD; Iva Petkovska, MD; Liina Poder, MD; Caroline Reinhold, MD, MSc; Elena L. Resnick, MD; Jessica B. Robbins, MD; Elizabeth A. Sadowski, MD; Evis Sala, MD, PhD; Andrew P. Sciallis, MD; Anup S. Shetty, MD; Erica B. Stein, MD; Karthik Subramaniam; John Vassallo; Carolyn L. Wang, MD; Ashish P. Wasnik, MD; Katie Widmeier; Amy Williams; Roderick J. Willmore, MD.

The planning committee, staff, authors and editors listed below have identified financial relationships or relationships to products or devices they or their spouse/life partner have with commercial interest related to the content of this CME activity:

Spencer C. Behr, MD has research support from General Electric Company and Cancer Targeted Technologies.
Manjiri Dighe, MD is on the speakers' bureau for, with research support from, Koninklijke Philips N.V.
Thomas A. Hope, MD has research support from General Electric Company.
Mark E. Lockhart, MD, MPH is a consultant/advisor John Wiley & Sons, Inc, and receives royalties/patents from Oxford University Press.

UNAPPROVED/OFF-LABEL USE DISCLOSURE

The EOCME requires CME faculty to disclose to the participants:

1. When products or procedures being discussed are off-label, unlabelled, experimental, and/or investigational (not US Food and Drug Administration [FDA] approved); and
2. Any limitations on the information presented, such as data that are preliminary or that represent ongoing research, interim analyses, and/or unsupported opinions. Faculty may discuss information about pharmaceutical agents that is outside of FDA-approved labelling. This information is intended solely for CME and is not intended to promote off-label use of these medications. If you have any questions, contact the medical affairs department of the manufacturer for the most recent prescribing information.

TO ENROLL

To enroll in the *Magnetic Resonance Imaging Clinics of North America* Continuing Medical Education program, call customer service at 1-800-654-2452 or sign up online at http://www.theclinics.com/home/cme. The CME program is available to subscribers for an additional annual fee of USD $250.

METHOD OF PARTICIPATION

In order to claim credit, participants must complete the following:

1. Complete enrolment as indicated above.
2. Read the activity.
3. Complete the CME Test and Evaluation. Participants must achieve a score of 70% on the test. All CME Tests and Evaluations must be completed online.

CME INQUIRIES/SPECIAL NEEDS

For all CME inquiries or special needs, please contact elsevierCME@elsevier.com.

Foreword

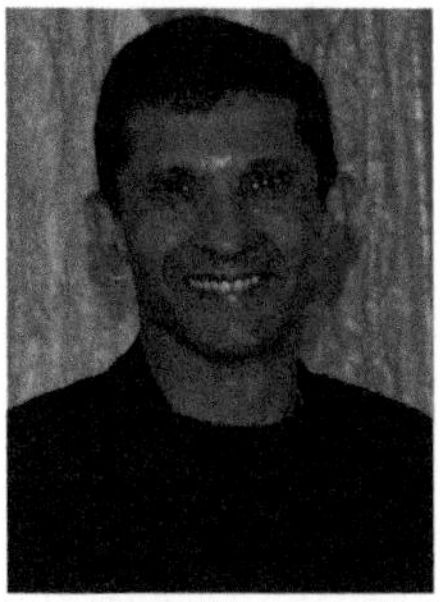

Suresh K. Mukherji, MD, MBA, FACR
Consulting Editor

This issue of *Magnetic Resonance Imaging Clinics of North America* is dedicated to the topic of MR imaging of the female pelvis. This is a very important topic that directly affects diagnosis, management, and treatment of numerous disorders. Ultrasound maintains its rightful place as the primary diagnostic imaging modality for women with pelvic symptoms and suspected gynecologic pathology. However, MR imaging provides detailed anatomic information that can direct management in a variety of disorders. MR imaging also enables tissue characterization essential to evaluation of uterine pathologies, sonographically indeterminate adnexal masses, and female pelvic emergencies. Dynamic MR imaging provides the unique opportunity to evaluate anatomically detailed muscular function. I want to personally thank all of the world-class authors for their outstanding contributions. The articles are superb, and I am very grateful for their tireless efforts.

I especially wish to thank Dr Kate Maturen for creating such an outstanding issue. Kate was one of my residents when I was at University of Michigan. There is no greater pleasure in academic medicine than watching your trainees succeed. Kate was always a "superstar" resident, and she is clearly destined to an outstanding academic career. I know very little about abdominopelvic imaging, so I can say with complete certainty I did nothing to contribute to her field of expertise! However, I am *thrilled* I have the privilege of being able to call such an outstanding radiologist a colleague and friend. Thank you, Kate!

Suresh K. Mukherji, MD, MBA, FACR
Department of Radiology
Michigan State University
846 Service Road
East Lansing, MI 48824, USA

E-mail address:
mukherji@rad.msu.edu

Magn Reson Imaging Clin N Am 25 (2017) xv
http://dx.doi.org/10.1016/j.mric.2017.05.001

Preface

Be an Advocate for Women's Health: Get a Pelvic MRI

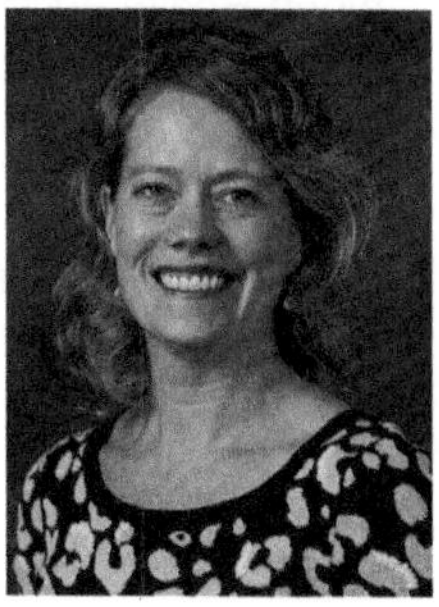

Katherine E. Maturen, MD, MS
Editor

Ultrasound maintains its rightful place as the primary diagnostic imaging modality for women with pelvic symptoms and suspected gynecologic pathology. Ultrasound is safe, inexpensive, and widely available, and often addresses the clinical question succinctly. But sometimes we need more. This issue is intended to expand the reader's understanding of the complementary role of MR imaging to ultrasound in the female pelvis, and the additional information this advanced modality can provide. An analogy can be made to neuroimaging: when head CT is not enough, MR imaging is widely accepted as the noninvasive next step. Likewise, when a gynecologic process is poorly seen or incompletely characterized by ultrasound, MR imaging is the natural next step. This concept is increasingly recognized by both gynecologists and radiologists, and it is my hope that the excellent review articles in this issue will help to spread the word further. We owe it to our patients to maximize the diagnostic value of MR imaging, by adapting and refining pelvic imaging protocols and developing expertise in interpretation.

MR imaging provides detailed anatomic information that can direct management in congenital uterine anomalies, disorders of placentation, and a variety of lesions of the perineum. MR imaging also enables tissue characterization essential to evaluation of benign uterine abnormalities, sonographically indeterminate adnexal masses, and triage of female pelvic emergencies. For pelvic floor disorders, dynamic imaging protocols illustrate muscular function in concert with anatomic detail fundamental to treatment planning. Finally, MR imaging pairs exquisite spatial and contrast resolution with functional imaging (including DWI, dynamic or multiphasic post contrast acquisitions, and even PET coregistration), enabling preoperative staging and treatment planning of locally advanced gynecologic cancers. The potential of MR imaging to contribute to gynecologic oncology care has yet to be fully actualized internationally, but its value for staging and surveillance of locally advanced cervical, endometrial, and vulvar cancers is acknowledged in the National Comprehensive Cancer Network Guidelines and the American College of Radiology Appropriateness Criteria, as well as important European consensus guidelines.

I am grateful for the time and expertise of the authors who have contributed the well-written and beautifully illustrated articles for this issue. Many of the authors are mentors, colleagues, and friends. Their work expertly demonstrates the great importance of subspecialty gynecologic imaging. Several of the authors are members of the Society of Abdominal Radiology Uterine and Ovarian Cancer Disease Focused Panel, and I would like to acknowledge both the society and the members of the panel for their efforts in moving the field forward. On a personal level, I would like to thank Dr Shruti Jolly, a talented radiation oncologist at the University of Michigan, who specializes in gynecologic cancer, as well as all of the

Magn Reson Imaging Clin N Am 25 (2017) xvii–xviii
http://dx.doi.org/10.1016/j.mric.2017.03.014
1064-9689/17/© 2017 Published by Elsevier Inc.

other members of the UM Gynecologic Oncology tumor board. They have taught me most of what I know about these diseases and helped to direct the course of my career by involving me in their clinical work. I would also like to thank my ever-supportive husband, Geoff, and our wonderful children, Iris and Julian, for their indulgence toward my work on this and other projects.

Finally, and most importantly, this issue of *Magnetic Resonance Imaging Clinics of North America* is dedicated to women's health care providers, honoring their commitment both to their patients and to maintaining widespread accessibility of high-quality gynecologic and reproductive health care.

Katherine E. Maturen, MD, MS
Departments of Radiology
and Obstetrics & Gynecology
University of Michigan Health Systems
1500 E Medical Center Drive, UH B1D530
Ann Arbor, MI 48109, USA

E-mail address:
kmaturen@umich.edu

MR Imaging of the Female Perineum

Clitoris, Labia, and Introitus

Monica D. Agarwal, MD, Elena L. Resnick, MD,
Jennifer Ni Mhuircheartaigh, MBBCh,
Koenraad J. Mortele, MD*

KEYWORDS

• MR imaging • Perineum • Clitoris • Introitus • Labia • Female

KEY POINTS

- A variety of common and uncommon pathologies affect the clitoris, labia, and introitus.
- These can be better evaluated by knowledge of the normal anatomy and optimized MR imaging techniques to facilitate observation of these entities.
- This is important to avoid unnecessary surgeries for benign conditions and to assist with surgical planning.

INTRODUCTION

MR imaging is an ideal technique to evaluate the female perineal structures owing to its excellent soft tissue contrast differentiation, high sensitivity to detect fluid, and multiplanar imaging capability.[1–3] In this article, we specifically focus on the evaluation of the clitoris, labia, and introitus. We discuss the normal anatomy of these structures, techniques to optimize their MR imaging evaluation, and several common and uncommon entities that may affect them. Knowledge of these conditions can prevent unnecessary surgeries in benign entities and assist with preoperative planning when surgery is needed.

NORMAL ANATOMY

The female perineal anatomy is complex.[4] The mons pubis is adipose tissue that overlies the pubic symphysis and separates inferiorly into thick skin folds, which are the labia majora,[4] bilateral anterior structures at the medial borders of the thighs.[3] The labia minora arise at the medial borders of the labia majora in the midline.[3,4] The anterior borders of the labia minora fuse at the level of the clitoral glans, forming the clitoral dorsal hood or prepuce.[3,4]

The clitoris is a pyramidal structure with the distal urethra and vagina as a core in the midline.[4,5] It is deep to the labia minora and the bulbospongiosus and ischiocavernosus muscles.[5] The clitoris and the perineal neurovascular bundles are large, paired terminations of the pudendal neurovascular bundles.[5] The clitoris is composed of erectile tissue (paired crura, bulbs, and corpora) and a nonerectile tip (glans),[3–6] as detailed below (**Fig. 1**).

Crura

- Parallel and medial to the ischiopubic rami
- Each tapers posteriorly to a thin line that becomes continuous with the ischiocavernosus muscle (dark on MR imaging)

The authors have nothing to disclose.

Abdominal Imaging Section, Department of Radiology, Beth Israel Deaconess Medical Center, 330 Brookline Avenue, Boston, MA 02215, USA
* Corresponding author. Beth Israel Deaconess Medical Center, 330 Brookline Avenue, Ansin 225, Boston, MA 02215.
E-mail address: kmortele@bidmc.harvard.edu

Magn Reson Imaging Clin N Am 25 (2017) 435–455
http://dx.doi.org/10.1016/j.mric.2017.03.011

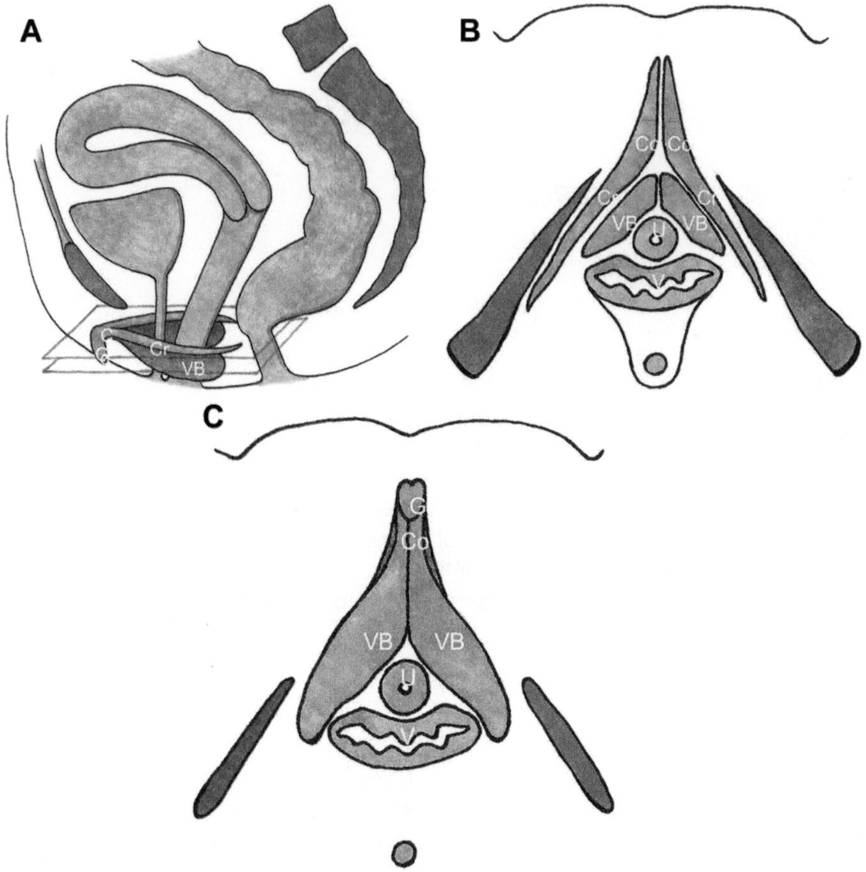

Fig. 1. (*A*) Sagittal diagram of pelvis including clitoris. Paired erectile tissue of the crura cranially (Cr) and vestibular bulbs caudally (VB) combine to form the corpora (Co). Glans (G) extends inferiorly from the corpora and is partially external. (*B*) Axial diagram of the cranial aspect of the clitoris. Paired Cr laterally, VB medially, and Co comprise the pyramidal clitoris, surrounding the distal urethra (U) and vagina (V). (*C*) Axial diagram of caudal aspect of the clitoris. The bulk of the VB extends inferiorly into the labia and continue anteriorly as the Co. The glans extends further inferiorly, originating at the inferior margin of the Co.

- Each continues anteriorly as the bodies (corpora)

Bodies (Corpora)

- Formed by 2 corpora cavernosa within a fibrous envelope, separated by an incomplete septum
- Start posteriorly as the crura and join anteriorly as a single body
- Descends and folds back on itself in a "boomerang-like" shape (best seen on the sagittal view)
- Superior body is attached by the deep suspensory ligament to pubic symphysis undersurface
- Most caudal part is contiguous with the glans

Bulbs

- Paramedian erectile tissue, parallel to the crura
- Surround urethra and vagina anterolaterally
- Convene anteriorly at the commissure, ventral to the urethra and close to the body and glans
- There may be point(s) of communication between commissure of the bulbs and the clitoral bodies

Glans

- Nonerectile tissue
- Caudal end of the body
- Partly external
- Projects into the mons pubic fat
- Midline septum is evident

The ischiocavernosus muscles cover the crura and attach to the ischiopubic rami, aiding in clitoral erection in combination with the bulbospongiosus mucles.[4] There is no difference in clitoral morphology between premenopausal and postmenopausal women.[3]

OPTIMIZED MR IMAGING TECHNIQUES

In our practice, we place gauze between the labia for labial separation and better delineation of the clitoris and labia (**Fig. 2**). Our perineal MR imaging protocol consists of the following sequences (slice thickness/field of view):

- Sagittal T2-weighted imaging (T2WI) (4 mm/22 mm)
- Axial oblique fat-saturated (FS) T2WI, perpendicular to abnormality (4 mm/22 mm)
- Coronal oblique T2WI, parallel to abnormality (4 mm/22 mm)
- Axial T1-weighted imaging (T1WI) in/out phase (5 mm/34 mm)
- Axial diffusion-weighted imaging (4 mm/22 mm)
- Axial oblique 3D T1WI FS precontrast (same angle and coverage as the axial oblique T2WI FS) (3 mm/24 mm)
- Axial oblique 3D T1WI FS post contrast—2 phases post timing run (3 mm/24 mm)

For imaging of the introitus, we administer 60 mL of ultrasound gel into the vagina via a Foley catheter and add an axial T2WI high-resolution sequence, which can be obliqued to cover the mass or region of interest only.

Clitoral anatomy is best seen in the axial plane with sagittal and coronal planes providing additional details, such that all components can be seen on MR imaging, with each plane providing a different representation of the structure.[6] Sagittal planes demonstrate the angled "boomerang-shaped" clitoral body and glans at the undersurface of the pubic symphysis.[6] The coronal plane demonstrates the 2 corpora uniting into a single body and terminating in the glans clitoris as well as depicting the labia minor and majora.[6]

Applying fat saturation highlights the cavernous tissue owing to its increased vascularity.[5,6] The clitoris enhances avidly on postcontrast T1WI, although the clitoral bulb enhances slightly less than the remainder of the clitoris.[3,5] The labia minora enhance more than the labia majora.[3]

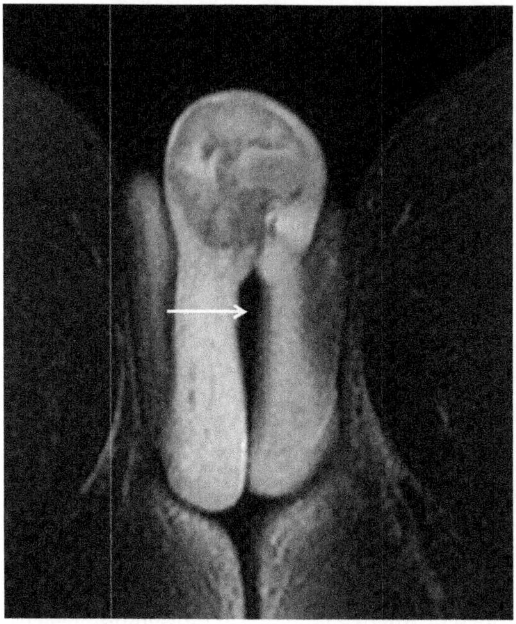

Fig. 2. Gauze (*arrow*) is placed between the labia minora for better delineation of the clitoris and labia.

BENIGN PERINEAL TUMORS

An array of neoplasms can affect the perineal structures, posing a diagnostic challenge owing to their rarity, as well as imaging and histologic overlap.[4] Aggressive angiomyxomas (AAM) and cellular angiofibromas are among the more common mesenchymal neoplasms.[4] Angiomyofibroblastoma (AMF), a related but less invasive soft tissue neoplasm that occurs in the same region and patient population, is a differential diagnostic consideration.[4] Additional benign tumors that are discussed include nodular fasciitis, vaginal fibroepithelial polyps, and nonneoplastic cysts.

Aggressive Angiomyxoma

AAM is a benign myxoid neoplasm affecting women in their third to fifth decades of life.[1,4,7,8] It has been reported rarely in men.[9] Patients may present with a mass, but AAMs are often asymptomatic and can become large, sometimes measuring more than 10 cm at presentation.[8,10,11] A large intrapelvic component may not appreciated on clinical examination, and these can often be mistaken for a lipoma, perineal hernia, or Bartholin gland cyst.[7,10] These masses tend to be slow growing.[1] Metastases are rare but have been reported.[12]

The mass arises from the connective tissues of the perineum or lower pelvis, rarely from perineal or pelvic viscera.[13] Grossly, it appears as a rubbery, gelatinous mass.[1,14] Histologically, the tumor is hypocellullar with stellate and spindle-shaped mesenchymal cells embedded in a loose myxoid stroma.[1,7,8]

Imaging is important to determine the anatomic extent and relationship to the pelvic floor, perineal tissues, and pelvic viscera to optimize the surgical approach.[4] On MR imaging, the mass is isointense or hypointense to muscle on T1WI.[1,8,13] On T2WI, the mass is hyperintense owing to high myxomatous content[15] with a characteristic "swirled" or "whorled" appearance, attributed to stretching of the fibrovascular stroma and disorganized vascular network within the tumor.[1,4,8,13] On postcontrast

T1WI, the tumor enhances avidly, sometimes revealing the swirled pattern, demonstrating their hypervascular nature (**Fig. 3**).[1,4,8,10,13] In 1 study, AAMs demonstrated high signal intensity on diffusion-weighted imaging with ADC values of more than 2×10^{-3} mm^2/s.[10]

Because AAMs tend to grow around and displace pelvic structures without penetration or invasion, patients can have extensive tumor above the pelvic floor with normal sexual, urinary, and anal sphincter function.[4,8,13] The tumor does not generally cause rectal, vaginal, urethral, or vascular obstruction.[13]

Surgery with wide local excision is the treatment of choice for AAM.[1,8,10] MR imaging is important for surgical planning to determine whether the tumor traverses the pelvic diaphragm, which allows the surgeon to determine if a perineal, abdominal, or combined approach to resection is needed.[4,8,13] Complete resection of AAMs is often not possible, hence the term "aggressive," denoting the high rate of local recurrence after resection (36%–72%).[4,7,16] The high local recurrence rate may be owing to diagnostic difficulty before the initial surgery, limiting complete preoperative assessment of tumor extent.[13] Additionally, the intimate relationship of the tumor to pelvic viscera with extension above and below the pelvic diaphragm makes complete resection difficult.[13] Most recurrences are likely owing to inadequate resection and residual tumor.[7,13] Patients often require multiple resections with wide margins to achieve control or cure.[4] Recurrence may occur, even with negative surgical margins.[11,17] Long-term follow-up is warranted owing to late recurrence in some cases.[10,18]

In AAMs that are estrogen and progesterone receptor positive, tamoxifen, raloxifene, and gonadotropin-releasing hormone agonists have been used as neoadjuvant therapy to shrink the tumor and minimize the radicality of surgery and as a treatment for recurrence.[1,10,11,16,19,20]

Angiomyofibroblastoma

AMF was characterized as a separate entity from AAM in 1992.[21] It affects the vulvar region of women ages 23 to 71, with a mean age of 42.[22] As with AAM and cellular angiofibroma, AMF often presents as a painless mass.[4] It tends to be well-circumscribed as opposed to the infiltrative nature of AAM.[4,21] AMFs range in size from 0.5 to 12.0 cm in diameter, with most less than 5 cm.[4,21] AMFs arise in the superficial soft tissues of the vulva, whereas AAMs often extends into the deep pelvic structures as described, particularly at recurrence.[21]

Histologically, AMF is characterized by alternating hypercellular and hypocellular zones with abundant vessels, predominantly capillaries.[21]

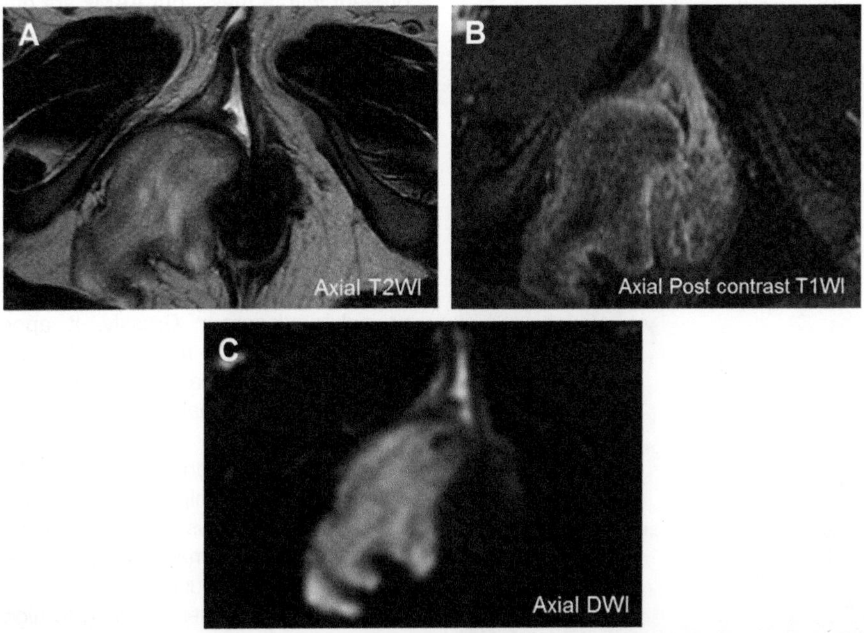

Fig. 3. Aggressive angiomyxoma. A 45-year-old woman presenting with a vulvar mass. Axial T2-weighted imaging (*A*) demonstrates hyperintensity with a characteristic swirled or whorled pattern. On postcontrast imaging (*B*), the mass is avidly enhancing owing to hypervascularity. Axial diffusion weighted imaging (*C*) demonstrates restricted diffusion.

AMF is distinguished from AAM by its circumscribed borders, greater cellularity, and more numerous vessels, among other histologic features, which are beyond the scope of this article.[21]

On MR imaging, Mortele and colleagues[23] described AMF to be hypointense and heterogeneous on T1WI with areas of hyperintensity representing interspersed fat contents. On T2WI, the mass may not be well seen owing to hyperintensity of the mass and the surrounding fat, depending on the location.[23] On postcontrast imaging, there is strong, homogenous enhancement owing to hypervascularity.[23] Local surgical excision is often curative and postoperative recurrence is rare, in contrast with AAM.[4,21]

Cellular Angiofibroma

Cellular angiofibroma, also known as AMF-like tumor, was first characterized as a distinct histologic entity in 1997.[22] It is rare, found in various anatomic sites, such as the perineum, vulva, genital tract, and inguinal regions.[24,25] Initially thought to only occur in women, it has been described in men in the scrotum and inguinal canal.[25,26] It occurs in men and women approximately equally.[26,27] Women are more affected in the fifth decade (ages 39–50), whereas men are mainly affected in the seventh decade.[22,26,27] Cellular angiofibromas have a small size (<3 cm) and are usually well-circumscribed, like AMFs.[22] The term cellular angiofibroma was given to highlight the principal histologic components: the cellular spindle cell stromal component and the prominent thick walled blood vessels.[22] There are scarce mature adipocytes.

On MR imaging, it is a circumscribed mass, isointense to muscle on T1WI.[24,26] On T2WI, it has heterogeneous signal intensity depending on the amount of collagenous stoma, myxoid matrix, spindle cell component, and fat.[24] Often, cellular angiofibroma demonstrates lower signal intensity on T2WI owing to fibrous tissue, fibrosis in the wall, abundant blood vessels, and lack of myxoid tissue.[24,26] It may have a T2 hypointense rim.[24] On postcontrast T1WI, it is highly vascular and avidly enhancing with solid, homogenous enhancement (**Fig. 4**).[24,26]

Treatment consists of simple local excision with clear margins.[24,25] Most literature cites that these do not recur,[22,24] although we have seen a case of recurrence in our institution, attributed to malignant degeneration. Thus, close postoperative monitoring and long-term follow-up is recommended; suspected recurrence should be imaged and explored.[25]

AAM, AMF, and cellular angiofibroma are compared in **Table 1**.

Nodular Fasciitis

Nodular fasciitis was initially named pseudosarcomatous fibromatosis.[28] This entity has variously been known as pseudosarcomatous fasciitis, infiltrative

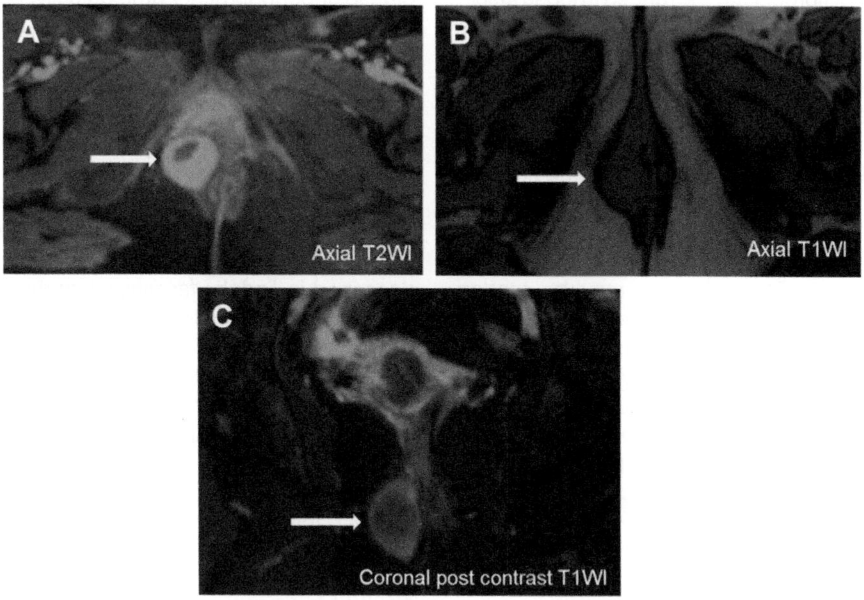

Fig. 4. Cellular angiofibroma. A 37-year-old woman presenting with a vulvar mass (*white arrow*). Axial T2-weighted imaging (T2WI) (*A*) demonstrates a hyperintense lesion, although T2 characteristic vary depending on the composition, and these are often hypointense on T2WI. The lesion has low signal intensity on T1-weighted imaging (*B*). The mass avidly enhances on postcontrast imaging owing to hypervascularity (*C*).

Table 1
Comparison of aggressive angiomyxoma, cellular angiofibroma, and angiomyofibroblastoma

Clinical Features	Aggressive Angiomyxoma	Cellular Angiofibroma	Angiomyofibroblastoma
Age (y)	3rd to 5th decade (often 35–40)	Women: 5th decade (39–50); men: 7th decade	Young to older women (ages 23–71; mean 42)
Sex	F>>M	F = M	F>>M
Presentation	Painless mass, effects of pressure on adjacent structures	Painless mass	Painless mass
Size of lesion	3–10 cm (often >5 cm at presentation)	<3 cm	0.5–12 cm (often <5 cm)
Behavior	Infiltrative	Well circumscribed	Well circumscribed
MR imaging			
T1W1	Isointense or hypointense to muscle	Isointense to muscle	Hyperintense (fat)
T2WI	Hyperintense (swirled or whorled pattern)	Heterogenous, often lower T2 signal intensity	Hyperintense (fat)
Post contrast	Avidly enhances (may have whorled pattern)	Avidly enhances	Avidly enhances
Treatment	Surgical excision; often recurs; metastases have been reported	Surgical excision is often curative; rare recurrence or malignant degeneration	Surgical excision is often curative; rare recurrence

Abbreviations: F, female; M, male; T1WI, T1-weighted imaging; T2WI, T2-weighted imaging.

fasciitis, and proliferative fasciitis, reflecting the limited understanding of this benign, self-limiting condition, despite it being the most common tumor of fibrous tissue.[29] Nodular fasciitis results from a proliferation of fibroblasts,[30] arranged in loose fascicles with a myxoid stroma and multinucleated giant cells.[31] Rapid growth of the lesion, a high mitotic rate and high cellularity can raise concern for a sarcoma both on imaging and pathology.[32]

The condition is typically seen in younger adults; 85% of patients are under 50 years of age.[33] It is rare in the pediatric population, however, accounting for 10% of cases.[34] Clinically, the lesions present as a rapidly growing mass developing over several weeks.[32] These lesions may be tender but tend to be small, less than 5 cm.[35] The lesions may be subcutaneous, within the fascia or intramuscular.[36] Rare cases of intravascular lesions have been described.[37] The most common site of involvement is the upper extremity (46%),[30] but it also commonly involves the head/neck, trunk, and lower extremity.[36] Cases of vulvar involvement have been published.[38] Spontaneous resolution can occur and lesions may respond to intralesional steroid injection. Surgical excision can be performed with a very low rate of recurrence, even with only partial excision.[39]

Lesions may be predominantly fibrous, cellular, or myxoid and, as a result, a variety of MR imaging appearances can be seen.[36] Lesions tend to be isointense to hyperintense to muscle on T1WI and hyperintense to fat on T2WI.[36,40] There is usually hyperenhancement, although this may be diffuse or peripheral.[30] Pathologically, nodular fasciitis is an unencapsulated but well-demarcated lesion; however, it can be focally infiltrative,[31] manifesting on MR imaging as lesional extension along fascial planes or a "fascial tail" (**Fig. 5**). In addition, aggressive features such as spread between compartments, bony changes, and intraarticular involvement have been described.[40] Calcification or ossification are rarely seen on radiographs.[41] The "inverted target" sign has been described in nodular fasciitis when there is hyperintense signal centrally on T2WI correlating with an area of relative hypoenhancement after contrast administration.[40,42] Nodular fasciitis is one of the few benign lesions that can demonstrate central necrosis (along with ancient schwannomas).[30] The appearances are not specific, however, and biopsy is typically necessary to exclude a sarcoma or other aggressive malignancy.

Vaginal Fibroepithelial Polyp

Vaginal fibroepithelial polpys, also known as fibroepithelial stromal polyps or mesodermal stromal polyps, develop in women during their reproductive

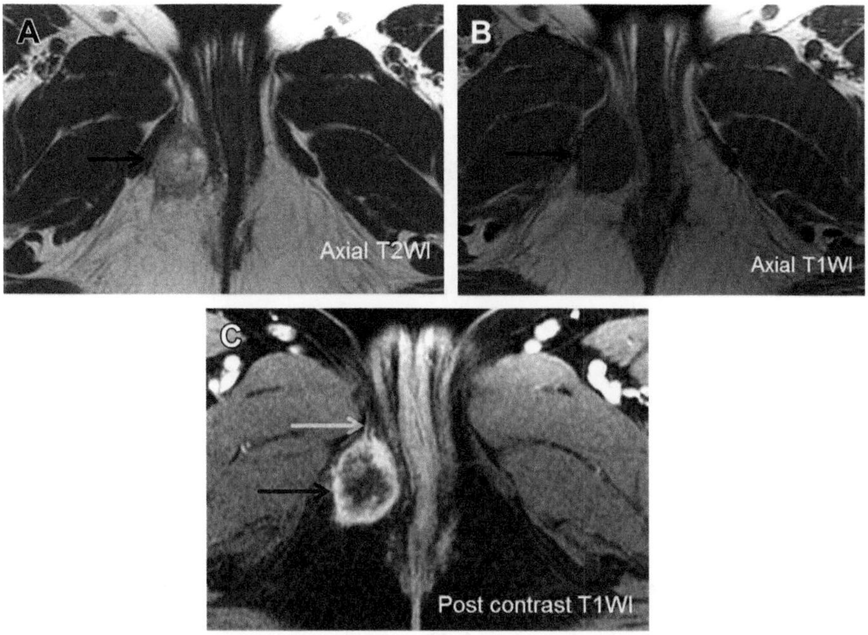

Fig. 5. Nodular fasciitis (*black arrow*). A 20-year-old woman presenting with a vulvar mass. Axial T2-weighted imaging (*A*) demonstrates a heterogeneously hyperintense mass, which is homogenously hypointense on T1-weighted imaging (*B*). On postcontrast imaging (*C*), the lesion demonstrates peripheral enhancement with a "fascial tail" (*white arrow*), linear extension along the fascia.

years, predominantly affecting the vagina, less commonly the vulva, and rarely the cervix.[43] They seem to have a hormonal association, because they are often found in patients who are pregnant at diagnosis, during tamoxifen therapy, or other hormone usage.[43,44]

Patients most commonly present with a painless mass,[45] although other presentations include skin tags, discharge, and vaginal bleeding.[43] They are usually less than 2 cm in diameter, but can measure up to 12 cm.[43,45] Lesions may be solitary or less commonly multiple and bilateral.[43] Bilaterality is more frequently encountered in pregnancy.[43]

On gross pathologic examination, fibroepithelial polyps are often pedunculated with polypoid stromal proliferation.[43] Histologically, they are covered with squamous epithelium.[43] The fibrovascular stroma is typically edematous with collagen fibers.[43] Fat may be present and it usually has a vascular component, generally toward the lesion center.[43]

On MR imaging, fibrous tissues presents as stratiform hypointense areas on T2WI.[43] At the center of the attachment site, there may be clustered fatty tissue, which appears as a linear hyperintense area on T1WI.[43] Most of the remainder of the lesion demonstrates increased signal intensity on T2WI owing to edematous stroma with less fibrosis and cellularity.[43] Phase shift T1-weighted gradient echo imaging or equivalent T1WI with fat suppression may demonstrate intralesional fat more clearly.[43] The lesion enhances on postcontrast T1WI (**Fig. 6**).

Surgical excision is often curative, although local recurrence can occur with incomplete excision.[43] Because they may be hormonally responsive, some recur in pregnancy; others regress during the postpartum period.[43] Metastases have not been reported.

Nonneoplastic Cysts (Bartholin Gland Cyst, Skene Gland Cyst, Clitoral Epidermal Inclusion Cyst)

Nonneoplastic cysts affecting the perineum have a similar MR imaging appearance to cysts seen elsewhere in the body (**Fig. 7**). They are characteristically strongly hyperintense on T2WI, hypointense on T1WI, with no or very thin peripheral enhancement.[4,46] If there is internal hemorrhage or mucin/protein within the cyst, they may appear hyperintense on T1WI.[4,46] Any of these can become infected, often causing imaging changes of wall thickening and/or peripheral enhancement.[2]

Cysts can be differentiated based on location (**Fig. 8**). If a line is drawn from the coccyx to the inferior aspect of the pubic symphysis

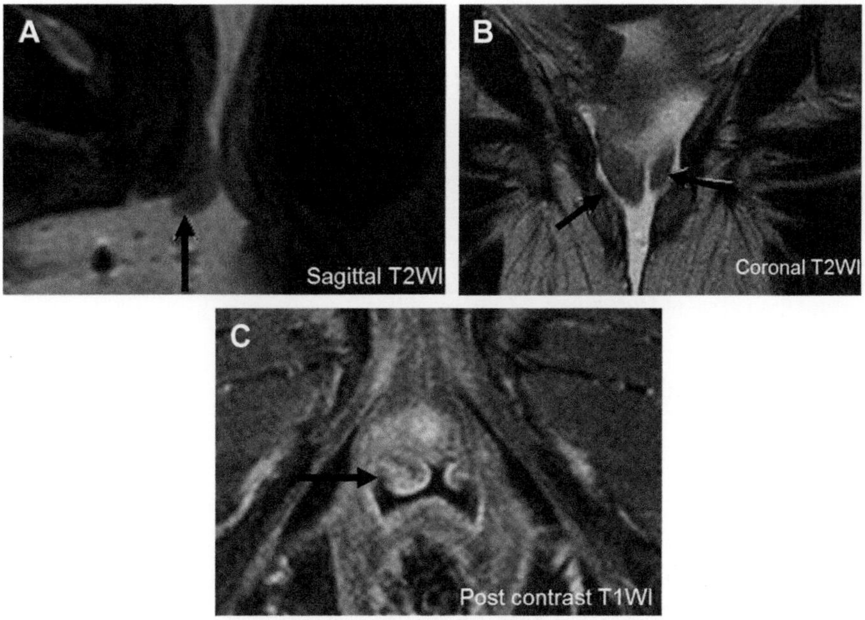

Fig. 6. Vaginal fibroepithelial polyp (*black arrows*). A 70-year-old woman with a vaginal mass. Sagittal (*A*) and coronal (*B*) T2-weighted imaging demonstrates intermediate signal polypoid masses with a stratiform appearance at the introitus (*black arrows*). The larger lesion enhances on T1-weighted imaging post contrast (*C*).

(pubococcygeal line), Bartholin gland cysts and Skene gland cysts occur below the line. Gartner duct cysts occur above or at the line at the anterolateral aspect of the vagina and are therefore not discussed in this article.[4,47] Bartholin gland cysts occur at the posterolateral wall of the introitus, whereas Skene gland cysts are anterior to the introitus and more medial, because they are associated with the urethra.[4]

Clitoral epidermal inclusion cysts have a similar MR imaging appearance as Bartholin gland and Skene gland cysts, but are located within the clitoris.

Bartholin gland cysts (see **Fig. 7**A–C)[2,4,46–48]

- The Bartholin gland is the female homologue of the male Cowper gland.
- Bilateral gland ducts open into the posterolateral aspects of the introitus.
- Ductal obstruction, which may be owing to a stone or stenosis resulting from prior infection, trauma, or inspissated mucus, leads to secretion retention and cyst formation.
- Most common vulvar cysts.
- Develop in 2% of women during their lifetime, usually second to third decade of life.
- Often asymptomatic, but may present with mild dyspareunia.
- 1 to 4 cm, but can become larger with repeated sexual stimulation.
- Pain may indicate enlargement or infection (most commonly *Neisseria gonorrhoeae*).
- Symptomatic cysts are treated with marsupialization or surgical excision with or without antibiotics, if infected.
- Incision and drainage for abscess with definitive treatment after resolution.
- Rarely, squamous cell carcinoma or adenocarcinoma can develop in a Bartholin gland duct or cyst, respectively (look for a solid component).
- Adenoid cystic carcinoma, more commonly seen in salivary glands, is a rare, slow-growing complication of Bartholin gland cyst with a tendency for local invasion, treated with vulvectomy and bilateral inguinal and femoral node dissection.[2]

Skene gland cysts (see **Fig. 7**D–F)[47–49]

- Gland ducts are paired structures lateral to the external urethral meatus.
- Open directly into the urethral lumen, anterior to the introitus.
- Cysts result from duct obstruction, similar to Bartholin gland cysts.
- Differentiate from urethral diverticulum, which tends to be in a midurethral location.
- Often asymptomatic.
- May cause recurrent urinary tract infection or urethral obstruction.
- May require drainage or excision if infected.

Clitoral epidermal inclusion cysts (see **Fig. 7**G–I)[50–53]

Clitoral epidermal inclusion cysts are occasionally spontaneous[52,54] or can occur after

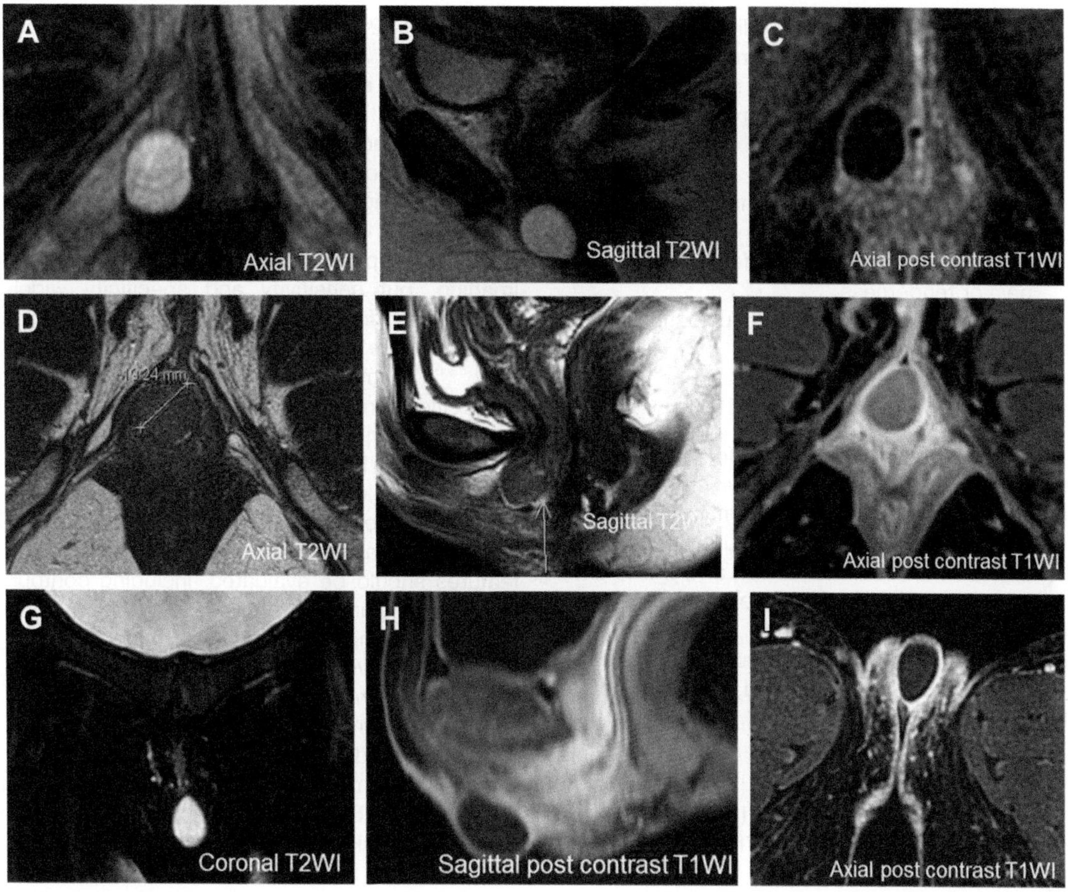

Fig. 7. Nonneoplastic cysts. Bartholin gland cyst at the posterolateral aspect of the introitus, which is hyperintense on axial (*A*) and sagittal (*B*) T2-weighted imaging (T2WI) and does not enhance on axial postcontrast T1-weighted imaging (T1WI) (*C*). Skene gland cyst anterior to the introitus, adjacent to the urethra. Internal proteinaceous content makes it hypointense on axial (*D*) and sagittal (*E, arrow*) T2WI. It does not enhance on axial postcontrast T1WI with mild central intrinsic T1 hyperintensity (*F*). Clitoral epidermal inclusion cyst, which is hyperintense on coronal T2WI (*G*), hypointense on sagittal T1WI (*H*), and does not enhance on axial postcontrast T1WI (*I*).

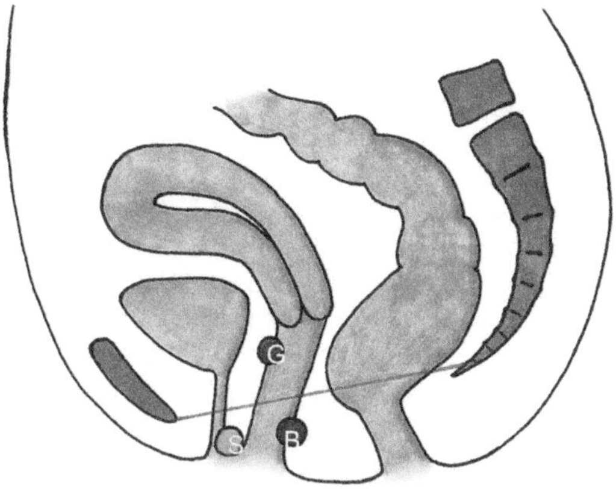

Fig. 8. Sagittal diagram of perineal nonneoplastic cysts. Gartner duct cysts (G) arise from the anterior vaginal wall above the pubococcygeal line. Skene's gland cysts (S) and Bartholin gland cysts (B) arise below the pubococcygeal line, the former more anteriorly in a periurethral distribution, and the latter posterolateral to the lower vagina.

accidental clitoral trauma.[55] However, they are most often seen with prior clitoral surgery and are the most common long-term complication of female genital mutilation, which is more commonly practiced in African countries.[50,53,54] According to the World Health Organization, female genital mutilation is defined as all procedures that involve partial or total removal of female external genitalia and/or injury to the female genital organs for nonmedical reasons.[51,56] Other complications of female genital mutilation include wound infection and labial adhesion.[50]

- May be more common than previously thought, possibly underreported in the literature.[51]
- Slow growing, intradermal or subcutaneous lesions with a wall composed of true epidermis.
- Result from embedding of epidermal keratinized squamous epithelial cells and

sebaceous glands into the line of the clitoral circumcision scar; the epidermal cells proliferate within the closed space to form a cyst.[53]

- Often contain sebaceous material on gross examination.
- Usually asymptomatic, but may be associated with dyspareunia, micturition disturbances, vulvar pain, or vaginal discharge.
- May become inflamed or infected, leading to pain or tenderness.
- Treatment is surgery with enucleation of the cyst.

MALIGNANT PERINEAL TUMORS

Vulvar carcinoma is the predominant malignant tumor in the female perineum, of which more than 85% are squamous cell carcinoma.[4] Other less common pathologic subtypes include adenocarcinoma, sarcoma, basal cell cancer, and extramammary Paget disease.[4] Other malignancies involving the perineum include metastases and secondary involvement of the vulva or perineum owing to direct local spread from adjacent structures.

Vulvar Carcinoma

Vulvar cancer accounts for 3% to 5% of primary gynecologic malignancies.[57,58] The disease has a bimodal distribution with more than one-half of cases occurring in women over the age of 70 years and less than 20% in women younger than 50.[4] However, the incidence in young women is increasing as the prevalence of human papilloma virus increases.[4,59]

Patients may present with a palpable mass, pruritus, bleeding, and/or discharge.[4] Vulvar cancer tends to be slow growing, involving the labia in two-thirds of cases.[4] It is locally infiltrative and may extend to the urethra, anorectum, and introitus/vagina; rarely is the bladder.[60] Extension beyond the pelvis is rare.[4]

MR imaging plays a crucial role to determine the location of the tumor, pelvic side wall involvement, and spread to the adjacent pelvic organs, including the bladder, rectum, introitus, and lymph nodes, assisting in depicting anatomy for surgical and radiation planning.[4,61] The most important prognostic factors to determine survival are tumor size, depth of invasion, and presence or absence of inguinofemoral nodal metastases,[4,57,58,62] which have been incorporated into the International Federation of Gynecology and Obstetrics staging system.[63] Accurate nodal staging can impact surgical approach and radiotherapy planning.[58]

Most vulvar cancers demonstrate low signal intensity on T1WI and moderate to high signal intensity on T2WI (**Fig. 9**).[4,58] After contrast administration, they variably enhance.[4] The T2WI characteristics have been found to be the most useful to delineate the tumor, estimate size, and assess invasion of adjacent structures.[4,58,64] Small primary tumors and more plaquelike tumors may be missed on MR imaging,[58] although using a smaller field of view and thinner sections may assist with identification.[58] Lymph nodes are easily surveyed on MR imaging, but sensitivity and specificity widely vary, ranging from 40% to 80%, with a high-false negative rate to detect malignant adenopathy.[58,65,66] However, because MR imaging is highly specific, there are few false-positive findings, and if a node is enlarged, the surgeon should have a high suspicion that it is involved.[58] One study found that a short to long axis diameter of greater than or equal to 0.75 for prediction of lymph node metastases yielded an accuracy of 85%, although other features should be evaluated, including contour, loss of fatty hilum, cystic change, and signal intensity similar to that of the primary tumor.[4,64]

Historically, vulvar carcinoma had been treated with radical vulvectomy and inguinofemoral lymph node resection en bloc,[4] the consequences of which included external genitalia disfiguration, wound infection, tissue breakdown, and long-term lymphedema.[4] Surgical treatment now consists of wide local excision for a lateral lesion and accompanying unilateral inguinofemoral lymphadenectomy, only if depth of stromal invasion is more than 1 mm, in attempts to decrease morbidity.[4] Central lesions near the introitus, clitoris, and perineum still require radical vulvectomy and bilateral lymphadenectomy, but with separate incisions.[4,67,68] Five-year survival rates are 96% in patients with negative inguinal lymph nodes, decreasing to 80% with 1 to 2 positive nodes, and sharply diminishing to 12% in patients with more than 2 positive nodes.[4] Of all recurrences, 67% are detected clinically during the first 2 years after initial treatment,[4] occurring in the vulva (57%), groin (22%), pelvis (4%), or distant sites (23%).[4,69]

Vulvectomy, either alone or in combination with inguinal lymph node dissection, with subsequent photon therapy, is done for vulvar cancers with involvement of the clitoris.[50] The treatment for clitoral involvement by malignancy alone is clitorodectomy.[50]

Anorectal and Secondary Cancers Involving the Introitus

Despite a rich supply of vessels and lymphatics, metastases to the perineum are rare.[1] The MR imaging appearance of metastases often reflect the MR imaging appearance of the primary tumor

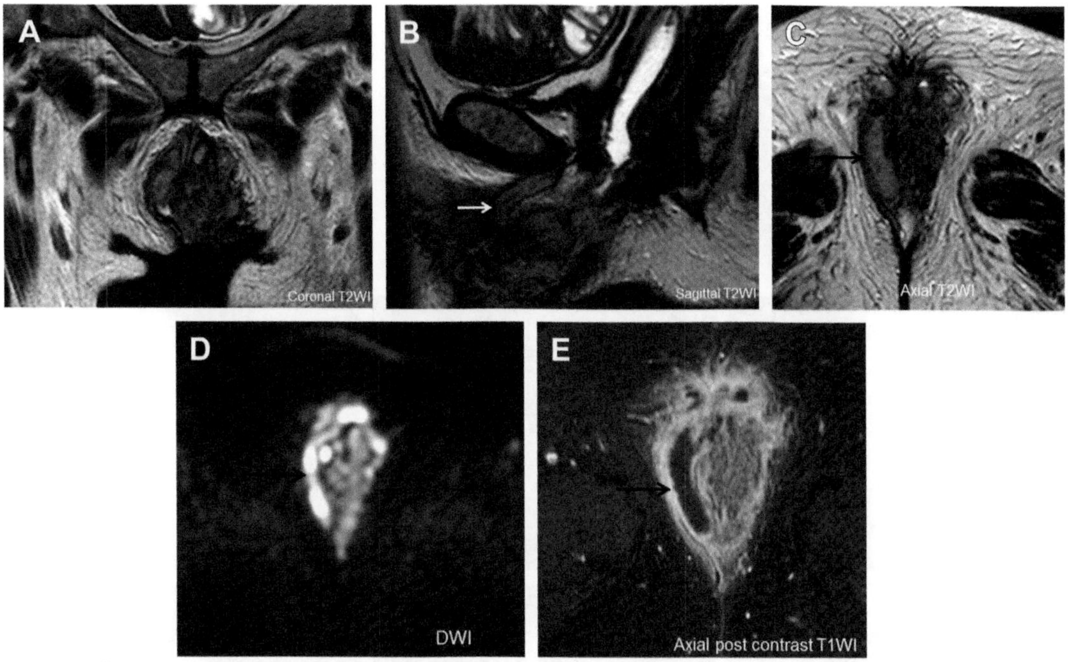

Fig. 9. Vulvar carcinoma complicated by abscess. A 70-year-old woman with a vulvar mass. Coronal (*A*), sagittal (*B*), and axial (*C*) T2-weighted imaging (T2WI) demonstrate an ill-defined vulvar mass with intermediate T2 signal intensity. It has restricted diffusion on axial diffusion-weighted imaging (*D*). The mass demonstrates enhancement on axial postcontrast T1-weighted imaging (*E*). A rim-enhancing fluid collection with restricted diffusion at the right aspect of the mass (*black arrow* in *C–E*) is a small abscess. The clitoral body (*white arrow*) is nicely seen on the sagittal T2WI (*B*). (*Courtesy of* Dr Christophe Balliauw, MD, Jessa Hospital, Belgium.)

(**Fig. 10**).[61] As with vulvar carcinoma, the T2WI best delineates the extent of disease within and beyond the vagina.[61]

In advanced disease or if there is local relapse after treatment, bladder and rectal cancer can involve the vagina.[61] In rectal adenocarcinomas, masses involving the vagina are often low signal intensity on T1WI and intermediate to high signal intensity on T2WI, depending on the mucinous content.[61]

Most anal cancers are squamous cell carcinomas and the rest are adenocarcinomas[4,70] or melanoma. Carcinomas demonstrate hypointensity on T1WI and intermediate signal intensity on T2WI.[4] After treatment, recurrent cancer may display more advanced local disease with involvement of adjacent organs.[4,71] Anal cancers of any size that invade adjacent organs are staged as T4.[72]

Metastases from extrapelvic or extragenital cancers are rare, most commonly from breast and colon adenocarcinoma.[61,73]

INFECTIOUS AND INFLAMMATORY CONDITIONS

Periclitoral Abscess

Periclitoral abscess is a rare condition with few reported cases.[74] As with epidermal inclusion cysts, most cases are related to patients who have been subject to female genital mutilation.[74,75] In such cases, periclitoral abscess formation follows from infection of an inclusion cyst.[51,74] However, spontaneous periclitoral abscesses occur without prior local surgery, but because these cases are rare, it is difficult to associate these with specific causes.[74]

As of 2012, only 18 reports of spontaneous periclitoral abscesses have been reported in the English literature.[74] In most cases, the etiology was unclear.[74] One speculated mechanism for development was defect of the squamous stratified epithelium that normally prevents pathogen entrance.[74] Several microorganisms that cause purulent infections have been isolated in published cases, namely, *Staphylococcus*, *Streptococcus bovis*, *Diptheriae* species, and *Bacteroides* species.[74,76,77] A periclitoral abscess arising as a complication of an existing pilonidal sinus tract of the should also be taken into consideration when a clinician is searching for an etiology.[74] These patients may have multiple recurrences until excision of the pilonidal sinus tract provides definitive treatment.[74]

MR imaging findings are similar to those of abscesses elsewhere in the body (**Fig. 11**). The lesion is often hypointense on T1WI, heterogeneously

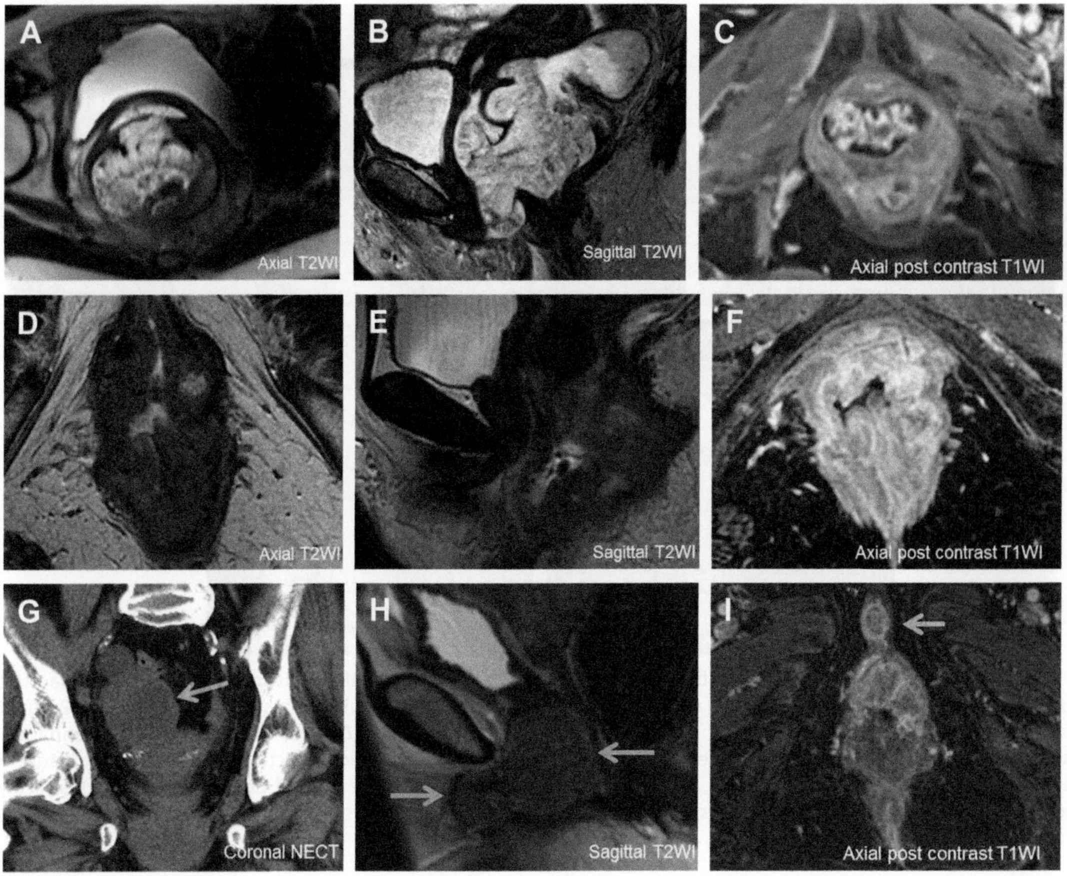

Fig. 10. Metastatic disease to the introitus and clitoris. Rectal cancer involving the introitus on axial T2-weighted imaging (T2WI) (*A*), Sagittal T2WI (*B*) and axial postcontrast T1-weighted imaging (T1WI) (*C*). Anal cancer involving the introitus on axial T2WI (*D*), sagittal T2WI (*E*), and axial postcontrast T1WI (*F*). Ovarian cancer involving the clitoris (*white arrows*) on coronal nonenhanced computed tomography (*G*), sagittal T2WI (*H*), and axial postcontrast T1WI (*I*).

hyperintense on T2WI, with thick rim enhancement. There may be surrounding T2 hyperintensity owing to edema in the surrounding adjacent structures.

There is no established management for periclitoral abscess, and it is often based on personal experience.[74] Treatment options include conservative management with antibiotics only until spontaneous drainage or resolution, simple incision, or local excision of the abscess cavity.[74] If encountered, a pilonidal tract should be excised to reduce the risk of recurrence.[74]

Perianal Fistula Involving the Labia

A fistula is an abnormal connection between 2 structures or organs or between an organ and body surface.[78] A perianal fistula is a connection between the anal canal and perineal skin surface.[79] Although the prevalence is low (0.01%), it causes significant morbidity.[78] Most patients present with discharge (65% of cases), but local pain is also common.[78,79] In anovaginal fistulas, patients may pass gas and feces through the vagina and have recurrent vaginal infections.[4]

Perianal fistulas are generally believed to be primarily related to anal gland sepsis or secondarily caused by conditions such as Crohn's disease, tuberculosis, trauma, pelvic malignancy, pelvic infection, diverticulitis, obstetric trauma, or radiation.[4,78] They have a strong tendency to recur, often requiring multiple surgical treatments.[78,80]

Most extend within the intersphincteric space to the skin[4,81,82]; however, 30% may pass through both the internal and external sphincters to enter the ischioanal space.[4,81] In some cases, perianal fistulas can extend into the supralevator space, above the levator ani muscle insertion,[4] or anteriorly into the labia majora. Differentiating between fistula and abscess and between intersphincteric and transphincteric disease has important management implications.[4,83]

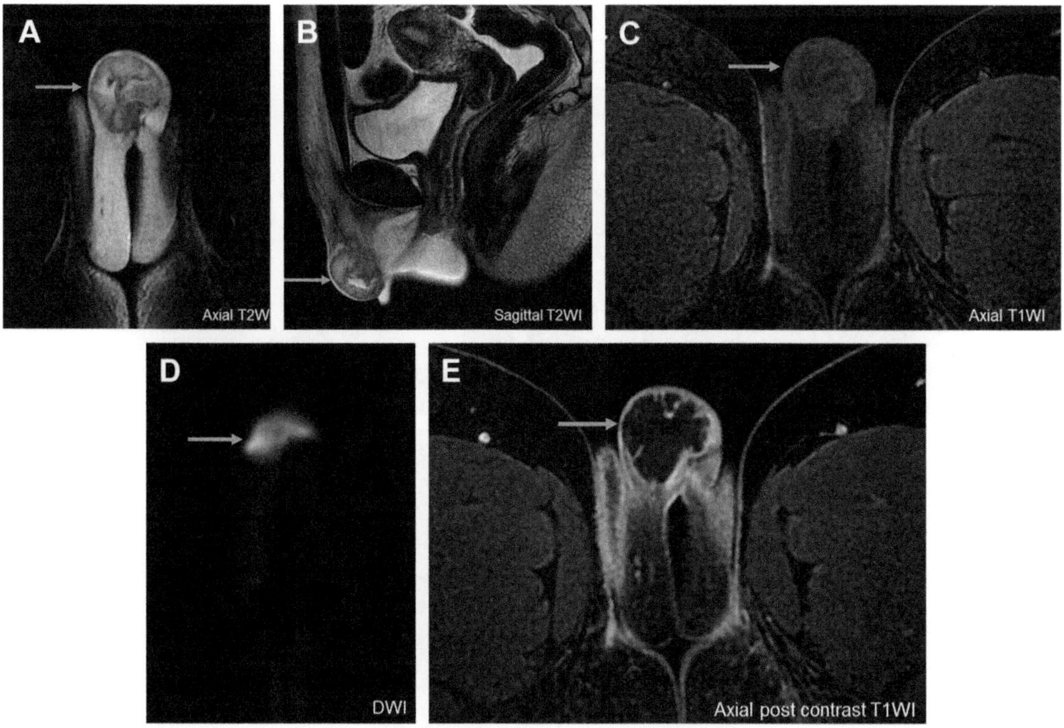

Fig. 11. Periclitoral abscess (*arrows*). A 19-year-old woman with labial swelling. Axial (*A*) and sagittal (*B*) T2-weighted imaging demonstrates a heterogeneously hyperintense mass, which is isointense to muscle on axial T1-weighted imaging (T1WI) (*C*). It demonstrates restricted diffusion (*D*). On axial postcontrast T1WI, it demonstrates rim enhancement (*E*).

MR imaging provides a noninvasive modality for the evaluation of perianal fistulizing disease with high spatial resolution to assist in surgical planning to decrease postoperative recurrence and risk of fecal incontinence.[4,78] It provides precise information on anal canal anatomy, the anal sphincter complex, and the relationship of the fistula to the perineal and pelvic floor structures.[78,82] It also allows for precise definition of the fistula tract and any secondary fistulas and abscesses, which contribute to the high recurrence rate.[78,84]

Precontrast T1WI provides an excellent anatomic overview of the sphincter complex, levator plate, and ischiorectal fossa.[78] However, fistulous tracts, inflammation, and abscesses all appear low to intermediate signal intensity on T1WI, with the same signal intensity as the sphincters and levator ani muscles, limiting differentiation.[78,82] Immediately postoperatively, hemorrhage will appear bright on T1WI, helping to differentiate blood products from residual tracks.[78] On T2WI, there is better contrast between the hyperintense fluid in the tract and the hypointense fibrous wall of the fistula, allowing adequate differentiation of the anatomic boundaries between the internal and external sphincters.[78]

On gadolinium-enhanced fat-suppressed T1WI, gadolinium is helpful to differentiate pus-filled active fistula from healing tract undergoing granulation, both of which can be hyperintense on T2WI.[4] Active fistulas demonstrate wall enhancement, whereas scar tissue formation within a healing tract enhances (**Fig. 12**).[4,78]

As with abscesses elsewhere, abscesses related to perianal fistulas appear as hyperintense on T2WI with rim enhancement and central hypoenhancement owing to pus.[4,78,82] Chronic fistulas and scar tissue appear as low signal intensity on T1WI and T2WI and do not enhance with gadolinium.[78,85]

Infected Bartholin Gland Cyst

Infected Bartholin gland cysts exhibit characteristics of cysts with central hypointensity on T1WI and hyperintensity on T2WI (**Fig. 13**), with additional findings of wall thickening with peripheral enhancement in many cases.[2]

Lichen Sclerosus

Lichen sclerosus and lichen planus are chronic inflammatory conditions affecting the vulva with

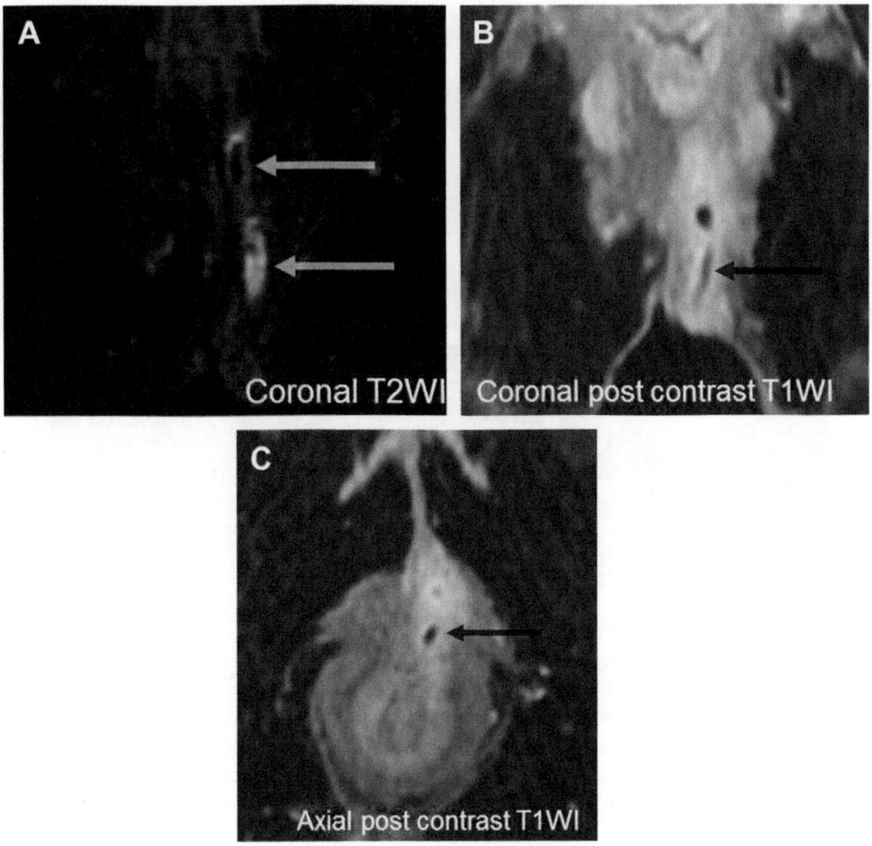

Fig. 12. Perianal fistula extending into the left labia majora (*arrows*). Coronal T2-weighted imaging (*A*) demonstrates a T2 hyperintense tract arising at the 1 o'clock position with rim enhancement on coronal (*B*) and axial (*C*) postcontrast T1-weighted imaging. This is consistent with an active transsphincteric perianal fistula with undrained fluid. It passes anteroinferiorly into the rectovaginal septum, opening to the perineal skin at the labia.

significant morbidity.[86] The cause of lichen sclerosus is unknown, but the possibility of an autoimmune etiology has been raised.[87,88] Most cases are seen in prepubertal girls or postmenopausal women.[87,88] Patients have a varied clinical presentation with itching occurring in most cases, but some women will endorse burning, soreness, and pain.[86,87] Some pediatric cases resolve in puberty,[87] but the disease can persists for decades, although the course may wax and wane.[86]

The classic presentation is a "figure of 8"–shaped white plaque around the vulva and anus.[87] It has generally been thought that lichen sclerosus does not affect the vagina, differentiating it from lichen planus, which does,[87] although a few cases of vaginal involvement by lichen sclerosus have been reported.[87,89] Other findings include atrophy, fissures, erosions, and ecchymoses with loss of genital architecture in advanced cases with subsequent effacement of the labia minora and clitoris.[87] The risk of developing squamous cell carcinoma in longstanding lichen sclerosus is 5%.[87,88]

Imaging is not typically used in the evaluation of lichen sclerosus, which is a vulvar skin disease that is readily diagnosed clinically. The MR imaging appearance is nonspecific, with diffuse hypointensity in the perineal area on T2WI, extending into the labia majora (**Fig. 14**). After gadolinium administration, there is low-level regional contrast enhancement, which may reflect fibrosis and chronic inflammation. The radiologist should look for evidence of urethral or introital obstruction in advanced cases.

Management may require a multidisciplinary approach and active patient involvement.[86] First-line treatment is potent topical corticosteroids.[86–88] Supportive measures and adjunct therapies, such as testosterone, progesterone, tacrolimus, surgery, and phototherapy, may improve patient outcomes.[86,88] Surgery should be reserved for symptomatic patients who have failed other treatments, because there is a high recurrence rate after surgery.[88]

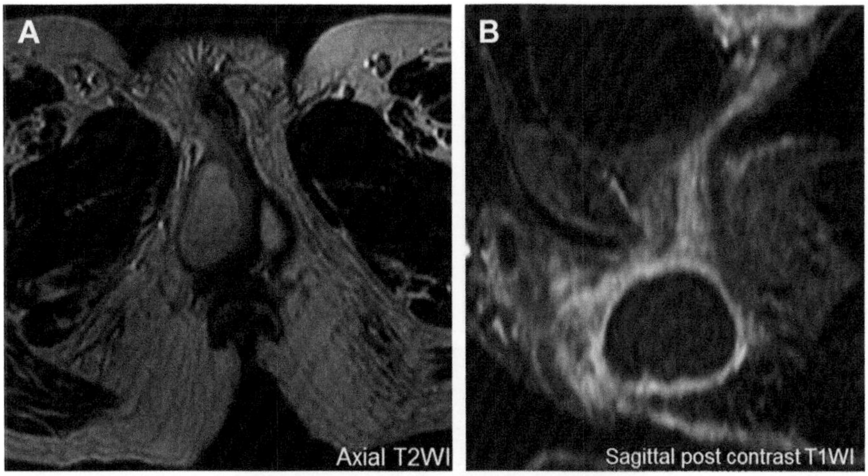

Fig. 13. Infected Bartholin gland cyst. Mass at the posterolateral aspect of the introitus, which is hyperintense on axial T2-weighted imaging (*A*). After contrast administration (*B*), the lesion demonstrates thick, irregular wall enhancement with adjacent inflammation, consistent with superinfection.

VASCULAR DISORDERS

Labial Venous Varicosities

Labial venous varicosities, which may result in labial and vulvar thrombophlebitis, can develop during pregnancy or the postpartum period.[4,90] Varicosities may be a pregnancy complication resulting from venous compression owing to the gravid uterus, usually shrinking in the postpartum period, although they may persist thereafter.[4,91–93]

In determining the cause of thromboembolism of labial venous varicosities, consideration should be given to tamoxifen use for breast cancer,[94,95] a history of thromboembolism, cardiovascular disease, malignancy, surgery, trauma, and any recent cancer treatment, such as chemotherapy.[4]

MR imaging and Doppler ultrasound imaging are both reliable to establish diagnosis of thrombosis of labial venous varicosities, although MR imaging provides a larger field of view to assess extent of thrombosis (**Fig. 15**).[4] MR imaging demonstrates hyperintensity on T1WI and T2WI in acute occlusive thrombus within an expanded vessel.[4]

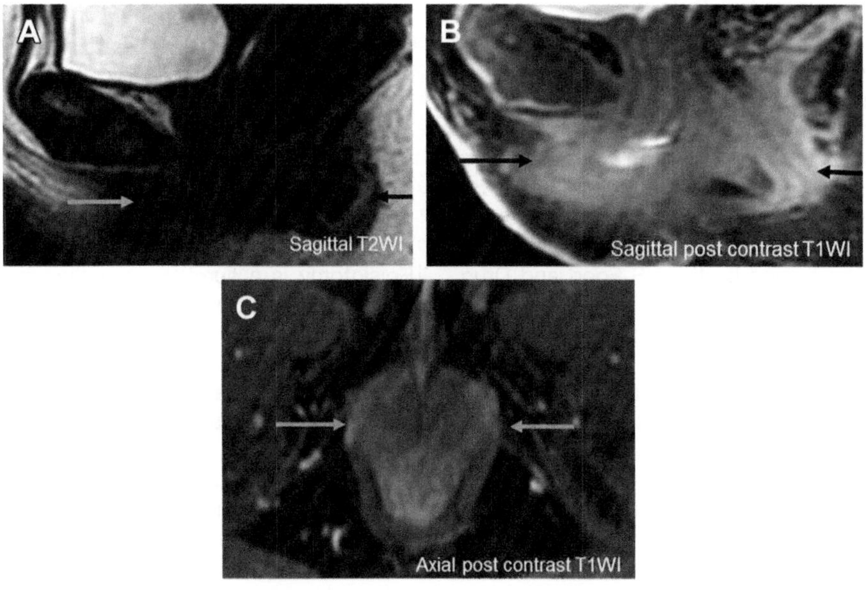

Fig. 14. Lichen sclerosus (*white* and *black arrows*). A 60-year-old woman with vaginal pruritus. Sagittal T2-weighted imaging (*A*) demonstrates an ill-defined, hypointense area at the perineum. On sagittal (*B*) and axial (*C*) postcontrast imaging, the area diffusely enhances.

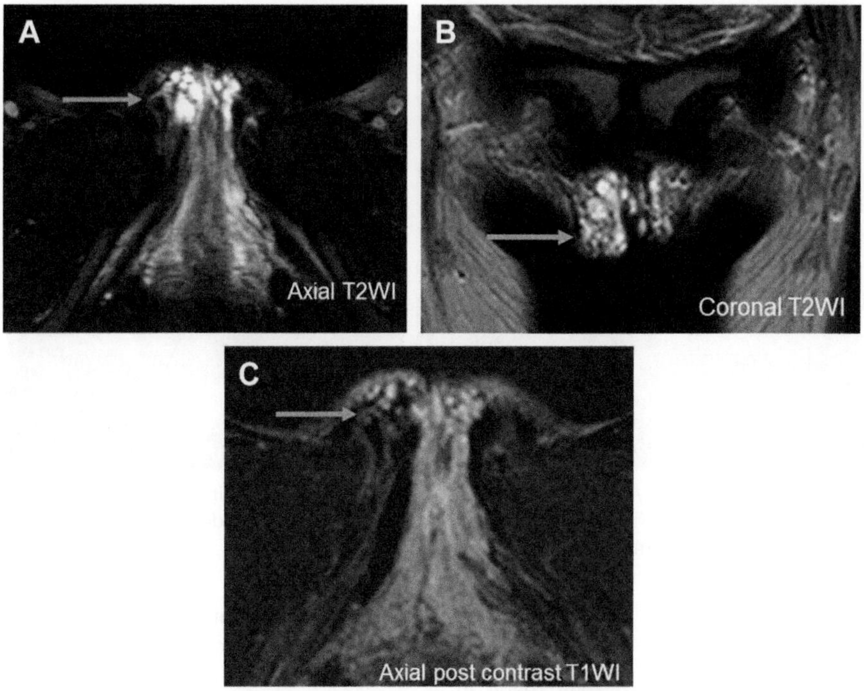

Fig. 15. Labial venous varicosities (*arrows*). A 25-year-old woman with vulvar heaviness. Axial (*A*) and coronal (*B*) T2-weighted imaging (T2WI) demonstrates prominent tortuous dilated vascular structures in the labia majora, right more than left. On axial postcontrast T1-weighted imaging (T1WI) (*C*), these demonstrate progressive enhancement. Acute thrombus would be hyperintense on T1WI and T2WI with vascular expansion and often perivascular inflammation.

Perivascular inflammation is a helpful ancillary finding in acute thrombosis.[4,96,97]

IATROGENIC ABNORMALITIES

Silicone Injections in the Labia

Augmentation of the buttocks is a popular procedure, despite a high complication rate.[98] US Food and Drug Administration–approved methods include liposuction for reduction and reshaping the buttocks, augmentation with autologous fat grafting with or without liposuction, and gluteal implants.[98] Buttock augmentation with silicone injections is not approved by the US Food and Drug Administration.[98] Unfortunately, there have been reports of unlicensed, nonmedically trained persons injecting industrial grade, nonmedical silicone into the buttocks or other areas.[98] This can lead to serious complications, including death.[98,99] It is assumed that most cases are performed illicitly or abroad.[98]

On MR imaging, silicone granulomas appear as hypointense on T1WI with hyperintense on short tau inversion recovery sequences or T2WI (**Fig. 16**).

Silicone migration along tissue planes to remote sites, including the labia, and/or into lymph nodes is a complication.[98] Other reported complications include injection site reactions, granuloma formation, ulceration, cellulitis, and embolism resulting in acute pneumonitis.[98] Silicone emboli can occur with intravascular injection.[98,100] Symptoms may be delayed for months to years after the procedure, further making the diagnosis difficult.[98] Complications are more likely to occur with industrial grade, impure, or adulterated silicone, and with large-volume injections.[98,100–103]

Episiotomy

Episiotomy is a surgical procedure in which the vaginal orifice is enlarged by a perineal incision during the last part or second stage of labor or delivery in an attempt to increase the diameter of the vaginal outlet to facilitate the baby's birth.[104,105] Suggested maternal benefits include reduction in third-degree tears, preservation of pelvic floor, and perineal muscle relaxation, leading to improved sexual function and a decreased risk of urinary or fecal incontinence, and easier repair compared with a laceration because an episiotomy is a surgical incision.[104] Hypothesized adverse effects include unavoidable extension of the incision into the anal sphincter or rectum,

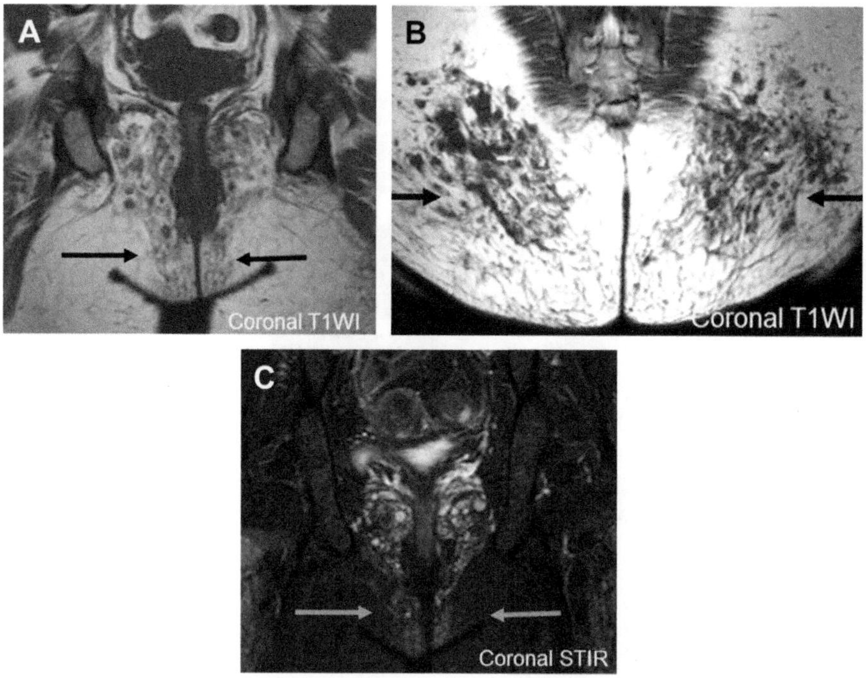

Fig. 16. Free silicone injections in the gluteus and labia (*arrows*). A 45-year-old woman with procedure in Brazil. Coronal T1-weighted imaging demonstrate multiple T1 hypointense nodules anteriorly at the labia (*A*) and posteriorly at the gluteus (*B*). These are hyperintense on the coronal short-tau inversion recovery (STIR) sequence (*C*).

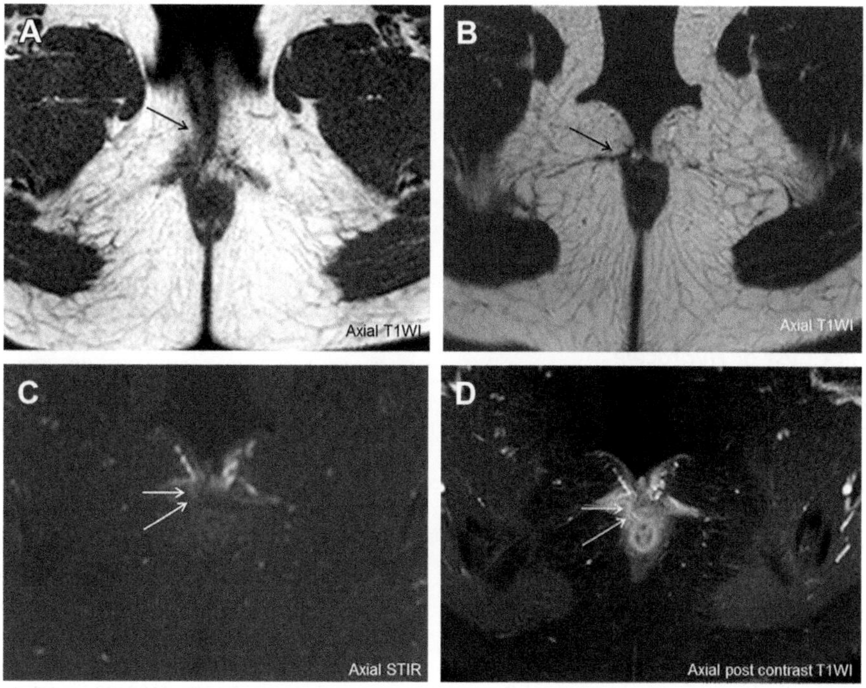

Fig. 17. Episiotomy scar (*arrows*). Incontinence and flatus after giving birth. Axial T1-weighted imaging (T1WI) (*A* and *B*) demonstrate a linear T1 hypointense scar extending from the anal external sphincter through the perineum. There is no fluid within it on the axial short-tau inversion recovery (STIR) sequence (*C*) to suggest a perianal fistula. The scar mildly enhances on axial postcontrast T1WI (*D*). (*Courtesy of* Dr Christophe Balliauw, MD, Jessa Hospital, Belgium.)

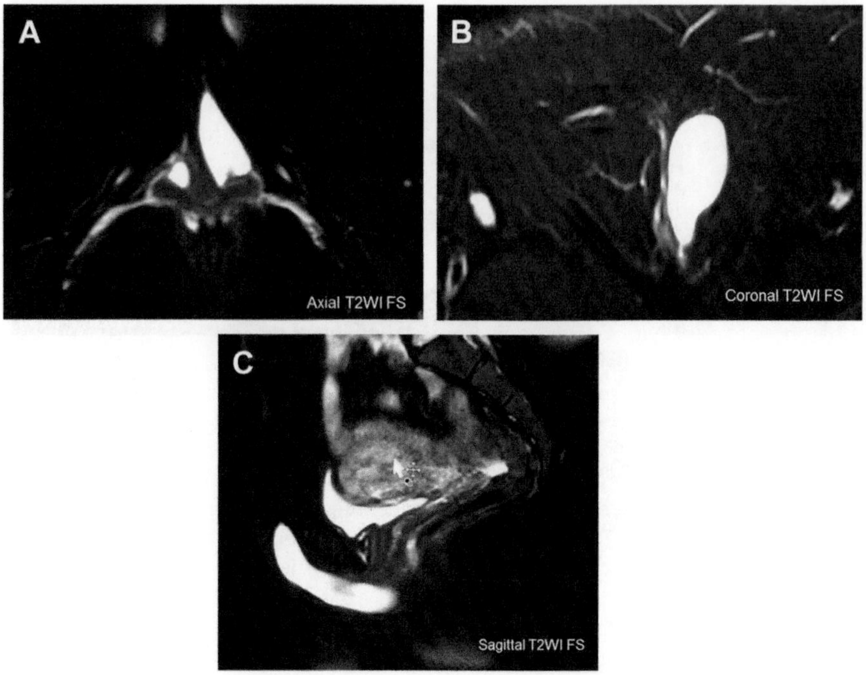

Fig. 18. Canal of Nuck cyst. Axial (*A*), coronal (*B*), and sagittal (*C*) T2-weighted, fat-saturated images demonstrate a T2 hyperintense fluid collection, extending into the left labia majora.

unsatisfactory anatomic results, vaginal prolapse, rectovaginal fistula, fistula in ano, increased hematoma, pain in the episiotomy region, infection and/or dehiscence, and sexual dysfunction.[104]

On MR imaging, an episiotomy appears as a linear tract extending from the introitus through the perineum on T1WI (**Fig. 17**). An old scar will be hypointense on short tau inversion recovery sequence imaging or T2WI and will not contain fluid. The scar mildly enhances on postcontrast T1WI, consistent with fibrous scar tissue.

DEVELOPMENTAL CONDITION

Canal of Nuck Cyst or Hydrocele

Hydrocele of the canal of Nuck is uncommon.[4] The round ligament is attached to the uterus with a small protrusion of the parietal peritoneum accompanying the round ligament through the inguinal ring into the inguinal canal (corresponding to the processus vaginalis in men).[4] Failure of obliteration results in an indirect inguinal hernia or a hydrocele of the Canal of Nuck, which can extend into the labium majora.[4,106] Patients typically present with a fluctuating painless swelling in the inguinolabial region.[4] Cysts or hydroceles rarely exceed 3 cm in diameter.[4]

Graded compression with the ultrasound transducer can display the canal extending from the abdominal cavity to the labia majora.[4] If intestinal contents are seen with the Valsalva maneuver or coughing during ultrasound imaging, it may help to differentiate a cyst from the more common inguinal hernia.[4] MR imaging demonstrates the extent of the hydrocele as a thin-walled, T2 hyperintense cystic mass in the inguinolabial region (**Fig. 18**).[4,106,107]

SUMMARY

A variety of common and uncommon pathologies affect the clitoris, labia, and introitus. These can be better evaluated by knowledge of the normal anatomy and optimized MR imaging techniques to facilitate observation of these entities. This is important to avoid unnecessary surgeries for benign conditions and to assist with surgical planning.

REFERENCES

1. Tappouni RF, Sarwani NI, Tice JG, et al. Imaging of unusual perineal masses. AJNR Am J Neuroradiol 2011;196(4):W412–20.
2. Siegelman ES, Outwater EK, Banner MP, et al. High-resolution MR imaging of the vagina. Radiographics 1997;17(5):1183–203.
3. Suh DD, Yang CC, Cao Y, et al. Magnetic resonance imaging anatomy of the female genitalia in premenopausal and postmenopausal women. J Urol 2003;170(1):138–44.

4. Hosseinzadeh K, Heller MT, Houshmand G. Imaging of the female perineum in adults. Radiographics 2012;32(4):E129–68.
5. O'Connell HE, Sanjeevan KV, Hutson JM. Anatomy of the clitoris. J Urol 2005;174(4):1189–95.
6. O'Connell HE, DeLancey JO. Clitoral anatomy in nulliparous, healthy, premenopausal volunteers using unenhanced magnetic resonance imaging. J Urol 2005;173(6):2060–3.
7. Fetsch JF, Laskin WB, Lefkowitz M, et al. Aggressive angiomyxoma: a clinicopathologic study of 29 female patients. Cancer 1996;78(1):79–90.
8. Sinha R, Verma R. Case 106: aggressive angiomyxoma. Radiology 2007;242(2):625–7.
9. Hong RD, Outwater E, Gomella LG. Aggressive angiomyxoma of the perineum in a man. J Urol 1997;157(3):959–60.
10. Surabhi VR, Garg N, Frumovitz M, et al. Aggressive angiomyxomas: a comprehensive imaging review with clinical and histopathologic correlation. AJNR Am J Neuroradiol 2014;202(6):1171–8.
11. Elkattah R, Sarkodie O, Otteno H, et al. Aggressive angiomyxoma of the vulva: a precis for primary care providers. Case Rep Obstet Gynecol 2013;2013:183725.
12. Siassi RM, Papadopoulos T, Matzel KE. Metastasizing aggressive angiomyxoma. N Engl J Med 1999;341(23):1772.
13. Outwater EK, Marchetto BE, Wagner BJ, et al. Aggressive angiomyxoma: findings on CT and MR imaging. AJNR Am J Neuroradiol 1999;172(2):435–8.
14. Kaur A, Makhija PS, Vallikad E, et al. Multifocal aggressive angiomyxoma: a case report. J Clin Pathol 2000;53(10):798–9.
15. Siegelman ES, Outwater EK. Tissue characterization in the female pelvis by means of MR imaging. Radiology 1999;212(1):5–18.
16. Giles DL, Liu PT, Lidner TK, et al. Treatment of aggressive angiomyxoma with aromatase inhibitor prior to surgical resection. Int J Gynecol Cancer 2008;18(2):375–9.
17. Chan YM, Hon E, Ngai SW, et al. Aggressive angiomyxoma in females: is radical resection the only option? Acta Obstet Gynecol Scand 2000;79(3):216–20.
18. Kiran G, Yancar S, Sayar H, et al. Late recurrence of aggressive angiomyxoma of the vulva. J Low Genit Tract Dis 2013;17(1):85–7.
19. McCluggage WG, Jamieson T, Dobbs SP, et al. Aggressive angiomyxoma of the vulva: dramatic response to gonadotropin-releasing hormone agonist therapy. Gynecol Oncol 2006;100(3):623–5.
20. Fine BA, Munoz AK, Litz CE, et al. Primary medical management of recurrent aggressive angiomyxoma of the vulva with a gonadotropin-releasing hormone agonist. Gynecol Oncol 2001;81(1):120–2.
21. Fletcher CD, Tsang WY, Fisher C, et al. Angiomyofibroblastoma of the vulva. A benign neoplasm distinct from aggressive angiomyxoma. Am J Surg Pathol 1992;16(4):373–82.
22. Nucci MR, Granter SR, Fletcher CD. Cellular angiofibroma: a benign neoplasm distinct from angiomyofibroblastoma and spindle cell lipoma. Am J Surg Pathol 1997;21(6):636–44.
23. Mortele KJ, Lauwers GJ, Mergo PJ, et al. Perineal angiomyofibroblastoma: CT and MR findings with pathologic correlation. J Comput Assist Tomogr 1999;23(5):687–9.
24. Baek C-K, Lim JS, Bae YS. Cellular angiofibroma of the perianal space: MR imaging and pathologic correlation. J Korean Soc Magn Reson Med 2011;15(3):262–6.
25. Canales BK, Weiland D, Hoffman N, et al. Angiomyofibroblastoma-like tumors (cellular angiofibroma). Int J Urol 2006;13(2):177–9.
26. Koo PJ, Goykhman I, Lembert L, et al. MRI features of cellular angiomyofibroma with pathologic correlation. J Magn Reson Imaging 2009;29(5):1195–8.
27. Iwasa Y, Fletcher CD. Cellular angiofibroma: clinicopathologic and immunohistochemical analysis of 51 cases. Am J Surg Pathol 2004;28(11):1426–35.
28. Konwaler BE, Keasbey L, Kaplan L. Subcutaneous pseudosarcomatous fibromatosis (fasciitis). Am J Clin Pathol 1955;25(3):241–52.
29. Weiss SW, Goldblum JR, Enzinger FM. Enzinger and Weiss's soft tissue tumors. 4th edition. St Louis (MO): Mosby; 2001.
30. Walker EA, Fenton ME, Salesky JS, et al. Magnetic resonance imaging of benign soft tissue neoplasms in adults. Radiol Clin North Am 2011;49(6):1197–217, vi.
31. Tomita S, Thompson K, Carver T, et al. Nodular fasciitis: a sarcomatous impersonator. J Pediatr Surg 2009;44(5):e17–19.
32. Fletcher CDM, Organization WH. WHO classification of tumours of soft tissue and bone. 4th edition. Lyon (France): International Agency for Research on Cancer (IARC); 2013.
33. Leung LY, Shu SJ, Chan AC, et al. Nodular fasciitis: MRI appearance and literature review. Skeletal Radiol 2002;31(1):9–13.
34. Price EB Jr, Silliphant WM, Shuman R. Nodular fasciitis: a clinicopathologic analysis of 65 cases. Am J Clin Pathol 1961;35:122–36.
35. Naidu A, Lerman MA. Clinical pathologic conference case 3: nodular fasciitis. Head Neck Pathol 2011;5(3):276–80.
36. Chaudhry AA, Baker KS, Gould ES, et al. Necrotizing fasciitis and its mimics: what radiologists need to know. AJNR Am J Neuroradiol 2015;204(1):128–39.

37. Kim ST, Kim HJ, Park SW, et al. Nodular fasciitis in the head and neck: CT and MR imaging findings. AJNR Am J Neuroradiol 2005;26(10):2617–23.
38. O'Connell JX, Young RH, Nielsen GP, et al. Nodular fasciitis of the vulva: a study of six cases and literature review. Int J Gynecol Pathol 1997;16(2): 117–23.
39. Hutter RV, Stewart FW, Foote FW Jr. Fasciitis. A report of 70 cases with follow-up proving the benignity of the lesion. Cancer 1962;15:992–1003.
40. Coyle J, White LM, Dickson B, et al. MRI characteristics of nodular fasciitis of the musculoskeletal system. Skeletal Radiol 2013;42(7):975–82.
41. Broder MS, Leonidas JC, Mitty HA. Pseudosarcomatous fasciitis: an unusual cause of soft-tissue calcification. Radiology 1973;107(1):173–4.
42. Wang XL, De Schepper AM, Vanhoenacker F, et al. Nodular fasciitis: correlation of MRI findings and histopathology. Skeletal Radiol 2002;31(3):155–61.
43. Kato H, Kanematsu M, Sato E, et al. Magnetic resonance imaging findings of fibroepithelial polyp of the vulva: radiological-pathological correlation. Jpn J Radiol 2010;28(8):609–12.
44. McCluggage WG. A review and update of morphologically bland vulvovaginal mesenchymal lesions. Int J Gynecol Pathol 2005;24(1):26–38.
45. Khalil AM, Nahhas DE, Shabb NS, et al. Vulvar fibroepithelial polyp with myxoid stroma: an unusual presentation. Gynecol Oncol 1994;53(1):125–7.
46. Kier R. Nonovarian gynecologic cysts: MR imaging findings. AJNR Am J Neuroradiol 1992;158(6): 1265–9.
47. Hahn WY, Israel GM, Lee VS. MRI of female urethral and periurethral disorders. AJNR Am J Neuroradiol 2004;182(3):677–82.
48. Walker DK, Salibian RA, Salibian AD, et al. Overlooked diseases of the vagina: a directed anatomic-pathologic approach for imaging assessment. Radiographics 2011;31(6):1583–98.
49. Ryu J, Kim B. MR imaging of the male and female urethra. Radiographics 2001;21(5):1169–85.
50. Al-Shebaily MM, Qureshi VF. Malignancies in clitoris: a review of literature on etiology, diagnosis, pathology and treatment strategies. Int J Cancer Res 2008;4(4):110–26.
51. Rouzi AA. Epidermal clitoral inclusion cysts: not a rare complication of female genital mutilation. Hum Reprod 2010;25(7):1672–4.
52. Schober MS, Hendrickson BW, Alpert SA. Spontaneous clitoral hood epidermal inclusion cyst mimicking clitoromegaly in a pediatric patient. Urology 2014;84(1):206–8.
53. Asante A, Omurtag K, Roberts C. Epidermal inclusion cyst of the clitoris 30 years after female genital mutilation. Fertil Steril 2010;94(3):1097.e1-3.
54. Anderson-Mueller BE, Laudenschlager MD, Hansen KA. Epidermoid cyst of the clitoris: an unusual cause of clitoromegaly in a patient without history of previous female circumcision. J Pediatr Adolesc Gynecol 2009;22(5):e130–132.
55. Celik N, Yalcin S, Gucer S, et al. Clitoral epidermoid cyst secondary to blunt trauma in a 9-year-old child. Turk J Pediatr 2011;53(1):108–10.
56. World Health Organization. Female genital mutilation: report of a technical working group. Geneva (Switzerland): Family and Reproductive Health; 1996.
57. Homesley HD. Management of vulvar cancer. Cancer 1995;76(10 Suppl):2159–70.
58. Sohaib SA, Richards PS, Ind T, et al. MR imaging of carcinoma of the vulva. AJNR Am J Neuroradiol 2002;178(2):373–7.
59. Hampl M, Deckers-Figiel S, Hampl JA, et al. New aspects of vulvar cancer: changes in localization and age of onset. Gynecol Oncol 2008;109(3):340–5.
60. Ghurani GB, Penalver MA. An update on vulvar cancer. Am J Obstet Gynecol 2001;185(2):294–9.
61. Parikh JH, Barton DP, Ind TE, et al. MR imaging features of vaginal malignancies. Radiographics 2008;28(1):49–63 [quiz: 322].
62. Homesley HD. Lymph node findings and outcome in squamous cell carcinoma of the vulva. Cancer 1994;74(9):2399–402.
63. van der Steen S, de Nieuwenhof HP, Massuger L, et al. New FIGO staging system of vulvar cancer indeed provides a better reflection of prognosis. Gynecol Oncol 2010;119(3):520–5.
64. Kataoka MY, Sala E, Baldwin P, et al. The accuracy of magnetic resonance imaging in staging of vulvar cancer: a retrospective multi-centre study. Gynecol Oncol 2010;117(1):82–7.
65. Grey AC, Carrington BM, Hulse PA, et al. Magnetic resonance appearance of normal inguinal nodes. Clin Radiol 2000;55(2):124–30.
66. Bipat S, Fransen GA, Spijkerboer AM, et al. Is there a role for magnetic resonance imaging in the evaluation of inguinal lymph node metastases in patients with vulva carcinoma? Gynecol Oncol 2006; 103(3):1001–6.
67. Rouzier R, Haddad B, Dubernard G, et al. Inguinofemoral dissection for carcinoma of the vulva: effect of modifications of extent and technique on morbidity and survival. J Am Coll Surg 2003; 196(3):442–50.
68. Kirby TO, Rocconi RP, Numnum TM, et al. Outcomes of stage I/II vulvar cancer patients after negative superficial inguinal lymphadenectomy. Gynecol Oncol 2005;98(2):309–12.
69. Salom EM, Penalver M. Recurrent vulvar cancer. Curr Treat Options Oncol 2002;3(2):143–53.
70. Deans GT, McAleer JJ, Spence RA. Malignant anal tumours. Br J Surg 1994;81(4):500–8.
71. Roach SC, Hulse PA, Moulding FJ, et al. Magnetic resonance imaging of anal cancer. Clin Radiol 2005;60(10):1111–9.

72. Kochhar R, Plumb AA, Carrington BM, et al. Imaging of anal carcinoma. AJNR Am J Neuroradiol 2012;199(3):W335–44.
73. Lindeque BG. The role of surgery in the management of carcinoma of the vagina. Baillieres Clin Obstet Gynaecol 1987;1(2):319–29.
74. Koussidis GA. Gynecologic rarities: a case of periclitoral abscess and review of the literature. Am J Obstet Gynecol 2012;207(5):e3–5.
75. Dave AJ, Sethi A, Morrone A. Female genital mutilation: what every American dermatologist needs to know. Dermatol Clin 2011;29(1):103–9.
76. Sur S. Recurrent periclitoral abscess treated by marsupialization. Am J Obstet Gynecol 1983; 147(3):340.
77. Kent SW, Taxiarchis LN. Recurrent periclitoral abscess. Am J Obstet Gynecol 1982;142(3):355–6.
78. de Miguel Criado J, del Salto LG, Rivas PF, et al. MR imaging evaluation of perianal fistulas: spectrum of imaging features. Radiographics 2012; 32(1):175–94.
79. Sainio P. Fistula-in-ano in a defined population. Incidence and epidemiological aspects. Ann Chir Gynaecol 1984;73(4):219–24.
80. Lilius HG. Fistula-in-ano, an investigation of human foetal anal ducts and intramuscular glands and a clinical study of 150 patients. Acta Chir Scand Suppl 1968;383:7–88.
81. Parks AG, Gordon PH, Hardcastle JD. A classification of fistula-in-ano. Br J Surg 1976;63(1):1–12.
82. Morris J, Spencer JA, Ambrose NS. MR imaging classification of perianal fistulas and its implications for patient management. Radiographics 2000;20(3):623–35 [discussion: 635–7].
83. Makowiec F, Jehle EC, Starlinger M. Clinical course of perianal fistulas in Crohn's disease. Gut 1995; 37(5):696–701.
84. Seow C, Phillips RK. Insights gained from the management of problematical anal fistulae at St. Mark's Hospital, 1984-88. Br J Surg 1991;78(5):539–41.
85. Bartram C, Buchanan G. Imaging anal fistula. Radiol Clin North Am 2003;41(2):443–57.
86. Schlosser BJ, Mirowski GW. Lichen sclerosus and lichen planus in women and girls. Clin Obstet Gynecol 2015;58(1):125–42.
87. Lambert J. Pruritus in female patients. Biomed Res Int 2014;2014:541867.
88. Smith YR, Haefner HK. Vulvar lichen sclerosus: pathophysiology and treatment. Am J Clin Dermatol 2004;5(2):105–25.
89. Zendell K, Edwards L. Lichen sclerosus with vaginal involvement: report of 2 cases and review of the literature. JAMA Dermatol 2013;149(10): 1199–202.
90. Veltman LL, Ostergard DR. Thrombosis of vulvar varicosities during pregnancy. Obstet Gynecol 1972;39(1):55–6.
91. Ninia JG, Goldberg TL. Treatment of vulvar varicosities by injection-compression sclerotherapy and a pelvic supporter. Obstet Gynecol 1996;87(5 Pt 1):786–8.
92. Scultetus AH, Villavicencio JL, Gillespie DL, et al. The pelvic venous syndromes: analysis of our experience with 57 patients. J Vasc Surg 2002;36(5):881–8.
93. Bell D, Kane PB, Liang S, et al. Vulvar varices: an uncommon entity in surgical pathology. Int J Gynecol Pathol 2007;26(1):99–101.
94. Meier CR, Jick H. Tamoxifen and risk of idiopathic venous thromboembolism. Br J Clin Pharmacol 1998;45(6):608–12.
95. Hernandez RK, Sorensen HT, Pedersen L, et al. Tamoxifen treatment and risk of deep venous thrombosis and pulmonary embolism: a Danish population-based cohort study. Cancer 2009; 115(19):4442–9.
96. Rapoport S, Sostman HD, Pope C, et al. Venous clots: evaluation with MR imaging. Radiology 1987;162(2):527–30.
97. Westerbeek RE, Van Rooden CJ, Tan M, et al. Magnetic resonance direct thrombus imaging of the evolution of acute deep vein thrombosis of the leg. J Thromb Haemost 2008;6(7):1087–92.
98. Frank SJ, Flusberg M, Friedman S, et al. CT appearance of common cosmetic and reconstructive surgical procedures and their complications. Clin Radiol 2013;68(1):e72–78.
99. Ali A. Contouring of the gluteal region in women: enhancement and augmentation. Ann Plast Surg 2011;67(3):209–14.
100. Lopiccolo MC, Workman BJ, Chaffins ML, et al. Silicone granulomas after soft-tissue augmentation of the buttocks: a case report and review of management. Dermatol Surg 2011;37(5):720–5.
101. Cardenas Restrepo JC, Munoz Ahmed JA. Large-volume lipoinjection for gluteal augmentation. Aesthet Surg J 2002;22(1):33–8.
102. Bruner TW, Roberts TL 3rd, Nguyen K. Complications of buttocks augmentation: diagnosis, management, and prevention. Clin Plast Surg 2006;33(3):449–66.
103. Hage JJ, Kanhai RC, Oen AL, et al. The devastating outcome of massive subcutaneous injection of highly viscous fluids in male-to-female transsexuals. Plast Reconstr Surg 2001;107(3):734–41.
104. Carroli G, Mignini L. Episiotomy for vaginal birth. Cochrane Database Syst Rev 2009;(1):CD000081.
105. Kettle C, Hills RK, Ismail KM. Continuous versus interrupted sutures for repair of episiotomy or second degree tears. Cochrane Database Syst Rev 2007;(4):CD000947.
106. Park SJ, Lee HK, Hong HS, et al. Hydrocele of the canal of Nuck in a girl: ultrasound and MR appearance. Br J Radiol 2004;77(915):243–4.
107. Safak AA, Erdogmus B, Yazici B, et al. Hydrocele of the canal of Nuck: sonographic and MRI appearances. J Clin Ultrasound 2007;35(9):531–2.

MR Imaging of the Pelvic Floor

Gaurav Khatri, MD[a], Alberto Diaz de Leon, MD[b], Mark E. Lockhart, MD, MPH[c,*]

KEYWORDS

• Dynamic pelvic floor MR imaging • MR defecography • Pelvic prolapse • Pelvic mesh

KEY POINTS

- Pelvic floor dysfunction typically affects multiple compartments of the pelvic floor.
- Knowledge of pelvic floor anatomy is important, and MR imaging allows for direct visualization of anatomic defects.
- Instillation of rectal contrast and defecation of the rectal gel during the examination are imperative for adequate MR defecography technique.
- Multiple attempts at defecation and/or Valsalva should be performed in order to elicit maximal prolapse.
- Pelvic floor MR imaging should include evaluation of anatomic defects and postsurgical changes including those pertaining to previously placed synthetic materials.

INTRODUCTION

Pelvic floor disorders affect approximately 25% of women over the age of 20 years[1] and up to 50% of women beyond 50 years old in the United States,[2] with negative impact on quality of life in a significant number of those affected.[3] Patients with pelvic floor dysfunction may present with pelvic pressure from pelvic organ prolapse, urinary or fecal incontinence, defecatory dysfunction, and/or chronic pelvic pain. Risk factors include female gender, advanced age, parity, childbirth, hysterectomy, obesity, connective tissue disorders, smoking, trauma to the pelvic floor, and other conditions that may result in chronic increase in intraabdominal pressure.[4] More than 500,000 surgical procedures are performed in the United States annually for pelvic organ prolapse and urinary incontinence,[5] and the lifetime risk of undergoing a single surgical procedure for either one of these conditions by the age of 80 years is 11%.[6] The direct cost of urinary incontinence in the United States for women in 1995 was estimated at $12 billion.[7] Importantly, the reoperation rate for recurrent prolapse is nearly 30%[6]; repeat intervention is often performed for occult components of disease that may have not been apparent on initial physical examination.

Physical examination may not be adequate as the sole means to evaluate pelvic floor dysfunction.[8,9] Imaging can help identify or better grade pelvic floor dysfunction given the complex and multifactorial nature of the condition, which often involves multiple compartments of the pelvic floor.[10–12] Fluoroscopic defecography has traditionally been used for imaging of pelvic floor dysfunction in the physiologic upright sitting position[13]; however, it involves exposure to ionizing radiation and does not allow for direct visualization of the pelvic floor anatomy. Depending on the specific technique used, it may not evaluate all 3 pelvic floor components or may require ingestion of oral contrast or instillation of contrast in the bladder and vagina.

The authors have nothing to disclose.

[a] Division of Body MRI, Department of Radiology, University of Texas Southwestern Medical Center, 5323 Harry Hines Boulevard, Dallas, TX 75390, USA; [b] Division of Abdominal Imaging MRI, Department of Radiology, University of Texas Southwestern Medical Center, 5323 Harry Hines Boulevard, Dallas, TX 75390, USA; [c] Division of Abdominal Imaging, Department of Radiology, University of Alabama at Birmingham, JTN 344, 619 19th Street South, Birmingham, AL 35249, USA
* Corresponding author.
E-mail address: mlockhart@uabmc.edu

Magn Reson Imaging Clin N Am 25 (2017) 457–480
http://dx.doi.org/10.1016/j.mric.2017.03.003

Dynamic MR imaging of the pelvis for evaluation of pelvic floor descent was first described by Yang and colleagues[14] in 1991 and has since developed into an important tool for both anatomic and functional evaluation of the pelvic floor. Multiplanar capabilities and high inherent contrast resolution of MR imaging allow for direct visualization of pelvic organs as well as the muscular anatomy of the pelvic floor. Furthermore, all 3 compartments of the pelvic floor can be evaluated in unison without additional patient preparation. High cost, supine positioning during imaging, and substantial variability of pelvic MR imaging measurements[15] have been deterrents to universal adoption of dynamic MR imaging of the pelvic floor. Although MR defecography may show a wide range of findings even in asymptomatic patients,[16] the degree of prolapse on MR imaging has been shown to be higher in symptomatic patients,[10] and MR imaging has been shown to alter surgical management in 67% of patients.[11] Recently published American College of Radiology imaging Appropriateness Criteria consider MR defecography with rectal contrast equivalent to fluoroscopic cystocolpoproctography for evaluation of suspected pelvic floor prolapse and urinary dysfunction. The criteria favor MR imaging for defecatory dysfunction and suspected recurrent prolapse, and for pelvic floor dysfunction following pelvic floor repair.[17] This article reviews pertinent pelvic floor anatomy, appropriate MR imaging techniques for evaluation of the pelvic floor, and findings encountered during interpretation of anatomic and functional pelvic floor MR imaging.

PELVIC FLOOR ANATOMY

A basic understanding of pelvic floor anatomy is essential for adequate anatomic and functional evaluation of the pelvic floor on MR imaging. For purposes of clinical evaluation, the female pelvis is classically divided into 3 compartments: the anterior compartment containing the bladder and urethra; the middle compartment containing the uterus, cervix, and vagina; and the posterior compartment containing the rectum and anal canal. These compartments are closely interrelated, and patients often present with multicompartment dysfunction.[10–12] The compartments of the pelvic floor are supported by a complex network of fascia, ligaments, and pelvic floor muscles that form 3 layers of support: the endopelvic fascia (superior), the pelvic diaphragm (middle), and the perineal membrane or urogenital diaphragm (inferior). The fascia and ligaments provide passive support, whereas the musculature of the pelvic diaphragm provides the underlying tone and can be recruited for active support.

Endopelvic Fascia

The endopelvic fascia is a sheet of connective tissue that extends across the pelvic floor from the bony pelvis on one side to the other and forms the superior-most layer of support of the pelvic floor. It covers the levator ani muscles and pelvic viscera. Various components of the endopelvic fascia are named according to their location. The pubocervical fascia between the bladder and vagina or cervix, the parametrium extending from the cervix to the lateral sidewalls, the paracolpium extending from the vagina to the pelvic sidewalls, and the rectovaginal fascia between the vagina and rectum may not be visible on standard MR imaging. Other components such as the urethral ligaments and perineal body are identifiable on MR imaging. The cardinal and uterosacral ligaments arise from condensations of the endopelvic fascia superiorly. Laterally, the endopelvic fascia coalesces to form the arcus tendineus along the bony pelvis, which serves as an attachment site for the muscles that form the pelvic diaphragm. The endopelvic fascia provides 3 levels of support in relation to vagina: level I (vaginal apex), level II (mid vagina), level III (distal vagina), and defects in each level may present with unique physical signs and symptoms.[18] Deficiencies within different portions of the fascia may determine the degree of prolapse in each compartment. For example, defects in the uterosacral ligaments or the paracolpium/parametrium may result in cervical or vaginal prolapse; tears in the pubocervical fascia or urethral ligaments may result in cystocele and urethral hypermobility; and defects in the perineal body or rectovaginal fascia may present with anterior rectocele or enterocele.[19]

Pelvic Diaphragm

The pelvic diaphragm provides the middle layer of support of the pelvic floor and consists of the ischiococcygeus muscles and the levator ani muscles. The levator ani is a vaselike or hourglass-shaped group of striated muscles composed of the iliococcygeus, pubococcygeus, and puborectalis muscles (**Fig. 1**). These muscles are well seen on MR imaging and normally maintain a convex appearance superiorly. The relatively thin iliococcygeus muscle attaches anteriorly to the pubic bone, laterally to the arcus tendineus, and inferiorly to the external anal sphincter. The thicker pubococcygeus muscle is more medially located relative to the iliococcygeus, it arises from the superior pubic rami and wraps around the bladder, urethra, vagina,

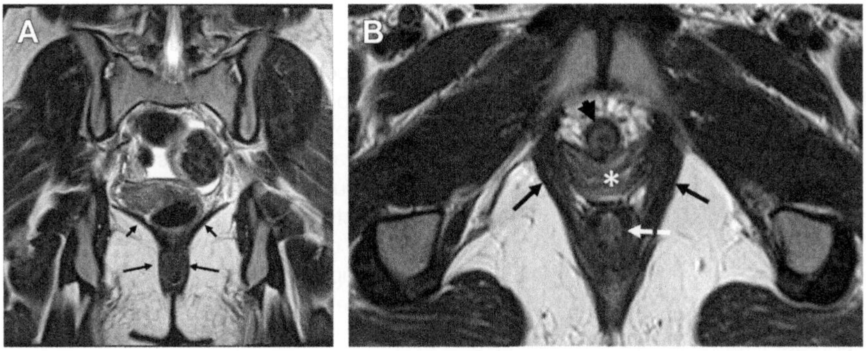

Fig. 1. Anatomy. (*A*) Coronal T2 TSE image at the level of the anus demonstrating vaselike morphology of the levator ani muscles, which are convex superiorly. The iliococccygeus and pubococcygeus muscles are difficult to differentiate from each other (*short arrows* in *A*), whereas the puborectalis (*long solid arrows* in *A*) is the more inferior muscle around the anus. (*B*) Axial T2 TSE image at the level of the pelvic floor hiatus. The puborectalis muscle (*long solid arrows* in *B*) attaches to the pubic bone anteriorly and makes a U- or V-shaped sling around the urethra (*arrowhead* in *B*), vagina (*asterisk* in *B*), and anus (*dashed arrow* in *B*).

and rectum. Posteriorly, the iliococccygeus and pubococcygeus form a thick condensation of tissue called the levator plate (**Fig. 2**), which inserts upon the sacrum and coccyx. The iliococccygeus and pubococcygeus muscles are difficult to differentiate on MR imaging owing to the overlap in fibers and morphology. The most caudal component of the levator ani muscle group is the puborectalis, which attaches anteriorly to the pubic symphysis and forms a U-shaped sling around the anorectum (see **Fig. 1**). The level of the puborectalis impression upon the posterior rectum demarcates the anorectal junction, and the margins of the puborectalis form the urogenital or pelvic floor hiatus. Superiorly, the puborectalis muscle fibers overlap with the pubococcygeus. The ischiococcygeus or the

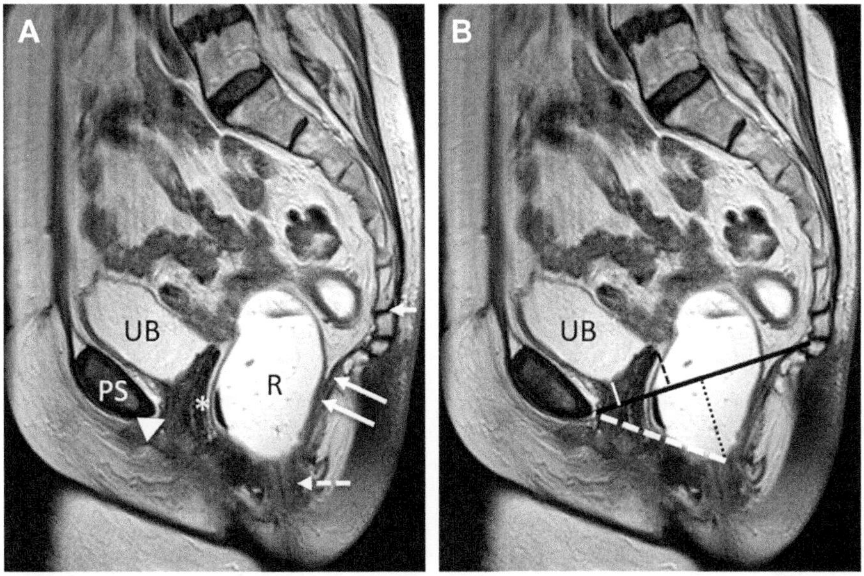

Fig. 2. Anatomy and references. Sagittal T2 TSE image (*A*) through the midline pelvis demonstrates normal pelvic anatomy, including musculoskeletal landmarks such as the pubic symphysis (PS), sacrococcygeal junction (*short solid arrow*), and the levator plate (*long solid arrows*) attaching upon the coccygeal segments. The urinary bladder (UB), urethra (*arrowhead*), vagina (*asterisk*), contrast-filled rectum (R), and anus (*dashed arrow*) are well seen. (*B*) Same sagittal T2 TSE image demonstrating the PCL (*solid black line* in *B*) extending from the inferior tip if the PS to the first coccygeal joint. Distance from the inferior most point of the UB (*solid white line*), and distance from the vaginal apex (*dashed black line*) are measured perpendicular to the PCL at rest. The H-line (*dashed white line*) is drawn from the inferior tip of the pubic symphysis to the anorectal junction. The M-line (*dotted black line*) is drawn perpendicularly down from the PCL to the posterior point of the H-line.

coccygeus muscle is a relatively minor part of the pelvic diaphragm, extending from the coccyx in the midline to the ischial spine bilaterally.[18,20] The pelvic diaphragm provides continuous tone to the pelvic floor, but can be contracted or relaxed actively. Atrophy or defects of the pelvic diaphragm, particularly the puborectalis, are well depicted on axial MR imaging (**Fig. 3**).

Perineal Membrane/Urogenital Diaphragm

The perineal membrane (also referred to as the urogenital diaphragm) forms the caudal-most layer of the pelvic floor and comprises primarily the deep transverse perineal muscle and connective tissue that extend from ischial rami laterally to the perineal body in the midline (**Fig. 4**). The perineal membrane attaches anteriorly to the pubic symphysis, giving the perineal membrane a triangular shape.

MR IMAGING TECHNIQUE

Dynamic MR imaging of the pelvic floor can be performed in an upright low field strength open magnet with the patient sitting on a modified MR imaging–safe commode,[21] or with the patient supine on a conventional high-field-strength magnet (1.5 T or 3 T). The sitting position is more physiologic; however, upright magnets are not readily available at most centers, making upright MR defecography difficult to perform. Alternatively, supine MR defecography can be performed with relative ease on most high-field-strength magnets. MR imaging with defecation in the sitting position may be preferred for evaluation of defecatory dysfunction in the posterior compartment[17]; however, Gufler and colleagues[22] showed no significant difference in depiction of prolapse in the anterior and middle compartment between supine MR imaging and upright colpocystoproctography. In contrast, Kelvin and colleagues[23] showed an underestimation of the extent of cystoceles and enteroceles on supine MR defecography relative to fluoroscopic cystocolpoproctography; they did, however, note that MR imaging had the advantage of directly visualizing all pelvic organs and musculature in a dynamic fashion. Multiple other studies have also compared upright fluoroscopic defecography or upright MR defecography with supine dynamic pelvic floor MR imaging with variable results. Most of these studies have not used defecation for the supine MR imaging protocol, thus confounding the true effect of positioning on degree of prolapse when comparing the examinations.[9,24–26] A recent study comparing MR defecography in both upright and supine positions in the same set of patients showed significantly lower position of the bladder and vagina at defecation during the upright MR imaging, but not of the anorectal junction[27]; however, imaging in the upright position immediately followed imaging in the supine position in that study, raising the possibility that pelvic floor fatigue could have played a role in eliciting a higher degree of prolapse on the latter examination. Kumar and colleagues[28] actually demonstrated a higher degree of prolapse in the anterior compartment when comparing supine MR imaging with defecation to another upright examination: standing voiding cystourethrogram (VCUG).

Regardless of supine or upright positioning, defecation has been shown to be imperative for dynamic assessment of the pelvic floor.[29–31] Functional imaging with defecation necessitates instillation of contrast material in the rectum.[32] Although the exact composition and volume of rectal contrast media vary widely in the literature,[21,33,34] ultrasound gel is the most commonly used agent due to sterility, relatively low cost, availability, and ease of instillation. The authors

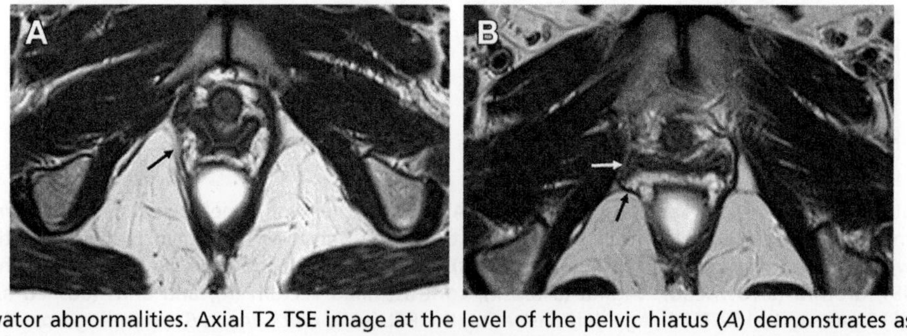

Fig. 3. Levator abnormalities. Axial T2 TSE image at the level of the pelvic hiatus (*A*) demonstrates asymmetric thinning of the right puborectalis muscle consistent with atrophy (*arrow* in *A*); however, the vagina still maintains its H-shape. Axial T2 TSE image at the level of the pelvic hiatus in another patient (*B*) demonstrates a defect in the right puborectalis muscle (*black arrow* in *B*), which appears scarred laterally. Note the lateral extension of the right side of the vagina through the defect (*white arrow* in *B*) and distortion of the H-shape.

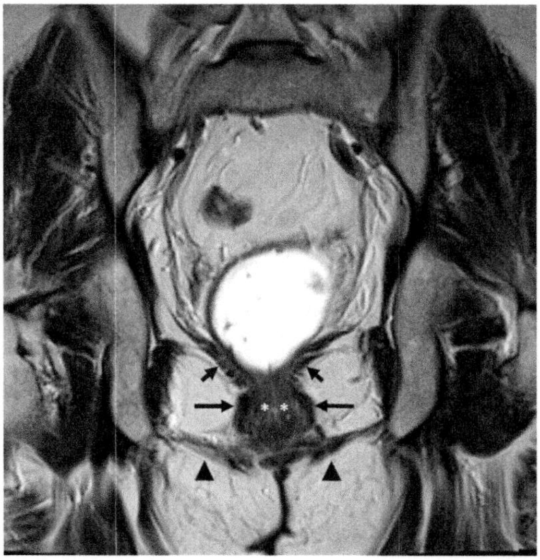

Fig. 4. Perineal membrane. Coronal T2 TSE image through the anal sphincter complex demonstrates the perineal membrane or urogenital diaphragm (*arrowheads*), which forms the third and most caudal layer of myofascial support of the pelvic floor stretching from the ischial tuberosities laterally to the perineal body in the midline (not shown). Note the pubococcygeus and iliococcygeus muscles (*short arrows*), the puborectalis muscle (*long arrows*), and the internal anal sphincter (*asterisks*).

use 120 mL of gel in order to avoid overdistention of the rectum while allowing adequate volume for defecation.[35] In their experience, smaller volumes of 60 mL are difficult for the patients to evacuate.

In addition to providing functional evaluation, MR imaging allows for direct visualization of multiple pelvic structures without having to opacify small bowel, bladder, or vagina with contrast. Furthermore, detailed evaluation of the pelvic floor levator muscles is possible on MR imaging.[20] Supine MR defecography, usually performed on a higher-field-strength magnet (1.5 T or 3 T), allows for higher resolution evaluation of the anatomy in comparison to lower-field-strength open magnets, which typically suffer from poor signal-to-noise as well as lower spatial and contrast resolution.[36] The higher resolution provided by supine high-field-strength MR imaging is also beneficial when evaluating previously placed urethral slings or pelvic mesh.[37]

Because of the unusual nature of MR defecography, referring physicians explain the examination to the patients during the clinic visit, and the authors provide patients with educational material about the examination before their arrival to the imaging center. The MR technologists brief the patients and attempt to relieve any anxiety about the examination upon arrival on the day of examination. They specifically coach the patients on how to perform the Kegel (squeeze), strain, and defecation maneuvers before taking the patient to the magnet room. Patients are also instructed to urinate upon arrival and then drink 16 ounces of water in an effort to achieve standardized mild bladder distention. The goal is to partially fill the bladder while avoiding overdistention because this may obscure prolapse in other compartments.[38,39] The MR imaging table is covered with disposable absorbent pads. Patients are positioned on the MR imaging table with their pelvis centered in an inflatable plastic enema ring. Ultrasound gel is instilled using a catheter tip syringe with patients in the lateral decubitus position, and the patients are then placed again in the supine position for imaging, with knees slightly flexed on a pillow or wedge for support. A multichannel phase-array surface coil is positioned over the patient's pelvis for MR image acquisition.

T2-weighted (T2w) turbo spin echo (TSE) images in sagittal, axial, and coronal planes and axial T1-weighted gradient echo (GRE) images can be acquired at rest to allow for anatomic evaluation. These should be followed by cine-type true fast imaging with steady state precession (TrueFISP) or single shot fast spin echo (SSFSE) in a single midsagittal plane for functional imaging performed during Kegel (squeeze), strain, and defecation. Although both sequences may perform acceptably, TrueFISP images have been shown to demonstrate higher degrees of prolapse in all 3 compartments than SSFSE images.[40] The authors advocate at least 3 attempts at defecation in order to elicit maximum degree of prolapse. The sagittal cine-type TrueFISP or SSFSE images should be repeated after defecation with a postdefecation strain maneuver, because this may sometimes show a higher degree of prolapse particularly when the patients are unable to completely empty the rectum during the defecation phases. If patients are not able to defecate after 3 attempts, they are instructed to defecate in the restroom and then immediately return to MR imaging for the postdefecation strain images. Optional sequences include cine-type TrueFISP or SSFSE images in coronal oblique or axial oblique planes, along the axis of the anal canal or the pubococcygeal line (PCL), respectively. These are helpful in visualizing para-midline defects that are occult in the single midsagittal plane. Although either 1.5-T or 3-T magnets may be used for MR defecography, the authors find certain sequences such as cine TrueFISP to be more robust with fewer artifacts at 1.5 T. A sample MR defecography protocol is detailed in **Table 1**.

Table 1
Sample 1.5-T MR defecography protocol

Sequence	Imaging Plane	Maneuver	FOV (cm)	Slice Thickness (mm)	TR (ms)	TE (ms)	Flip Angle (°)	Matrix
T2 TSE	Axial	Rest	26	5	3920	91	150	320 × 256
T2 TSE	Sagittal	Rest	26	5	4070	91	150	320 × 256
T2 TSE	Coronal	Rest	26	5	5120	91	150	320 × 256
T1 GRE OP/IP	Axial	Rest	26	5	140	2.3/4.6	55	256 × 208
Cine TrueFISP	Sagittal	Kegel	34	8	734.4	1.8	80	256 × 256
Cine TrueFISP ×3	Sagittal	Defecation	34	8	734.4	1.8	80	256 × 256
Cine TrueFISP	Axial Oblique	Defecation	33	8	742.6	1.8	80	256 × 256
Cine TrueFISP	Coronal Oblique	Defecation	33	8	946.4	1.8	80	256 × 256
Cine TrueFISP	Sagittal	Postdefecation strain	34	8	734.4	1.8	80	256 × 256

Abbreviations: FOV, field of view; OP/IP, opposed phase/in phase; TE, echo time; TR, repetition time.

MR IMAGING INTERPRETATION

In order to facilitate comprehensive and efficient evaluation of the pelvic floor, the authors use a data collection sheet, which is particularly helpful when a trainee or radiologist with relatively less experience is performing the initial interpretation. In addition, they use a standardized dictation template to report the examinations (**Box 1**). Reporting templates may differ between centers depending on the practice patterns of the referrers, but they should report anatomic findings and functional findings in all 3 pelvic floor compartments. It is imperative to include positive and pertinent negative elements that are deemed necessary by referring clinicians and radiologists, in an organized format. Further details regarding suggested elements to include in the report can be found in the later discussion, "What the referring physician needs to know."

Anatomic Evaluation

As mentioned previously, one of the advantages of dynamic MR imaging of the pelvic floor is that it also allows for high-resolution anatomic evaluation in multiple planes. Morphologic changes of the pelvic floor seen on MR imaging correlate with functional deficiencies, and there are significant differences in levator muscle volume, shape, and integrity between patients with incontinence or pelvic organ prolapse and asymptomatic individuals.[41–45] The levator muscles can be assessed for areas of asymmetric thickening or atrophy, focal defects, scarring (see **Fig. 3**), ballooning (**Fig. 5**), or focal eventration.[46] The inferior-most levator ani muscle, the puborectalis, may be thinner on the right than on the left when viewed in the axial plane, even in asymptomatic women, likely due to chemical shift artifact.[41,47] Lateral scarring or absence of the anterior attachment of the puborectalis to the pubic bone as seen on axial images may represent a tear (see **Fig. 3**B).[48] Puborectalis muscle tears may be unilateral or bilateral, and they may result from vaginal trauma or injury during childbirth, episiotomy, or other vaginal surgery. When bilateral, these may result in a "batwing shape" of the perineum at the level of the lower vagina and urethra due to absence of the pubovisceralis portion of the levator ani. The vagina may appear flat and protrude laterally into the muscle defects and lie close to the obturator internus muscle on the affected side (see **Fig. 3**B).[48] In addition to the puborectalis muscle, the anal sphincter complex should also be evaluated on axial images. The thick circular internal anal sphincter is typically intermediate in signal intensity on T2w images, whereas the more inferiorly located external sphincter is thinner and more hypointense. The levator muscles should also be evaluated for asymmetric defects, thinning, or bulging on the coronal images. These may correlate with findings of asymmetric prolapse on functional images. Sagittal images are useful to evaluate the integrity of the levator plate, which inserts on the coccygeal joints. The levator plate insertion may span multiple levels upon the coccyx, however, the dominant point of insertion should be noted.

Box 1
Dictation template

History: []

Technique: [] mL of [] was instilled into the rectum. Multiplanar MR imaging of the pelvis was performed using static axial T1-weighted, axial, coronal, sagittal T2-weighted, as well as dynamic multiplanar cine imaging during Kegel, defecation, and maximal strain after defecation. All images were obtained with patient in [] position.

IV Contrast: None

Comparison: None

Findings:

Anatomic Evaluation: [Prior hysterectomy/other surgery] [Levator muscle symmetry/asymmetry/atrophy/focal defects] [Prior bulking agent/urethral sling/vaginal mesh/SC mesh]

Levator plate insertion: []

Last nonmobile SC/coccygeal joint: []

[] is used as posterior point of reference for the PCL in this patient

Functional Evaluation: Patient [was/was not] able to defecate during the examination. [No/minimal/significant] rectal contrast remains after defecation.

Anterior Compartment

The bladder measures [] cm × [] cm × [] cm (volume [] mL).

Bladder base location relative to the PCL:

Rest: [] cm [above/below]

Defecation/Maximal strain: [] cm [above/below]

Findings are consistent with [no/grade 1/grade 2/grade 3] cystocele.

Urethral Angle:

Rest: [] degrees; defecation/maximal strain: [] degrees

This is consistent with [no/significant] urethral hypermobility.

Middle Compartment

Vaginal length: [] cm.

[Vaginal apex/cervix] location relative to PCL:

Rest: [] cm [above/below]

Defecation/maximal strain: [] cm [above/below]

This is consistent with [no/grade 1/grade 2/grade3] [vaginal/cervical/uterine] prolapse.

H line (levator hiatus)

Rest: [] cm (normal ≤6 cm).

Defection/maximal strain: [] cm.

M line (anorectal junction location relative to PCL)

Rest: [] cm (normal ≤2 cm below PCL)

Defecation/maximal strain: [] cm

Above findings are consistent with [normal/widened] levator hiatus and [normal/low lying] anorectal junction at rest with [no abnormal/grade 1/2/3] widening and [no abnormal/grade1/2/3] descent during defecation/maximal strain.

Posterior Compartment

Anorectal/levator-anus angle

Rest: [] degrees; Kegel: [] degrees; defecation/maximal strain: [] degrees.

This is consistent with [normal/narrowed/widened] resting angle with [expected narrowing/diminished narrowing] during Kegel and [expected widening/no change/paradoxic narrowing] during defecation/maximal strain.

Rectal Intussusception:

[No rectal intussusception/intrarectal intussusception/intraanal intussusception/extraanal intussusception] [if present, provide length of intussusception] seen.

Rectocele:

Rectocele size: [] cm anteroposterior.

Rectocele location: [upper/mid/distal vagina or along entire vaginal length]

[No/grade 1/2/3] rectocele [with/without] bulge along posterior vaginal wall

[Enterocele/peritoneocele/sigmoidocele]:

Distance below PCL: [] cm.

Distance below vaginal apex along posterior vaginal wall: [] cm.

[No/grade 1/2/3] [enterocele/peritoneocele/sigmoidocele] seen.

Other: None []

Impression:

1. [Anatomic findings including prior surgery or repair]
2. [Anterior compartment including cystocele/urethral mobility]
3. [Middle compartment including vagina/cervix/uterus]
4. [Normal/widened] levator hiatus and [normal/low lying] anorectal junction at rest with [no abnormal/grade 1/2/3] widening and [no abnormal/grade1/2/3] descent during defecation/maximal strain.
5. [Rectocele?]
6. [Rectal intussusception?]
7. [Enterocele/peritoneocele/sigmoidocele?]
8. [Normal/narrowed/widened] resting angle with [expected narrowing/diminished narrowing] during Kegel and [expected widening/no change/paradoxic narrowing] during defecation/maximal strain.

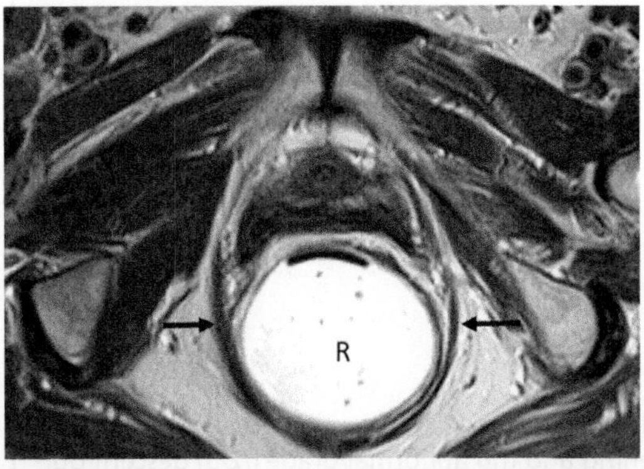

Fig. 5. Ballooning of levator muscles. Axial T2 TSE image demonstrates bulging of the pelvic floor hiatus. The puborectalis muscle is thinned and ballooned out laterally on either side (*arrows*) and the gel-filled rectum (R) occupies the widened pelvic floor hiatus. This appearance is in contrast to the normal appearance of the pelvic floor hiatus in **Fig. 1**B.

Anatomic evaluation should also report the presence or absence of the uterus and cervix and include assessment of other pelvic organs, such as the bladder, urethra, vagina, and rectosigmoid colon. The bladder may be thick-walled or trabeculated if the patient suffers from recurrent infections or bladder outlet obstruction.[49] The normal urethra should have a circular target-like morphology; however, this may be absent in postmenopausal women. In the setting of urinary incontinence, there may be distortion of the surrounding tissue, the urethra may appear flattened or may demonstrate funneling,[4] and there may be disruption of the urethral ligaments.[43] Morphologic alterations of the vagina may correlate with specific levels of defects in the pelvic floor support system. For example, a level I fascial defect as a result of detachment of the uterosacral ligament results in posterior sagging of the vagina bilaterally. The appearance is

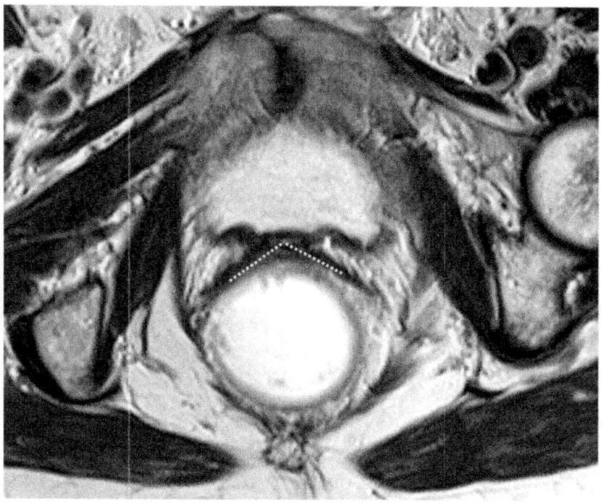

Fig. 6. Loss of level I fascial support. Axial T2 TSE image at the level of the upper vagina demonstrates posterior displacement of the lateral vagina on either side (*dotted line*). This appearance, termed the "chevron sign," results from loss of level I support of the endopelvic fascia.

termed the "chevron sign" (**Fig. 6**).[50] A level II defect of the middle third of the vagina along with puborectalis muscle defects may cause the vagina to lose its expected "H" shape and appear relatively flat on axial images (**Fig. 7**).[48] A paravaginal level II defect may result in posterior drooping of the urinary bladder resulting in the "saddlebag sign" if bilateral.[50] A level III endopelvic fascia defect due to deficiency of the urethral ligaments may result in widening of the retropubic space, sometimes termed the "mustache sign."[50]

Finally, in addition to assessment of native pelvic floor anatomy, MR imaging allows for evaluation of injected urethral bulking agents,

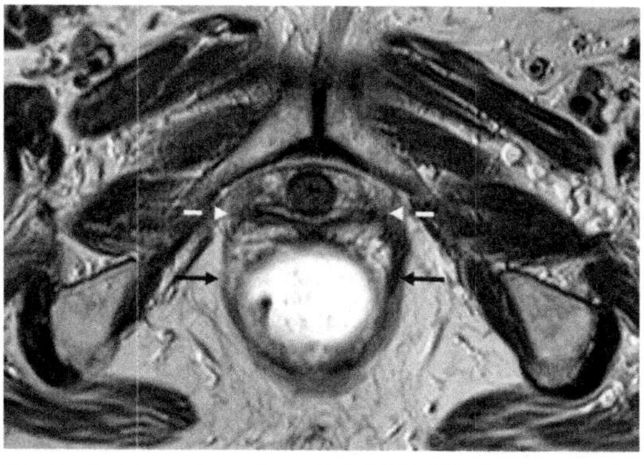

Fig. 7. Flattened vagina. Axial T2 TSE image at the level of the mid vagina demonstrates a flattened appearance of the vagina (*dashed arrows*) instead of the expected "H" or butterfly shape. This appearance is a result of a level II endopelvic fascia defect along with weakness of the puborectalis muscles bilaterally. The puborectalis muscles demonstrate outward bowing or ballooning (*solid arrows*).

previously placed urethral slings, and vaginal mesh.[37] Discussion of the various types and brands of bulking agents, slings, and mesh is outside the scope of this review, but the radiologist must be familiar with the typical appearances and locations of these synthetic materials. Urethral bulking agents are injected circumferentially within the spongiform tissue of the urethra and typically appear slightly hyperintense on T2w images (**Fig. 8**). These do not enhance, and on occasion, may demonstrate marked hyperintense signal on T2w images, mimicking urethral diverticula. Correlation with prior history of pelvic floor intervention is imperative to differentiate urethral diverticulum from bulking agent in these scenarios.

Urethral slings are generally placed at the level of the mid urethra. When the arms of the slings extend into the retropubic space, these are called retropubic slings (**Fig. 9**). They form a U or V shape around the urethra and extend superiorly and superficially to the anterior abdominal wall by traversing the retropubic space. A fat plane must be maintained between the sling and the urinary bladder. Loss of this fat plane with focal thickening of the bladder should raise suspicion for bladder wall erosion (**Fig. 10**). Patients with erosion may present with pain, infection, or irritative bladder symptoms. Transobturator slings extend laterally into the obturator foramina and do not involve the retropubic space, thus resulting in a low risk of bladder- or urinary-related complications and lower likelihood of major vascular injury. Nonetheless, transobturator slings are associated with higher rates of erosion, vaginal perforation, and groin pain as compared with retropubic slings.[37] From an imaging perspective, transobturator slings are more challenging to visualize on MR imaging.

Vaginal mesh kits are placed along the anterior and/or posterior vaginal walls, but mesh erosion rates as high as 18% have been reported.[51] The central body of vaginal mesh may appear as a hypointense bandlike structure on axial or sagittal T2w images along the vaginal wall; however, scar tissue can have a similar appearance and may mimic mesh (see **Fig. 10**). More peripherally, the arms of vaginal mesh kits may be seen extending posterolaterally to the sacrospinous ligaments, levator muscles, and inferiorly into the ischiorectal fossae (see **Figs. 9** and **10**). Sacrocolpopexy (SC) mesh has a distinct appearance as it extends from its superior attachment on the sacral promontory with slight rightward curvature to attach upon the vaginal apex (**Fig. 11**). It is generally placed in an extraperitoneal location, which results in the rightward bowed appearance. In the central pelvis, when viewed on cross section, SC mesh demonstrates homogeneous hypointense signal

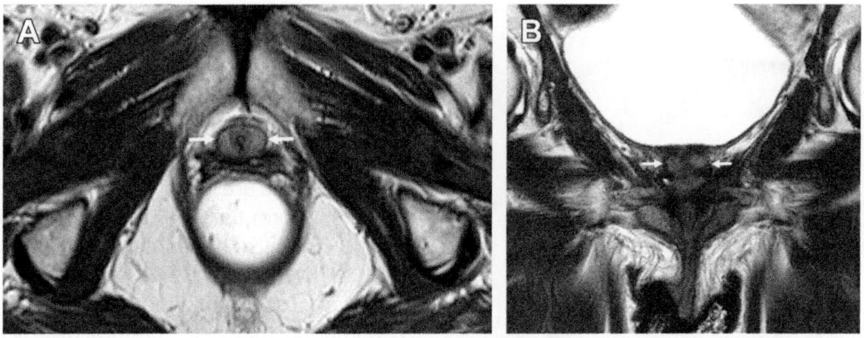

Fig. 8. Bulking agent. Axial T2 TSE image at the level of the mid urethra demonstrates circumferential increased signal intensity within the spongiform tissue (*arrows* in *A*). The appearance is consistent with urethral bulking agent. Coronal T2 TSE image in another patient demonstrates slightly hyperintense urethral bulking agent (*arrows* in *B*) surrounding the lumen below the bladder neck.

on T2w images and may be mistaken for bowel or a colonic diverticulum. Thickening and high signal intensity of the mesh on T2w images, or associated collections should suggest superimposed infection.

Slings, mesh, and their associated fibrotic reaction all appear hypointense on T2w images, and scarring may frequently mimic synthetic material. In addition to erosion or extrusion, other potential complications of mesh include infection, abscesses, or hematomas, some of which may not be visible on physical examination.[52]

Functional Evaluation

Establishment of appropriate landmarks on sagittal images is critical for functional evaluation of the anterior, middle, and posterior compartments of the pelvis. Multiple reference lines have been proposed in the literature,[53] with the midpubic line (MPL) and the PCL being the most common. The MPL is drawn through the long axis of the pubic symphysis and corresponds to the level of the hymen on physical examination.[54,55] The PCL corresponding to the level of the pelvic floor

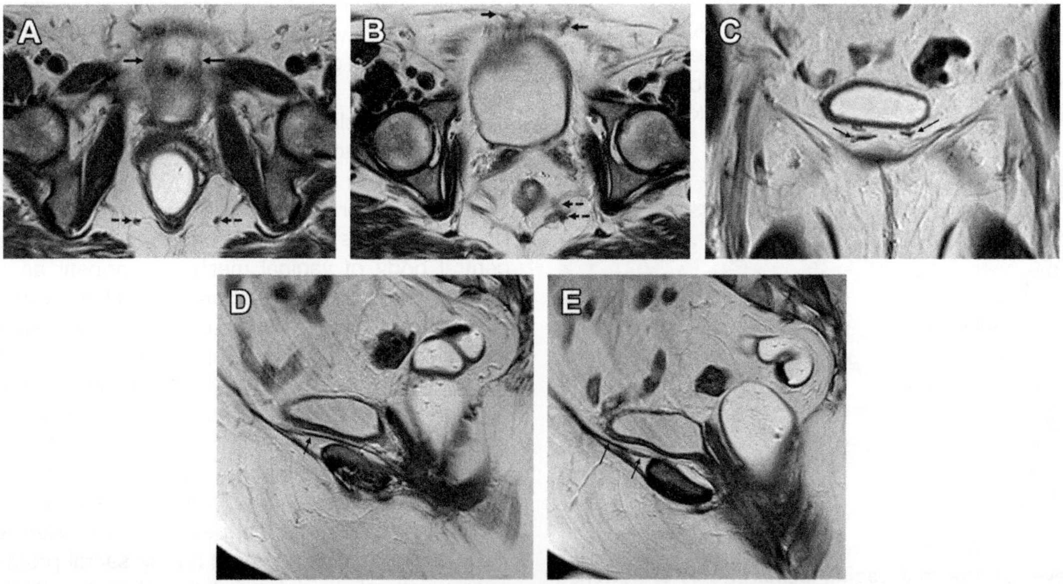

Fig. 9. Urethral sling. Axial T2 TSE images demonstrate the arms of the sling in the retropubic space extending toward the rectus sheath anteriorly (*solid arrows* in *A, B*). Arms of posterior vaginal mesh also seen in the ischioanal fossae (*dashed arrows* in *A*) and traversing the levator muscles on the left (*dashed arrow* in *B*). Coronal T2 TSE image demonstrates expected location and normal morphology of retropubic components of the urethral sling (*solid arrows* in *C*). The retropubic components are well seen on the sagittal images on either side of midline (*arrows* in *D, E*). In the retropubic space, a fat plane must be maintained between the sling and the urinary bladder.

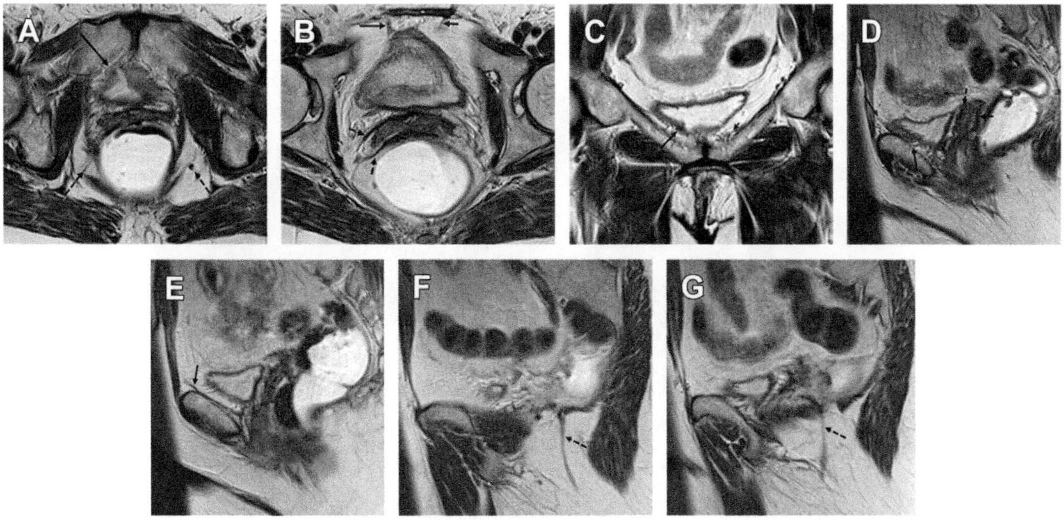

Fig. 10. Bladder wall erosion. Axial T2 TSE image at the bladder neck shows retraction of the urinary bladder in the expected location of the right arm of the retropubic sling (*solid arrow* in *A*). Arms of vaginal mesh are seen in the ischioanal fossae (*dashed arrows* in *A*). More cranially, right arm of the RP sling is in close proximity to the urinary bladder (*long solid arrow* in *B*), while the left arm is distant from the bladder (*short solid arrow* in *B*). Vaginal mesh segments along the anterior and posterior vaginal walls are seen as linear hypointense bands (*dashed arrows* in *B*); however, scar tissue can have this appearance. Coronal T2 TSE image demonstrates erosion of the right arm of the RP sling into the wall of the UB (*long arrow* in *C*), while there is a fat plane separating the left arm from the bladder (*short arrow* in *C*). Sagittal T2 TSE image to the right of midline demonstrates focal bladder wall thickening (*long solid arrows* in *D*) at site of sling erosion. Anterior and posterior vaginal mesh seen as linear T2 hypointense bands (*dashed arrows* in *D*), again difficult to differentiate from scar tissue. Left arm of the urethral sling in the RP space is separated from the bladder by a fat plane (*solid arrow* in *E*). Sagittal T2 TSE images through the left (*F*) and right (*G*) pelvis demonstrate arms of vaginal mesh (*dashed arrows* in *F, G*) extending through the levator muscles and sacrospinous ligaments into the ischioanal fossae.

is the most widely used reference line.[53] It was first defined by Yang and colleagues[14] as extending from the inferior tip of the pubic symphysis to the tip of the last coccygeal joint. Subsequent definitions have varied slightly in regards to their choice of posterior landmark used to draw the PCL.[53] The authors have found that the coccyx typically rotates inferiorly and posteriorly during straining and defecation. Because downward motion of the coccygeal tip would alter the location of the PCL, the authors advocate using the most inferior nonmobile sacrococcygeal or coccygeal joint as the posterior point of the PCL (see **Fig. 2**B). This strategy allows for a most stationary reference landmark that is consistent between rest and defecation. It is important to document which specific joint was used for drawing the PCL in each case. Staging prolapse on MR imaging with either the PCL or the MPL has shown variable agreement with patient symptoms and only poor or fair agreement with clinical staging.[55–57] Regardless, the choice of reference line should be made in consensus with radiologists and referring physicians. Functional evaluation is performed with reference to the PCL at the authors' institutions, as described within this article.

The "HMO" system is used to grade pelvic floor laxity and organ descent and includes evaluation of the "H-line," "M-line," and organ-specific prolapse.[58] The "H-line" is a measure of the width of the pelvic floor hiatus in the anteroposterior dimension and is measured from the inferior tip of the pubic symphysis to the posterior circular fibers of the anorectal junction (see **Fig. 2**B). Normal H-line at rest is $\leq$6 cm. The "M-line" is drawn perpendicularly down from the PCL to the posterior extent of the H-line at the posterior aspect of the anorectal junction (see **Fig. 2**B). It represents the degree of pelvic floor descent. The anorectal junction is demarcated by the impression of the horizontal fibers of the puborectalis muscle on the posterior wall of the rectum and can be identified by cross-referencing the axial images with a midline sagittal image. The M-line at rest is typically $\leq$2 cm. Degree of pelvic hiatus widening and floor descent is commonly graded based on a previously published grading scale[33] (**Table 2**). Excessive widening and descent of the pelvic floor have been termed the descending perineum syndrome, which is discussed later under abnormalities of the posterior compartment.

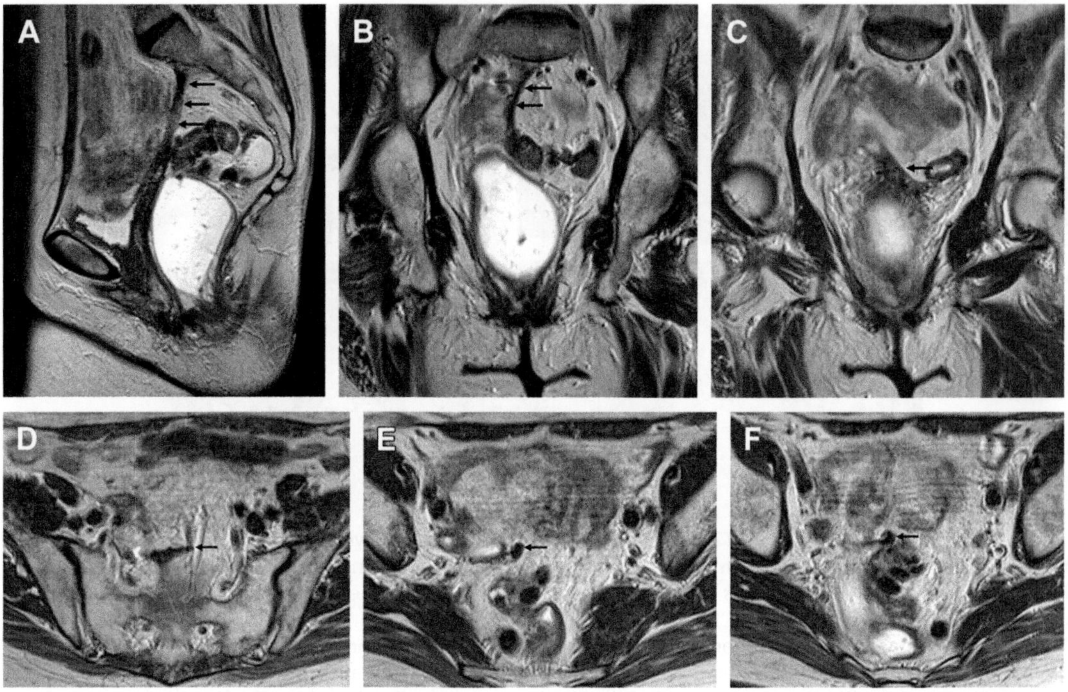

Fig. 11. SC mesh. Sagittal (*A*), coronal (*B, C*), and axial (*D–F*) T2 TSE images demonstrate typical T2 hypointense appearance of SC mesh (*arrows*) extending from the sacral promontory to the vaginal apex. Coronal images depict the expected slight rightward curvature due to extraperitoneal placement. Note the round hypointense configuration in cross section in the central pelvis on axial images that can mimic bowel or colonic diverticulum (*arrows* in *D–F*).

The "O" in the HMO system represents organ-specific prolapse. Organ prolapse is noted by measuring the lowest point of the organ along a line drawn perpendicular to the PCL and is graded according to the rule of 3's[24,33] (**Table 3**).

In addition to degree of prolapse, the authors measure the urethral angle to assess for urethral hypermobility in the anterior compartment. The anorectal angle and levator plate angle are measures of pelvic floor relaxation in the posterior compartment. The anorectal angle is generally measured between the anal canal and the posterior wall of the inferior rectum. A wide range of normal values has been proposed for the anorectal angle likely owing to the differences in measurement techniques and range in the literature from 93° to 127° at rest.[16,21,59,60] The anorectal angle should widen during defecation and narrow during Kegel generally by 15° to 20°.[21] However, the

Table 2
Grading of pelvic floor relaxation using H-line and M-line as measured during maximal straining or defecation

Grade	H-line, cm	M-line, cm
0 (normal)	<6	0–2
1 (mild)	6–8	2–4
2 (moderate)	8–10	4–6
3 (severe)	≥10	≥6

Data from Reiner CS, Weishaupt D. Dynamic pelvic floor imaging: MRI techniques and imaging parameters. Abdom Imaging 2013;38(5):903–11.

Table 3
Grading of pelvic organ prolapse relative to pubococcygeal line

Grade	Perpendicular Distance Caudal to PCL, cm
1 (mild)	<3
2 (moderate)	3–6
3 (severe)	>6

Data from Bertschinger KM, Hetzer FH, Roos JE, et al. Dynamic MR imaging of the pelvic floor performed with patient sitting in an open-magnet unit versus with patient supine in a closed-magnet unit. Radiology 2002;223(2):501–8; and Reiner CS, Weishaupt D. Dynamic pelvic floor imaging: MRI techniques and imaging parameters. Abdom Imaging 2013;38(5):903–11.

degree of change is variable.[16,59,60] In some cases, there is severe deformity of the rectal wall during defecation, and the authors have found accurate depiction of the anorectal angle difficult. For this reason, the authors measure the angle between the levator plate and the anal canal. They find that the well-visualized linear morphology of the levator plate on the sagittal images allows for easier and consistent depiction of the angle. They place a lower emphasis on the absolute value of the angle due to the variation in published normal values, but rather highlight the direction of change as normal (widening during defecation and narrowing during Kegel) or abnormal. Another angle that is often measured in the posterior compartment is the levator plate angle, which is measured between the levator plate and the PCL. The levator plate angle has been shown to be significantly higher during strain in patients with pelvic organ prolapse than in control subjects.[41] During strain or defecation, widening of the levator plate angle greater than 10° compared with baseline angle at rest indicates loss of pelvic floor support.[61]

Functional evaluation of the pelvic floor is described based on compartments: anterior, middle, and posterior.

Anterior compartment

Cystocele Descent of the bladder greater than 1 cm below the PCL is termed cystocele (**Fig. 12**).[14] Grading of cystoceles follows the rule of 3's[24,33] (see **Table 3**). Dynamic MR imaging in the supine position has been shown to have very high sensitivity (100%), positive predictive value (97%), and negative predictive value (100%) for cystoceles when compared with intraoperative findings.[62] Supine MR imaging with defecation may actually demonstrate a larger degree of cystocele than standing VCUG.[28] Clinically, cystoceles may present with a bulge along the anterior vaginal wall. In severe cases, the anterior vaginal wall may become effaced, and complete vaginal eversion may result. Large cystoceles can cause kinking of the urethra and lead to urinary obstruction. In such cases, the bladder may also occupy the entire pelvic floor hiatus and obscure defects in other compartments. Hence, it is best to avoid overdistention of the urinary bladder during MR defecography. In addition, when large cystoceles are seen without prolapse in other compartments, reimaging after bladder emptying should be considered in order to uncover potential prolapse in other compartments.

Urethral hypermobility In the authors' experience, many patients with anterior compartment prolapse also present with urethral hypermobility, defined as a urethral angle greater than 30° at rest, at strain, or an increase in urethral angle by at least 30° between rest and defecation.[63] Similar to findings on VCUG, the urethral angle on MR imaging is measured between the urethral axis and a vertical line drawn at the external meatus, which frequently intersects the inferior margin of the

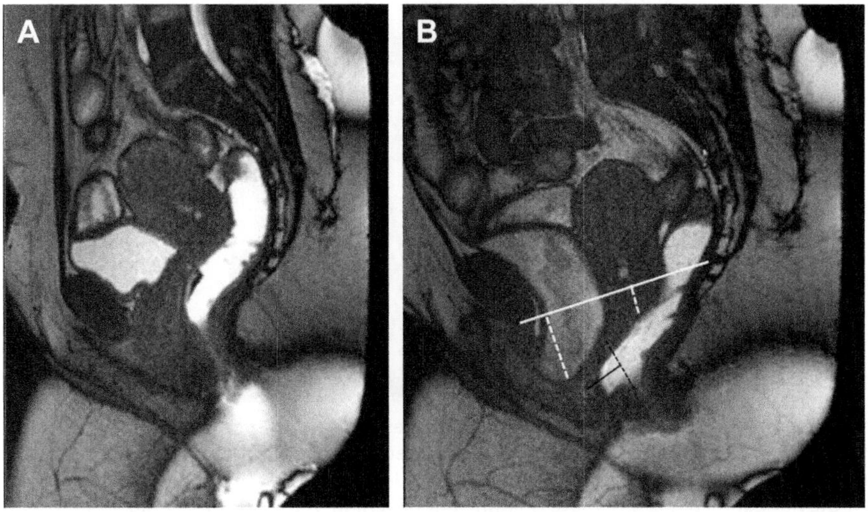

Fig. 12. Cystocele. TrueFISP images through the midline sagittal plane at rest (*A*) and during defecation (*B*) demonstrate extension of the bladder below the PCL (*solid white line* in *B*) during defecation. The cystocele size is measured perpendicularly down from the PCL (*long dashed white line* in *B*). Also noted on the defecation image is mild prolapse of the cervix (*short dashed white line* in *B*) below the PCL, and a small anterior rectocele. Rectocele size is measured in anteroposterior dimension (*solid black line*) relative to the expected location of the normal anterior rectal wall (*dashed black line*). AP, anteroposterior.

pubic symphysis.[63,64] The axis of the urethra may be well seen on midline sagittal T2w images at rest, but it can be more challenging to identify on the lower-resolution defecation images. In cases of a curved urethra, the authors estimate the urethral axis to be along a line drawn between the internal and external urethral meatus (**Fig. 13**). Identification of urethral hypermobility in asymptomatic patients is of uncertain clinical significance; however, urethral mobility can be the underlying cause for stress urinary incontinence (SUI). When detected in patients with SUI, urethral hypermobility may alter surgical management.[65,66] Changes in urethral angle in postoperative patients can also be used as a measure of outcome after surgical repair.[64] Potential causes for urethral hypermobility include pudendal nerve dysfunction, prior surgery, defect of muscle or fascia, prior pregnancy, vaginal delivery, obesity, and advanced age.[67]

Bladder outlet obstruction Bladder outlet obstruction may occur after surgical intervention for SUI with anti-incontinence procedures such as autologous slings, Burch suspension, Marshall-Marchetti-Krantz procedure, pubovaginal slings, transvaginal needle suspension, and tension-free vaginal tape; rates of urinary obstruction after these procedures range between 1% and 33%.[68] Severe urethral hypermobility can also cause kinking of the urethra, which may lead to obstruction. Other potential nonneurogenic causes include pelvic organ prolapse (bladder or other organs), primary bladder neck obstruction,

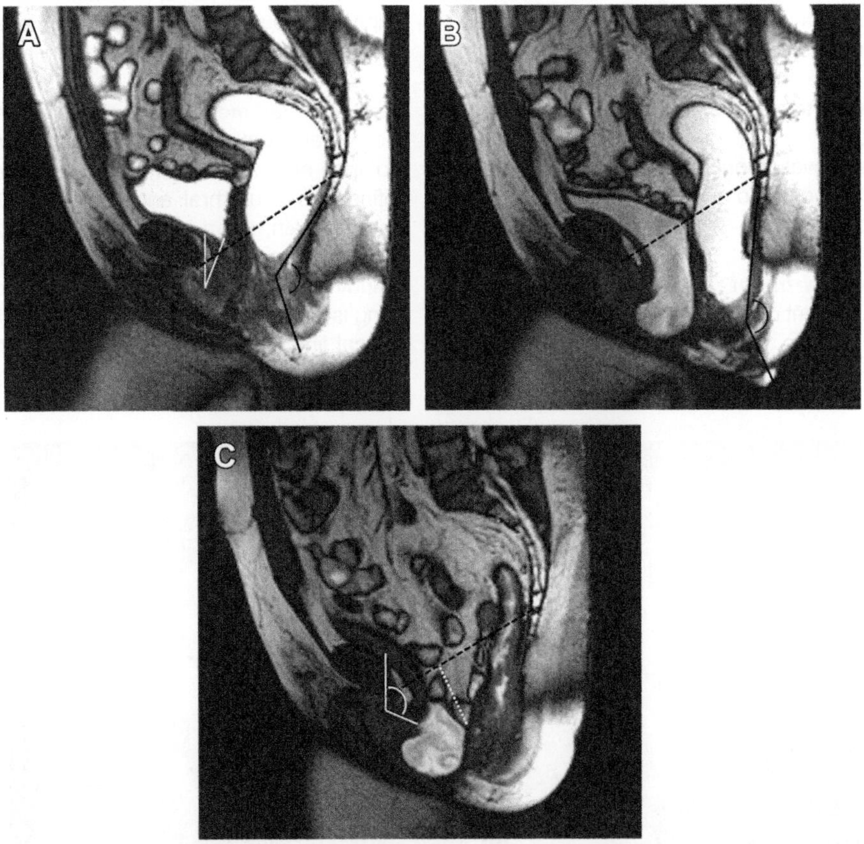

Fig. 13. Compartmental angles. Sagittal TrueFISP images at rest (*A*), early defecation (*B*), and end defecation after multiple attempts (*C*). Urethral angle (*white angle*) is measured between the urethral axis and a vertical line drawn at the external urethral meatus. The urethra demonstrates a "J-shape" at rest (*A*). At end defecation (*C*), the urethra rotates below the horizontal plane and there is significant widening of the urethral angle greater than 30° consistent with urethral hypermobility. The anorectal angle is measured between the posterior wall of the rectum or the levator plate and the axis of the anal canal (*black angle* in *A*). Although the anal canal is difficult to visualize in (*B*) and (*C*) due to patient motion out of the midline plane of imaging, there is clearly a more vertical orientation of the posterior rectal wall and levator plate leading to widening of the angle, as expected during defecation (*black angle* in *B*). Note the added benefit of multiple defecation attempts. Small bowel is seen extending below the PCL (*black dashed line*) only on the late end defecation acquisition, consistent with an enterocele (*dotted white line* in *C*).

or mass effect from benign or malignant causes.[68] Patients with bladder outlet obstruction may present with voiding hesitancy, positional voiding, manual splinting during voiding, or frank urinary retention requiring bladder catheterization.[4] Additional complaints may include recurrent infection and pain particularly when associated with erosion of synthetic material into the urethra or bladder. Bladder outlet obstruction due to prolapse may coexist with overactive bladder symptoms, and treatment of the prolapse (surgical or nonsurgical) may improve, but not completely cure, the overactive bladder symptoms.[69]

Although diagnosis of bladder outlet obstruction is difficult on MR imaging without a voiding phase during image acquisitions, a trabeculated or thick-walled urinary bladder is more likely to be seen in cases of bladder outlet obstruction or advanced prolapse.[49]

Middle compartment

The uterus, cervix, and vagina compose the middle compartment of the pelvis. Disruption of the uterosacral ligaments, potentially after hysterectomy, or tearing of the paracolpium or parametrium may result in middle compartment prolapse. Anterior and posterior vaginal wall bulging may result from disruption of the pubocervical and rectovaginal fasciae, respectively. Patients may present with pelvic pressure, pain, sensation of vaginal mass, dyspareunia, urinary retention, or back pain.[4] MR imaging has high sensitivity for vaginal vault or uterine prolapse.[62] Weakening of the paravaginal support structures may result in a more horizontal orientation of the vagina on sagittal images even at rest. The normal "H" shape of the vagina on axial images may be disrupted (see **Fig. 3**). During functional imaging, middle compartment prolapse is quantified by measuring the lowest point of the cervix (see **Fig. 12**), or the vaginal apex (**Fig. 14**) in the case of prior hysterectomy relative to the PCL. As with other organs, the grading of cervical prolapse is based on the rule of 3's[24,33] (see **Table 3**). Any distance of cervix or vaginal apex extension below the PCL classifies as prolapse. In severe cases of middle compartment prolapse, the vagina may be completely everted, and the uterus or cervix may be prolapsed outside the vaginal introitus.

Vaginal prolapse may obscure prolapse in other compartments on physical examination because a separate anterior or posterior vaginal bulge may be difficult to detect. Imaging may be helpful in this setting; however, severe prolapse of the uterus or presence of a large fibroid in a prolapsed uterus may conceal prolapse of other compartments even on imaging by completely occupying the pelvic floor hiatus. This may result in recurrent symptoms after middle compartment repair of prolapse due to "new" previously undetected anterior or posterior compartment prolapse, resulting in a need for repeat surgical intervention. Middle compartment prolapse can also predispose patients to enterocele or peritoneocele formation by increasing traction upon the posterior cul-de-sac and widening the potential space through which the peritoneal sac may herniate.

Posterior compartment

Enterocele Enterocele refers to herniation of peritoneal contents in the posterior cul-de-sac below the PCL and into the rectovaginal space. This typically results from disruption of the rectovaginal septum. Depending on the contents of the hernia sac, it may be more accurately described as an enterocele (small bowel) (**Fig. 15**), peritoneocele (peritoneal fat), sigmoidocele (sigmoid colon), or less commonly, cecocele (cecum) (see **Fig. 14**). Patients who have had a hysterectomy or other pelvic surgeries that disrupt the posterior vaginal support structures or displace the vagina anteriorly are at higher risk for enterocele formation.[38,70] Enteroceles may present as a posterior vaginal bulge; however, physical examination alone is often inadequate for enterocele detection.[38,70] Furthermore, when a posterior vaginal bulge is detected clinically, differentiation of enterocele from rectocele (anterior herniation of the rectum discussed later) is often difficult on physical examination. Because of direct visualization of intrapelvic structures, MR imaging not only enables differentiation between enterocele and rectocele[71] but also allows characterization of actual contents within the enterocele sac and provides an advantage over fluoroscopic defecography in this regard.[72] Reliable detection of small enteroceles with fluoroscopic defecography may require opacification of the small bowel with oral contrast, while MR imaging requires no additional patient preparation. Enteroceles typically manifest during the late stage of defecation after rectal emptying. Hence, it is important to perform postdefecation strain dynamic images because these may demonstrate enteroceles not seen on defecation images (**Fig. 16**). In cases where the patient is not able to empty the rectum on the table, they should be asked to evacuate in the restroom before acquisition of the postdefecation strain images. In cases of a persistently distended rectum, large uterus, or overdistended urinary bladder, bowel herniation may be seen below the PCL, but not into the rectovaginal space. Although this may not technically meet the definition of

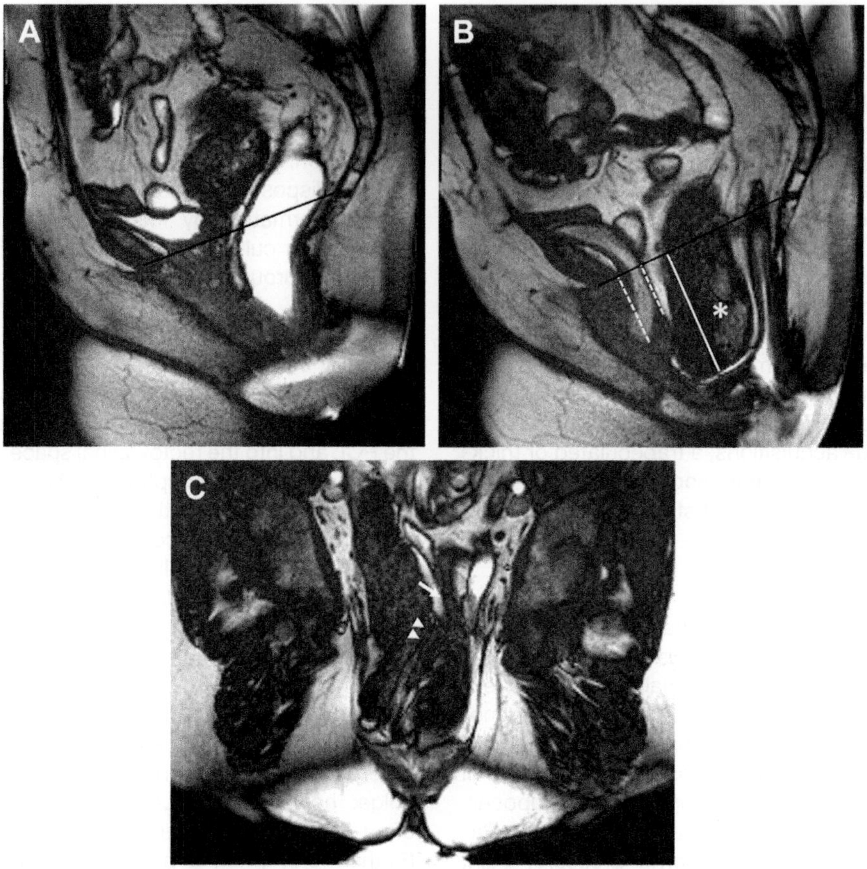

Fig. 14. Multicompartment prolapse. TrueFISP images through the midline sagittal plane at rest (*A*) and during defecation (*B*) demonstrate extension of the bladder below the PCL (*solid black line*) during defecation. The cystocele size (*long dashed white line*) is measured perpendicularly down from the PCL, as is prolapse of the vagina (*short dashed white line*). In addition, there is a large stool or gas-filled structure (*asterisk*) that prolapses into the rectovaginal space (*solid white line*) and compresses the anterior rectal wall. This was suspected to be either a distended redundant sigmoid colon or an atypical location of cecum. Correlation with coronal oblique images demonstrates the ileocecal valve (*arrowheads* in *C*) and terminal ileum (*long arrow* in *C*) extending into this structure, confirming a large cecocele.

enterocele, the authors alert the physicians to the possibility of an occult enterocele in these cases. The clinical utility of this finding remains to be determined. In some cases, large enteroceles may in fact prevent complete rectal emptying and result in defecatory dysfunction and feeling of incomplete evacuation due to mass effect upon the rectum.[73] Other enterocele-associated complaints may include bowel obstruction, vaginal pressure, dyspareunia, or low back pain.[4] Patients may report a dragging sensation in upright position due to stretching of herniated bowel mesentery within the enterocele sac that is relieved in the supine position.[70] Identification of enteroceles is important because it may impact surgical management,[74] in order to prevent bowel injury during rectocele repair with posterior colporrhaphy.[70] Size of enteroceles can be measured relative to the vaginal apex, but more commonly using a line drawn perpendicular to the PCL. Enteroceles are also graded according to the rule of 3's (see **Table 3**).[24,33]

Rectocele A rectocele is an outpouching of the rectal lumen, most typically along the anterior rectal wall. Depending on the size of the rectocele, it may result in a bulge along the posterior wall of the vagina. Rectoceles typically occur early in the defecation or strain process, but can be difficult to differentiate from enteroceles clinically. Rarely, outpouchings of the posterior rectal wall occur due to defects in the levator plate, resulting in posterior rectoceles.[13] Anterior rectoceles are quantified on sagittal images by measuring the anteroposterior extent of the outpouching relative to the expected margin of normal anterior rectal

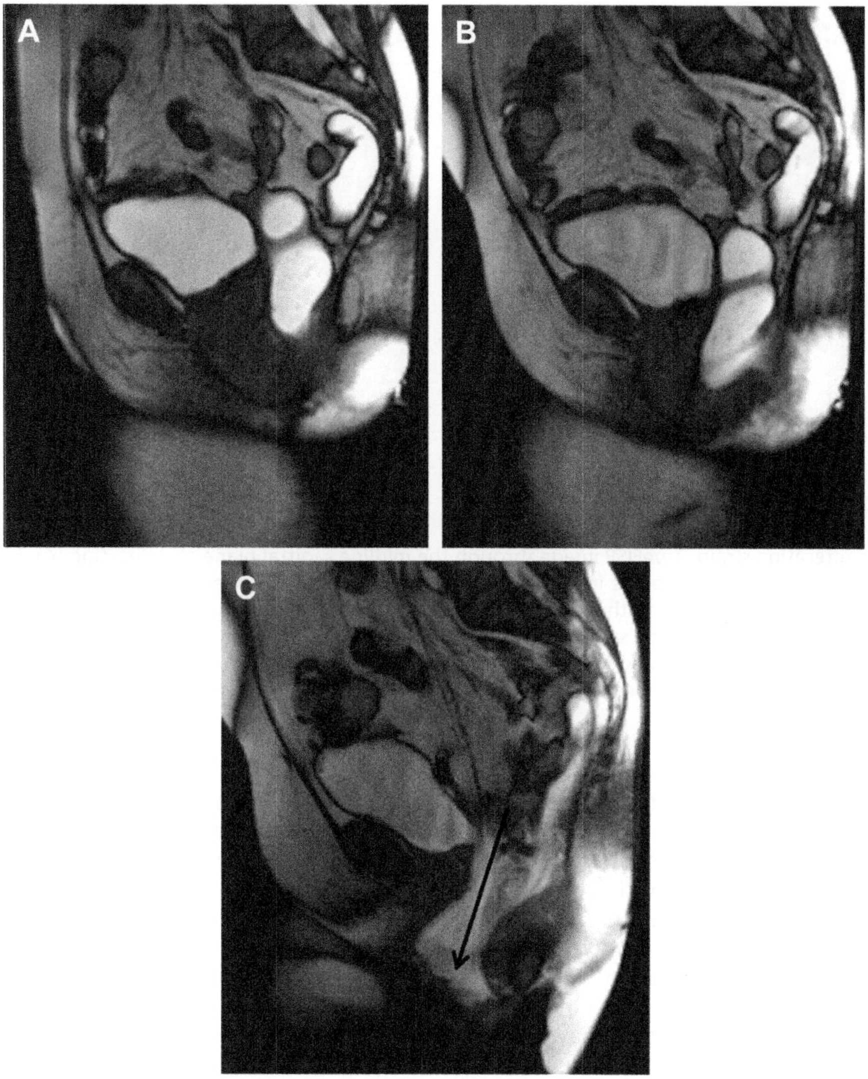

Fig. 15. Entereocele. TrueFISP images through the midline sagittal plane at rest (*A*), initial defecation (*B*), and late defecation (*C*). Early defecation image (*B*) demonstrates no significant prolapse. Late defecation image demonstrates a large hernia sac in the rectovaginal space that contains small bowel loops, consistent with an enterocele (*long arrow* in *C*).

wall (see **Figs. 12** and **16**). They are graded as small (<2 cm), moderate (2-4 cm), or large (>4 cm).[70] Rectoceles may be present in up to 80% of asymptomatic individuals, typically measuring up to 2 to 2.5 cm in this setting.[16,59,60] In general, rectoceles measuring greater than 2 cm should be considered significant.[75]

Patients with symptomatic rectoceles may present with incomplete defecation and may report a history of manual splinting at the posterior vaginal wall in order to evacuate. MR defecography may show retained rectal contrast in the rectocele in such cases. As reported above, differentiation between rectocele and enterocele may be difficult on physical examination, and MR defecography is particularly helpful in this setting.[71] Risk factors for rectocele formation include vaginal trauma from childbirth, surgery, chronic increased intraabdominal pressure, hysterectomy, and advanced age.[76]

Rectal intussusception Rectal intussusception refers to herniation of all layers of the rectal wall into the more distal rectum or anus. Depending on location of the prolapsed segment, it may be intrarectal, intraanal, or extraanal. Extraanal intussusception is called rectal prolapse and can be readily identified on clinical examination.

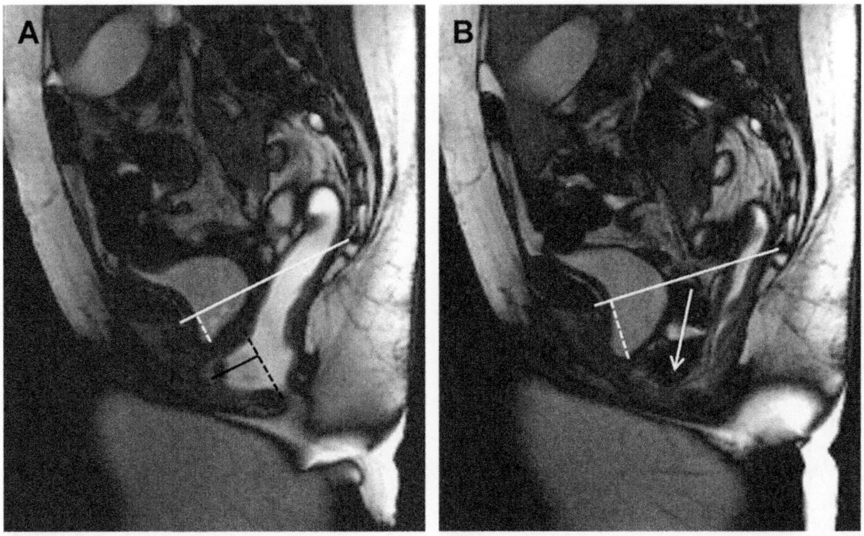

Fig. 16. Postdefecation strain. TrueFISP image through the midline sagittal plane at defecation (*A*) demonstrates a grade 1 cystocele (*dashed white line* in *A*) relative to the PCL (*solid white line* in *A*) along with a sizable rectocele (*black solid line* in *A*) relative to the expected location of normal anterior rectal wall (*dashed black line* in *A*). TrueFISP image through the midline sagittal plane during postdefecation strain (*B*) demonstrates at least grade 2 cystocele (*dashed white line* in *B*) and vaginal prolapse relative to the PCL (*solid white line* in *B*) as well as a moderate enterocele (*arrow* in *B*) demonstrating the utility of this additional acquisition.

Full-thickness rectal prolapse is differentiated from mucosal prolapse, which only involves the mucosal layer of the wall. Although true rectal intussusception is usually circumferential, partial-thickness mucosal prolapse can be limited to only a portion of the rectal wall. In some cases, rectal intussusception or prolapse may be a result of dyssynergic defecation or chronic straining, which can cause pudendal neuropathy. Pudendal nerve damage in this manner or from other factors such as injury during vaginal birth may result in weakness of the anal sphincter complex, which in turn may cause rectal prolapse in the setting of a mobile rectum.[77] MR defecography has been shown to have a sensitivity of 70% relative to fluoroscopic defecography for the detection of rectal intussusception; however, direct visualization of the rectal wall by MR imaging allows for differentiation between partial-thickness and full-thickness intussusception.[78] Partial-thickness mucosal prolapse may be treated conservatively or with transanal excision of the prolapsed mucosa, but full-thickness rectal intussusception may require a rectopexy.[77,79] Full-thickness circumferential intussusception on MR imaging may result in an "arrow" sign of the rectum during defecation (**Fig. 17**).

Rectal intussusception has been reported on imaging in 50% of asymptomatic volunteers.[60] Thus, when present on imaging, this finding needs to be correlated with symptom status. When symptomatic, the patient with rectal intussusception or prolapse may report constipation or obstructed defecation, rectal bleeding or passage of mucous, and fecal incontinence. Furthermore, rectal intussusception can be seen in 45% to 80% of patients with solitary rectal ulcer syndrome.[77]

Anal incontinence Anal incontinence is the loss of voluntary control of passage of stool or flatus via the anus. It has a prevalence rate of 11% to 15% within adults in the community.[80] It is typically an acquired condition that results from direct injury or deficiency of the sphincter complex, as can be seen with vaginal childbirth or prior episiotomy. It can also be a result of pudendal nerve dysfunction due to chronic straining, advanced age, or heavy smoking.[81] Deficiency of the internal sphincter typically manifests as passive incontinence at rest, whereas dysfunction of the external sphincter results in urge incontinence.[82] Both endoanal coil and external phased array coil MR imaging may be used to evaluate for atrophy or defects in the anal sphincter complex.[83] Patients with obstructed defecation may also present with overflow incontinence or postdefecation leakage. In these cases, imaging may help identify the cause for the underlying defecatory dysfunction, such as rectocele, enterocele, rectal intussusception, or dyssynergia, to determine appropriate management.[83] Hetzer and colleagues[11] demonstrated utility of MR defecography in the setting of fecal incontinence. In their study, MR defecography depicted rectal

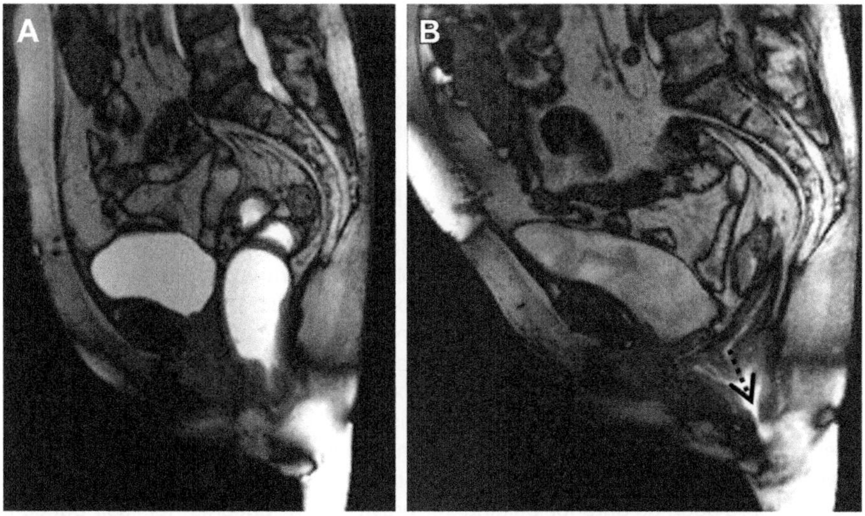

Fig. 17. Rectal Intussusception. TrueFISP image through the midline sagittal plane at rest (*A*) demonstrates expected gel in the rectum. TrueFISP image through the midline sagittal plane at defecation (*B*) demonstrates an "arrow" sign of the rectum consistent with full-thickness intussusception (intrarectal intussusception in this case).

descent of greater than 6 cm in 94% of patients, cystocele greater than 3 cm in 40% of patients, and vaginal prolapse of greater than 3 cm in 43% of patients. Rectoceles, enteroceles, and rectal prolapse were diagnosed in 34%, 32%, and 20% of patients with fecal incontinence, respectively. Interobserver agreement was good to excellent in the study, and the MR defecography findings altered surgical approach in 67% of patients.

Pelvic floor dyssynergia Pelvic floor dyssynergia, also referred to as dyssynergic defecation, anismus, spastic pelvic floor syndrome, or nonrelaxing puborectalis syndrome, is a functional condition characterized by paradoxic contraction of or inability to relax the puborectalis muscle during attempted defecation. Involuntary contraction of the striated muscle results in narrowing rather than widening of the anorectal angle due to anterior and upward traction of the levator plate (**Fig. 18**). Patients demonstrate prolonged and incomplete defecation as well as delay between the opening of the anal canal and initiation of defecation.[84] On anatomic images, the puborectalis muscle may appear

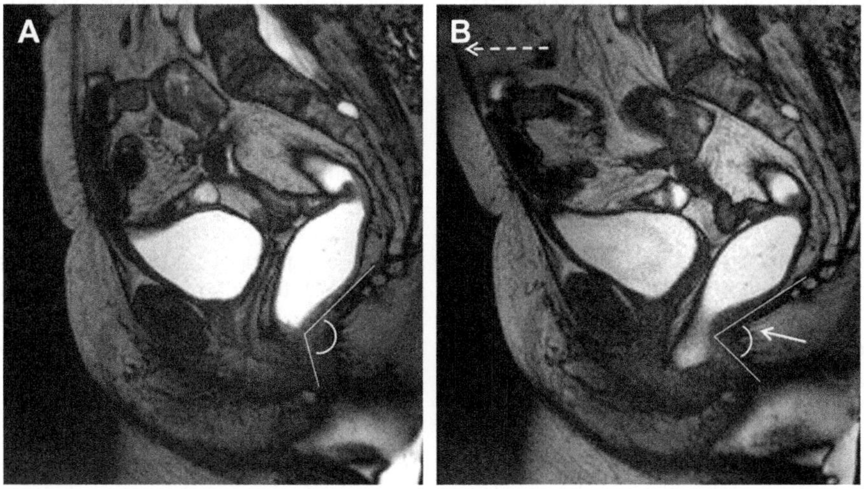

Fig. 18. Pelvic floor dyssynergia. TrueFISP image through the midline sagittal plane at rest (*A*) demonstrates normal anorectal or levator-anus angle. TrueFISP image through the midline sagittal plane at defecation (*B*) demonstrates descent of the rectum with a small anterior rectocele; however, there is contraction instead of relaxation of the levator plate (*solid arrow*) with resultant narrowing of the angle. Note anterior bulging of the ventral abdominal wall (*dashed arrow* in *B*) suggesting increased intraabdominal pressure during attempted defecation. The rectum does not empty.

hypertrophied with resultant prominent impression upon the anorectal junction. MR defecography demonstrates impaired evacuation, abnormal change in the anorectal angle, and paradoxic sphincter contraction more commonly in patients with dyssynergic defecation than in those without.[85]

In the authors' experience, impaired evacuation on MR defecography may sometimes be environmental due to unnatural surroundings or positioning. On occasion, patients may not comprehend technologists' instructions. Technologists should be trained to adequately coach and encourage patients during the procedure, especially during the defecation phase. Paradoxic levator contraction and anorectal angle narrowing seen during attempts at defecation when seen with signs of adequate increased intraabdominal pressure such as anterior bulging of the abdominal wall and descent of the rectum (see **Fig. 18**) may indicate true dyssynergia rather than inability to defecate due to "stage-fright" or inability to comprehend instructions. Anterior rectoceles may be seen in association with pelvic floor dyssynergia.[21] Identification of dyssynergia as a cause of incomplete defecation and exclusion of other functional or anatomic causes with MR defecography can impact management as patients with dyssynergia may be candidates for nonsurgical treatment with biofeedback therapy.

Descending perineal syndrome Descending perineal syndrome is characterized by excessive descent of the pelvic floor at rest and/or defecation. The condition results from loss of tone of the pelvic muscles and can be caused by injury or dysfunction of the pudendal nerve (secondary to trauma or delivery), or conditions that result in chronic straining.[86] Although descending perineal syndrome may affect the posterior compartment most commonly, it frequently involves all 3 compartments, resulting in diffuse perineal bulge and discomfort. Imaging may show a low-lying anorectal junction at rest indicating weakness and reduced tone of the pelvic floor myofascial support system.[87] This may be associated with levator muscle bulging that can be seen on axial and coronal images and implies a widened pelvic floor hiatus. The H-line and M-line will typically be elongated at rest and will demonstrate a further increase during defecation. There may be excessive widening of the anorectal or levator plate angles. When the entire pelvic floor is affected, there will be organ prolapse below the PCL in the anterior and middle compartments as well. There may be diminished elevation of the pelvic floor during Kegel (squeeze).[86] Patients often present with incomplete rectal emptying, which sets off a cycle of worsening straining and pelvic floor descent, eventually leading to incontinence. Additional complaints may include perineal discomfort and pain.[86]

PEARLS/PITFALLS/VARIANTS

Because of the potentially embarrassing nature of MR defecography, patient preparation before the examination is of utmost importance. It is helpful to build strong relationships with and educate referring physicians who in turn can discuss the examination with patients at preimaging clinic visits. In addition, resources such as trusted informational Web sites (http://www.radiologyinfo.org/en/info.cfm?pg=dynamic-pelvic-floor-mri) can be provided to patients for self-education before arrival to the radiology department. Finally, technologists must be trained well in order to coach patients through the examination.

It is important not to image the patient with an overdistended bladder or rectum, because these can both obscure prolapse in other compartments, as discussed previously in this review. If the bladder is overdistended or if there is a large cystocele occupying the pelvic hiatus, repeat images may be necessary after bladder emptying. Defecation images should be obtained at least 3 times in order to elicit maximum prolapse. A postdefecation strain series may be helpful to demonstrate occult enteroceles or other prolapse.

For detection of parasagittal defects or prolapse, acquisition of cine images in coronal or axial oblique planes may be necessary. Alternatively, coronal images may be obtained through the pelvis from anterior to posterior with the patient in maximal strain.

On occasion, patients may not defecate during the examination; this limits evaluation for prolapse and is particularly challenging in patients referred for defecatory dysfunction. Inability to defecate due to "stage-fright" or being in a nonphysiologic supine position can be difficult to differentiate from pelvic floor nonrelaxation or dyssynergia. Anterior bowing of the abdominal wall and descent of the pelvic floor can be used as signs of adequate effort, and lack of defecation in this setting may represent true abnormality. Patients may also be asked to leave the MR imaging table to defecate in a restroom, and postdefecation strain images should be obtained to assess for organ prolapse in those cases. In some cases, patients are not able to defecate even while in the restroom, confirming severe defecatory dysfunction.

WHAT THE REFERRING PHYSICIAN NEEDS TO KNOW

Although practice patterns vary by institution, patients referred for MR defecography typically have clinical signs or symptoms of pelvic floor dysfunction in at least one compartment, or they may have had prior intervention in the pelvic floor. A structured dictation template (see **Box 1**) should be used and should contain elements of both anatomic and functional evaluation. The authors suggest starting with a thorough anatomic evaluation of the pelvis and reporting postsurgical changes such as hysterectomy, or previously placed urethral bulking agent or slings or vaginal mesh. Regarding the functional evaluation, referring physicians are often evaluating for occult prolapse in compartments other than those seen on physical examination. They may suspect anatomic causes for the patient's symptoms, such as bladder prolapse and urethral kinking as cause for bladder outlet obstruction, or rectocele or rectal intussusception as a cause for defecatory dysfunction. Rectoceles and enteroceles/peritoneoceles are difficult to differentiate on clinical examination, but can be easily differentiated on MR imaging.[71] The contents of the peritoneocele sac are important to report, that is, fat-containing peritoneocele versus small bowel containing enterocele versus colon containing sigmoidocele or cecocele. A sigmoidocele with a severely redundant colon may require partial sigmoid resection in extreme cases, whereas an enterocele may be fixed with a sacrocolpopexy. Finally, in cases of defecatory dysfunction, it is important to be able to exclude anatomic causes and identify pelvic floor dyssynergia because patients with this diagnosis can be treated with biofeedback therapy rather than surgical intervention. In general, reports for MR defecography studies should mention positive as well as pertinent negative findings in each compartment of the pelvic floor.

SUMMARY

Dynamic pelvic floor MR imaging, particularly with defecation, has emerged as a powerful tool that allows high-resolution anatomic and functional evaluation of the pelvis. Variability in technique and interpretation methods, nonphysiologic positioning when performed supine, and relative high cost are deterrents to universal acceptance of this technique; however, the direct visualization of the pelvic contents and musculature, high inherent soft tissue and contrast resolution, lack of exposure to ionizing radiation, and relatively noninvasive nature are some of the benefits that make it an important complementary tool for assessment of pelvic floor dysfunction. Furthermore, given the large numbers of patients undergoing pelvic floor surgery, the ability to evaluate for complications of pelvic mesh, slings, or other interventions at no additional time or financial cost further strengthens its role.

REFERENCES

1. Nygaard I, Barber MD, Burgio KL, et al. Prevalence of symptomatic pelvic floor disorders in US women. JAMA 2008;300(11):1311–6.
2. Thom D. Variation in estimates of urinary incontinence prevalence in the community: effects of differences in definition, population characteristics, and study type. J Am Geriatr Soc 1998;46(4):473–80.
3. Mouritsen L, Larsen JP. Symptoms, bother and POPQ in women referred with pelvic organ prolapse. Int Urogynecol J Pelvic Floor Dysfunct 2003;14(2):122–7.
4. Bitti GT, Argiolas GM, Ballicu N, et al. Pelvic floor failure: MR imaging evaluation of anatomic and functional abnormalities. Radiographics 2014;34(2):429–48.
5. Weber AM, Abrams P, Brubaker L, et al. The standardization of terminology for researchers in female pelvic floor disorders. Int Urogynecol J Pelvic Floor Dysfunct 2001;12(3):178–86.
6. Olsen AL, Smith VJ, Bergstrom JO, et al. Epidemiology of surgically managed pelvic organ prolapse and urinary incontinence. Obstet Gynecol 1997;89(4):501–6.
7. Wilson L, Brown JS, Shin GP, et al. Annual direct cost of urinary incontinence. Obstet Gynecol 2001;98(3):398–406.
8. Kelvin FM, Hale DS, Maglinte DD, et al. Female pelvic organ prolapse: diagnostic contribution of dynamic cystoproctography and comparison with physical examination. Am J Roentgenol 1999;173(1):31–7.
9. Vanbeckevoort D, Van Hoe L, Oyen R, et al. Pelvic floor descent in females: comparative study of colpocystodefecography and dynamic fast MR imaging. J Magn Reson Imaging 1999;9(3):373–7.
10. Healy JC, Halligan S, Reznek RH, et al. Patterns of prolapse in women with symptoms of pelvic floor weakness: assessment with MR imaging. Radiology 1997;203(1):77–81.
11. Hetzer FH, Andreisek G, Tsagari C, et al. MR defecography in patients with fecal incontinence: imaging findings and their effect on surgical management. Radiology 2006;240(2):449–57.
12. Maglinte DD, Kelvin FM, Fitzgerald K, et al. Association of compartment defects in pelvic floor dysfunction. AJR Am J Roentgenol 1999;172(2):439–44.

13. Maglinte DD, Kelvin FM, Hale DS, et al. Dynamic cystoproctography: a unifying diagnostic approach to pelvic floor and anorectal dysfunction. AJR Am J Roentgenol 1997;169(3):759–67.
14. Yang A, Mostwin JL, Rosenshein NB, et al. Pelvic floor descent in women: dynamic evaluation with fast MR imaging and cinematic display. Radiology 1991;179(1):25–33.
15. Lockhart ME, Fielding JR, Richter HE, et al. Reproducibility of dynamic MR imaging pelvic measurements: a multi-institutional study. Radiology 2008; 249(2):534–40.
16. Schreyer AG, Paetzel C, Furst A, et al. Dynamic magnetic resonance defecography in 10 asymptomatic volunteers. World J Gastroenterol 2012;18(46): 6836–42.
17. Pannu HK, Javitt MC, Glanc P, et al. ACR appropriateness criteria pelvic floor dysfunction. J Am Coll Radiol 2015;12(2):134–42.
18. Strohbehn K. Normal pelvic floor anatomy. Obstet Gynecol Clin North Am 1998;25(4):683–705.
19. Garcia del Salto L, de Miguel Criado J, Aguilera del Hoyo LF, et al. MR imaging-based assessment of the female pelvic floor. Radiographics 2014;34(5): 1417–39.
20. Strohbehn K, Ellis JH, Strohbehn JA, et al. Magnetic resonance imaging of the levator ani with anatomic correlation. Obstet Gynecol 1996;87(2):277–85.
21. Mortele KJ, Fairhurst J. Dynamic MR defecography of the posterior compartment: indications, techniques and MRI features. Eur J Radiol 2007;61(3): 462–72.
22. Gufler H, Ohde A, Grau G, et al. Colpocystoproctography in the upright and supine positions correlated with dynamic MRI of the pelvic floor. Eur J Radiol 2004;51(1):41–7.
23. Kelvin FM, Maglinte DD, Hale DS, et al. Female pelvic organ prolapse: a comparison of triphasic dynamic MR imaging and triphasic fluoroscopic cystocolpoproctography. Am J Roentgenol 2000; 174(1):81–8.
24. Bertschinger KM, Hetzer FH, Roos JE, et al. Dynamic MR imaging of the pelvic floor performed with patient sitting in an open-magnet unit versus with patient supine in a closed-magnet unit. Radiology 2002;223(2):501–8.
25. Healy JC, Halligan S, Reznek RH, et al. Dynamic MR imaging compared with evacuation proctography when evaluating anorectal configuration and pelvic floor movement. AJR Am J Roentgenol 1997;169(3):775–9.
26. Lienemann A, Anthuber C, Baron A, et al. Dynamic MR colpocystorectography assessing pelvic-floor descent. Eur Radiol 1997;7(8):1309–17.
27. Iacobellis F, Brillantino A, Renzi A, et al. MR Imaging in diagnosis of pelvic floor descent: supine versus sitting position. Gastroenterol Res Pract 2016;2016: 6594152.
28. Kumar N, Khatri G, Sims R, et al. Supine Magnetic Resonance Defecography for Evaluation of Anterior Compartment Prolapse – Correlation with Standing Voiding Cystourethrogram. Paper presented at: American Roentgen Ray Society Annual Meeting. Washington, DC, 2013.
29. Flusberg M, Sahni VA, Erturk SM, et al. Dynamic MR defecography: assessment of the usefulness of the defecation phase. AJR Am J Roentgenol 2011; 196(4):W394–9.
30. Kumar N, Khatri G, Xi Y, et al. Valsalva Maneuvers versus Defecation for MRI Assessment of Multi-Compartment Pelvic Organ Prolapse. Paper presented at: American Roentgen Ray Society Annual Meeting. San Diego, 2014.
31. Foti PV, Farina R, Riva G, et al. Pelvic floor imaging: comparison between magnetic resonance imaging and conventional defecography in studying outlet obstruction syndrome. Radiol Med 2013; 118(1):23–39.
32. Pannu HK, Scatarige JC, Eng J. Comparison of supine magnetic resonance imaging with and without rectal contrast to fluoroscopic cystocolpoproctography for the diagnosis of pelvic organ prolapse. J Comput Assist Tomogr 2009;33(1):125–30.
33. Reiner CS, Weishaupt D. Dynamic pelvic floor imaging: MRI techniques and imaging parameters. Abdom Imaging 2013;38(5):903–11.
34. Solopova AE, Hetzer FH, Marincek B, et al. MR defecography: prospective comparison of two rectal enema compositions. AJR Am J Roentgenol 2008; 190(2):W118–24.
35. Khatri G, Bailey AA, Bacsu C, et al. Influence of rectal gel volume on defecation during dynamic pelvic floor magnetic resonance imaging. Clin Imaging 2015;39(6):1027–31.
36. Law YM, Fielding JR. MRI of pelvic floor dysfunction: review. AJR Am J Roentgenol 2008;191(6 Suppl): S45–53.
37. Khatri G, Carmel ME, Bailey AA, et al. Postoperative imaging after surgical repair for pelvic floor dysfunction. Radiographics 2016;36(4):1233–56.
38. Kelvin FM, Maglinte DD. Dynamic cystoproctography of female pelvic floor defects and their interrelationships. AJR Am J Roentgenol 1997;169(3): 769–74.
39. Kelvin FM, Maglinte DD, Benson JT, et al. Dynamic cystoproctography: a technique for assessing disorders of the pelvic floor in women. AJR Am J Roentgenol 1994;163(2):368–70.
40. Hecht EM, Lee VS, Tanpitukpongse TP, et al. MRI of pelvic floor dysfunction: dynamic true fast imaging with steady-state precession versus HASTE. AJR Am J Roentgenol 2008;191(2):352–8.
41. Hoyte L, Schierlitz L, Zou K, et al. Two- and 3-dimensional MRI comparison of levator ani structure, volume, and integrity in women with stress

incontinence and prolapse. Am J Obstet Gynecol 2001;185(1):11–9.
42. Lewicky-Gaupp C, Brincat C, Yousuf A, et al. Fecal incontinence in older women: are levator ani defects a factor? Am J Obstet Gynecol 2010; 202(5):491.e1-6.
43. Kim JK, Kim YJ, Choo MS, et al. The urethra and its supporting structures in women with stress urinary incontinence: MR imaging using an endovaginal coil. Am J Roentgenol 2003;180(4):1037–44.
44. Heilbrun ME, Nygaard IE, Lockhart ME, et al. Correlation between levator ani muscle injuries on magnetic resonance imaging and fecal incontinence, pelvic organ prolapse, and urinary incontinence in primiparous women. Am J Obstet Gynecol 2010; 202(5):488.e1-6.
45. Lammers K, Fütterer JJ, Inthout J, et al. Correlating signs and symptoms with pubovisceral muscle avulsions on magnetic resonance imaging. Am J Obstet Gynecol 2013;208(2):148.e1-7.
46. Pannu HK, Genadry R, Gearhart S, et al. Focal levator ani eventrations: detection and characterization by magnetic resonance in patients with pelvic floor dysfunction. Int Urogynecol J Pelvic Floor Dysfunct 2003;14(2):89–93.
47. Fielding JR, Dumanli H, Schreyer AG, et al. MR-based three-dimensional modeling of the normal pelvic floor in women: quantification of muscle mass. AJR Am J Roentgenol 2000;174(3):657–60.
48. DeLancey JO, Kearney R, Chou Q, et al. The appearance of levator ani muscle abnormalities in magnetic resonance images after vaginal delivery. Obstet Gynecol 2003;101(1):46–53.
49. Bai SW, Park SH, Chung DJ, et al. The significance of bladder trabeculation in the female lower urinary system: an objective evaluation by urodynamic studies. Yonsei Med J 2005;46(5):673–8.
50. Huddleston HT, Dunnihoo DR, Huddleston PM 3rd, et al. Magnetic resonance imaging of defects in DeLancey's vaginal support levels I, II, and III. Am J Obstet Gynecol 1995;172(6):1778–82 [discussion: 1782–4].
51. Maher C, Feiner B, Baessler K, et al. Surgical management of pelvic organ prolapse in women. Cochrane Database Syst Rev 2013;4:CD004014.
52. Giri SK, Wallis F, Drumm J, et al. A magnetic resonance imaging-based study of retropubic haematoma after sling procedures: preliminary findings. BJU Int 2005;96(7):1067–71.
53. Broekhuis SR, Futterer JJ, Barentsz JO, et al. A systematic review of clinical studies on dynamic magnetic resonance imaging of pelvic organ prolapse: the use of reference lines and anatomical landmarks. Int Urogynecol J Pelvic Floor Dysfunct 2009;20(6):721–9.
54. Singh K, Reid WM, Berger LA. Assessment and grading of pelvic organ prolapse by use of dynamic magnetic resonance imaging. Am J Obstet Gynecol 2001;185(1):71–7.
55. Woodfield CA, Hampton BS, Sung V, et al. Magnetic resonance imaging of pelvic organ prolapse: comparing pubococcygeal and midpubic lines with clinical staging. Int Urogynecol J Pelvic Floor Dysfunct 2009;20(6):695–701.
56. Fauconnier A, Zareski E, Abichedid J, et al. Dynamic magnetic resonance imaging for grading pelvic organ prolapse according to the International Continence Society classification: which line should be used? Neurourol Urodyn 2008;27(3):191–7.
57. Rosenkrantz AB, Lewis MT, Yalamanchili S, et al. Prevalence of pelvic organ prolapse detected at dynamic MRI in women without history of pelvic floor dysfunction: comparison of two reference lines. Clin Radiol 2014;69(2):e71–7.
58. Comiter CV, Vasavada SP, Barbaric ZL, et al. Grading pelvic prolapse and pelvic floor relaxation using dynamic magnetic resonance imaging. Urology 1999;54(3):454–7.
59. Bartram CI, Turnbull GK, Lennard-Jones JE. Evacuation proctography: an investigation of rectal expulsion in 20 subjects without defecatory disturbance. Gastrointest Radiol 1988;13(1):72–80.
60. Shorvon PJ, McHugh S, Diamant NE, et al. Defecography in normal volunteers: results and implications. Gut 1989;30(12):1737–49.
61. Fielding JR. MR imaging of pelvic floor relaxation. Radiol Clin North Am 2003;41(4):747–56.
62. Gousse AE, Barbaric ZL, Safir MH, et al. Dynamic half Fourier acquisition, single shot turbo spin-echo magnetic resonance imaging for evaluating the female pelvis. J Urol 2000;164(5):1606–13.
63. Walsh LP, Zimmern PE, Pope N, et al. Comparison of the Q-tip test and voiding cystourethrogram to assess urethral hypermobility among women enrolled in a randomized clinical trial of surgery for stress urinary incontinence. J Urol 2006;176(2): 646–9 [discussion: 650].
64. Showalter PR, Zimmern PE, Roehrborn CG, et al. Standing cystourethrogram: an outcome measure after anti-incontinence procedures and cystocele repair in women. Urology 2001;58(1):33–7.
65. Poon C, Zimmern PE. Transvaginal surgery for stress urinary incontinence owing to urethral hypermobility. In: Zimmern PE, Norton PA, Haab F, et al, editors. Vaginal surgery for incontinence and prolapse. London: Springer-Verlag; 2006. p. 91–107.
66. Toledo LG, Cabral PH, Casella ML, et al. Prognostic value of urethral mobility and Valsalva leak point pressure for female transobturator sling procedure. Int Braz J Urol 2012;38(5):667–73.
67. Stoker J, Halligan S, Bartram CI. Pelvic floor imaging. Radiology 2001;218(3):621–41.
68. Dmochowski RR. Bladder outlet obstruction: etiology and evaluation. Rev Urol 2005;7(Suppl 6):S3–13.

69. de Boer TA, Salvatore S, Cardozo L, et al. Pelvic organ prolapse and overactive bladder. Neurourol Urodyn 2010;29(1):30–9.
70. Kelvin FM, Maglinte DD, Hornback JA, et al. Pelvic prolapse: assessment with evacuation proctography (defecography). Radiology 1992;184(2):547–51.
71. Tunn R, Paris S, Taupitz M, et al. MR imaging in posthysterectomy vaginal prolapse. Int Urogynecol J Pelvic Floor Dysfunct 2000;11(2):87–92.
72. Lienemann A, Anthuber C, Baron A, et al. Diagnosing enteroceles using dynamic magnetic resonance imaging. Dis Colon Rectum 2000;43(2): 205–12 [discussion: 212–3].
73. Fielding JR. Practical MR imaging of female pelvic floor weakness. Radiographics 2002;22(2):295–304.
74. Klauschie JL, Cornella JL. Surgical treatment of vaginal vault prolapse: a historic summary and review of outcomes. Female Pelvic Med Reconstr Surg 2012;18(1):10–7.
75. Delemarre JB, Kruyt RH, Doornbos J, et al. Anterior rectocele: assessment with radiographic defecography, dynamic magnetic resonance imaging, and physical examination. Dis Colon Rectum 1994; 37(3):249–59.
76. Colaiacomo MC, Masselli G, Polettini E, et al. Dynamic MR imaging of the pelvic floor: a pictorial review. Radiographics. 2009;29(3):e35.
77. Felt-Bersma RJ, Tiersma ES, Cuesta MA. Rectal prolapse, rectal intussusception, rectocele, solitary rectal ulcer syndrome, and enterocele. Gastroenterol Clin North Am 2008;37(3):645–68, ix.
78. Dvorkin LS, Hetzer F, Scott SM, et al. Open-magnet MR defaecography compared with evacuation proctography in the diagnosis and management of patients with rectal intussusception. Colorectal Dis 2004;6(1):45–53.
79. Tsiaoussis J, Chrysos E, Glynos M, et al. Pathophysiology and treatment of anterior rectal mucosal prolapse syndrome. Br J Surg 1998;85(12):1699–702.
80. Macmillan AK, Merrie AE, Marshall RJ, et al. The prevalence of fecal incontinence in community-dwelling adults: a systematic review of the literature. Dis Colon Rectum 2004;47(8):1341–9.
81. Bharucha AE, Fletcher JG, Melton LJ 3rd, et al. Obstetric trauma, pelvic floor injury and fecal incontinence: a population-based case-control study. Am J Gastroenterol 2012;107(6):902–11.
82. Soffer EE, Hull T. Fecal incontinence: a practical approach to evaluation and treatment. Am J Gastroenterol 2000;95(8):1873–80.
83. Terra MP, Stoker J. The current role of imaging techniques in faecal incontinence. Eur Radiol 2006; 16(8):1727–36.
84. Halligan S, Bartram CI, Park HJ, et al. Proctographic features of anismus. Radiology 1995;197(3):679–82.
85. Reiner CS, Tutuian R, Solopova AE, et al. MR defecography in patients with dyssynergic defecation: spectrum of imaging findings and diagnostic value. Br J Radiol 2011;84(998):136–44.
86. Roos JE, Weishaupt D, Wildermuth S, et al. Experience of 4 years with open MR defecography: pictorial review of anorectal anatomy and disease. Radiographics. 2002;22(4):817–32.
87. Maglinte DD, Bartram CI, Hale DA, et al. Functional imaging of the pelvic floor. Radiology 2011;258(1): 23–39.

MR Imaging of Vulvar and Vaginal Cancer

Anup S. Shetty, MD[a,*], Christine O. Menias, MD[b]

KEYWORDS

• Vaginal cancer • Vulvar cancer • MR imaging • Female pelvic MR imaging • Body MR imaging

KEY POINTS

- Vulvar and vaginal cancer are uncommon gynecologic malignancies most commonly diagnosed on physical examination and pelvic biopsy.
- MR imaging provides excellent spatial and contrast resolution to locally stage these tumors, and detect posttreatment recurrence or complications.
- Although staging by the International Federation of Gynecology and Obstetrics is performed clinically, MR can assess for subtle involvement of adjacent organs and the pelvic sidewall.
- Optimizing the MR imaging protocol and technique is critical for optimal staging, particularly the use of endovaginal gel to distend the vaginal vault.
- Signal intensity, diffusion restriction, and enhancement are key imaging findings to detect and accurately stage vulvar and vaginal cancer.

INTRODUCTION

Primary vulvar cancer is an uncommon malignancy, representing 5% to 8% of all gynecologic malignancies in the United States.[1] Primary vaginal cancer is even rarer, accounting for only 2% to 3% of gynecologic malignancies, with secondary involvement including metastatic disease or direct extension of extravaginal tumors being far more frequent.[2,3] Human papillomavirus, particularly subtypes 16 and 18, has been implicated as a causative agent in both types of malignancy, resulting in an increasing incidence in the younger population.[4,5] Although infrequent, late-stage vulvar and vaginal cancers and the impacts of their treatment may result in disturbing physical and emotional consequences for patients, ranging from physical disfigurement to incontinence and sexual dysfunction. The American Cancer Society estimates that nearly 6000 women will be diagnosed with vulvar cancer and 4600 women will be diagnosed with vaginal cancer in 2016.[6,7]

Both vulvar and vaginal cancer are most frequently diagnosed with physical examination and pelvic biopsy. Vulvar cancer may present as a palpable vulvar mass often with pruritus, bleeding, and urinary symptoms, although it can be misdiagnosed as benign vulvar disease.[8] Vaginal cancer usually results in painless vaginal bleeding and discharge.[9] Although many vulvar and vaginal entities can be imaged by ultrasound and computed tomography (CT), MR imaging is the modality of choice to image complex vaginal and vulvar anatomy and pathology. Due to its superlative soft tissue contrast and high-resolution multiplanar imaging without ionizing radiation, MR is a superb modality for local staging of vaginal

Disclosure Statement: The authors have no commercial or financial conflicts of interest, or external sources of funding, to disclose.

[a] Mallinckrodt of Institute Radiology, Washington University School of Medicine, Campus Box 8131, 510 South Kingshighway Boulevard, St Louis, MO 63110, USA; [b] Department of Radiology, Mayo Clinic in Arizona, 1300 East Shea Boulevard, Scottsdale, AZ 85259, USA
* Corresponding author.
E-mail address: anup.shetty@wustl.edu

Magn Reson Imaging Clin N Am 25 (2017) 481–502
http://dx.doi.org/10.1016/j.mric.2017.03.013

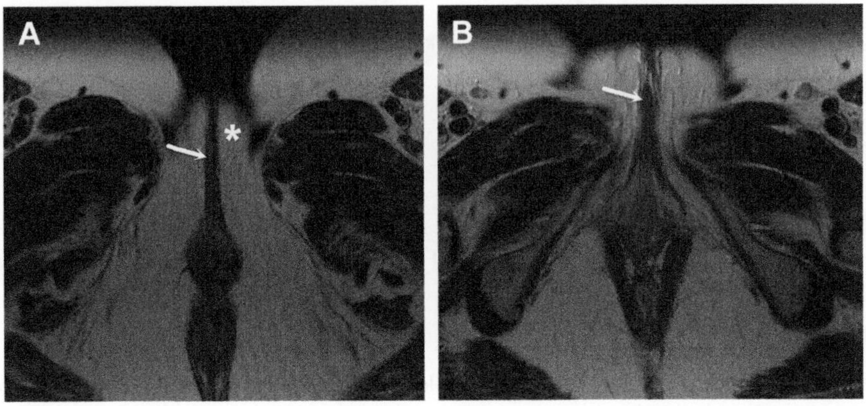

Fig. 1. Anatomy of the normal vulva on axial TSE T2-weighted imaging. (*A*) Normal appearance of the labia majora (*asterisk*) and labia minora (*arrow*). (*B*) Normal appearance of the clitoris (*arrow*).

and vulvar cancers and surveillance after treatment. Combined PET/MR imaging offers potential in the staging and surveillance in gynecologic malignancies, and future studies will likely demonstrate value in assessment of vulvar and vaginal carcinomas.[10,11]

This review focuses on anatomy of the vulva and vagina as depicted on MR imaging, the pathology of vulvar and vaginal carcinomas, MR imaging techniques for the female pelvis, MR imaging features of vulvar and vaginal cancers, and the differential diagnosis of these lesions and pitfalls in diagnosis.

ANATOMY

The urogenital triangle of the female perineum is defined by the pubic symphysis anteriorly, an imaginary line between the ischial tuberosities posteriorly, and the ischiopubic rami anterolaterally. The vulva is the triangular shaped structure of the female external genitalia, bounded superficially by the skin and deeply by the urogenital diaphragm, and consisting of the labia majora laterally and labia minora medially (**Fig. 1**). The vestibule surrounds the external urethral meatus and vaginal introitus, with the Bartholin glands positioned posterolateral on each side of the introitus that secrete lubricants into the vestibule.[12,13]

The vagina is a fibromuscular tube that extends from the introitus to the cervix (**Fig. 2**). The vaginal mucosa is T2 hyperintense, blending with vaginal secretions and any gel used to distend the vaginal cavity; in contrast to the T2 hypointense submucosal and muscularis layers. The adventitial layer of the

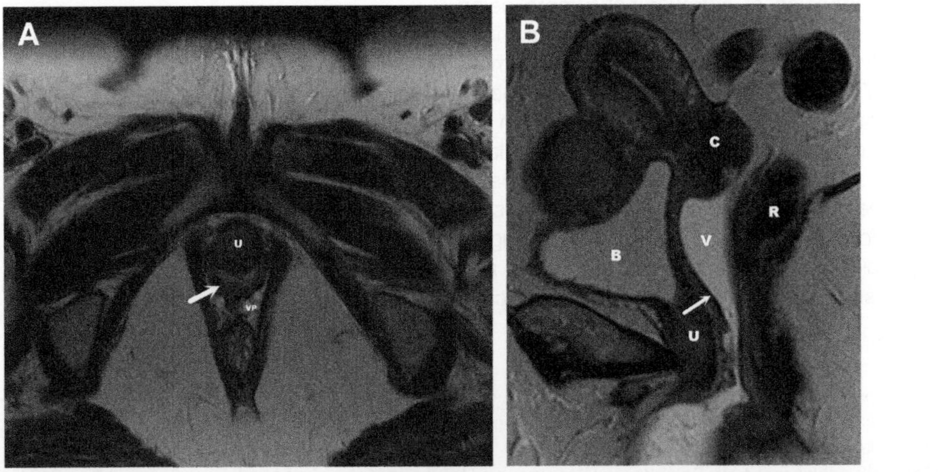

Fig. 2. Anatomy of the normal vagina on TSE T2-weighted MR imaging. Axial MR image (*A*) demonstrates the normal collapsed appearance of the vagina (*arrow*), T2-hyperintense appearance of the adventitial perivaginal venous plexus (VP), and urethral sphincter (U). Sagittal MR image with endovaginal gel (*B*) demonstrates normal appearance of the distended vagina (V) and T2 hypointense appearance of the vaginal submucosa and muscularis layers (*arrow*). The urinary bladder (B) and urethra (U) border the vagina anteriorly, rectum (R) posteriorly, and cervix (C) superiorly.

FIGO staging of vulvar cancer

FIGO Stage	Features
IA	Tumor <2 cm with <1 mm stromal invasion, confined to vulva or perineum
IB	Tumor >2 cm or with >1 mm stromal invasion, confined to vulva or perineum
II	Any size tumor extending to adjacent perineal structures (distal third of the urethra or vagina, anus), no positive nodes
IIIA	Any size tumor with positive lymph nodes (1–2 <5 mm or 1 >5 mm)
IIIB	Any size tumor with positive lymph nodes (3+ <5 mm or 2+ >5 mm)
IIIC	Any size tumor with positive nodes and extracapsular spread
IVA	Tumor invading upper two-thirds of urethra or vagina, bladder, rectum, or fixed to pelvic bone; or fixed or ulcerated regional positive lymph nodes
IVB	Distant metastases, including pelvic lymph nodes

FIGO staging of vaginal cancer

FIGO Stage	Features
I	Tumor limited to vaginal wall
II	Tumor involves paravaginal tissue without extension to pelvic side wall
III	Tumor extends to pelvic side wall
IVA	Tumor extends beyond true pelvis, or involves bladder and rectal mucosa
IVB	Distant metastases

vagina contains the vaginal venous plexus, which is T2 hyperintense and avidly enhances after intravenous gadolinium administration.

Lymphatic drainage of the vagina varies depending on the segment of vagina in question.[3] Drainage of the upper third of the vagina follows that of the uterine vessels, draining to obturator, internal iliac, and external iliac lymph nodes, followed by the para-aortic lymph nodes. Drainage of the lower third of the vagina follows that of vaginal vessels, draining to inguinal, femoral, and, less frequently, the mesorectal lymph nodes. The middle third of the vagina may drain via either or both routes. Sentinel lymph node mapping is often performed before surgery due to variability in this drainage pattern.[14]

Sequence	TR	TE	FOV	Matrix	Slice Thickness, mm	NSA
T2W coronal SSTSE	1000	81	400 × 400	320 × 320	8	1
T2W axial TSE	8240	115	350 × 260	448 × 512	6	2
T1W axial GRE on and out-of-phase	120	2.38	350 × 260	240 × 320	8	1
EPI axial DWI (b = 50, 500, 1000)	13,100	91	350 × 260	112 × 128	3	2
T2W sagittal TSE	5030	125	280 × 320	512 × 448	5	2
T2W axial TSE small FOV	5770	115	220 × 250	512 × 448	5	2
T2W coronal TSE	5500	115	350 × 350	512 × 512	6	2
T1W 3D FS spoiled GRE axial	4.66	2.38	350 × 260	540 × 640	3.5	1
Administer 0.1 mmol/kg intravenous gadolinium contrast at 2 mL/s, and wait 18 s						
T1W 3D FS spoiled GRE axial ×3	4.66	2.38	350 × 260	540 × 640	3.5	1
T1W 3D FS spoiled GRE sagittal	4.66	2.38	350 × 350	640 × 640	3.5	1
T1W 3D FS spoiled GRE coronal	4.66	2.38	410 × 410	540 × 640	3.5	1

Abbreviations: DWI, diffusion-weighted imaging; EPI, echo planar imaging; FOV, field of view in mm; FS, fat suppressed; GRE, gradient-recalled echo; NSA, number of signal averages; SSTSE, single-shot turbo spin echo; TE, echo time; TR, repetition time; TSE; turbo spin echo; T1W, T1 weighted; T2W, T2 weighted.

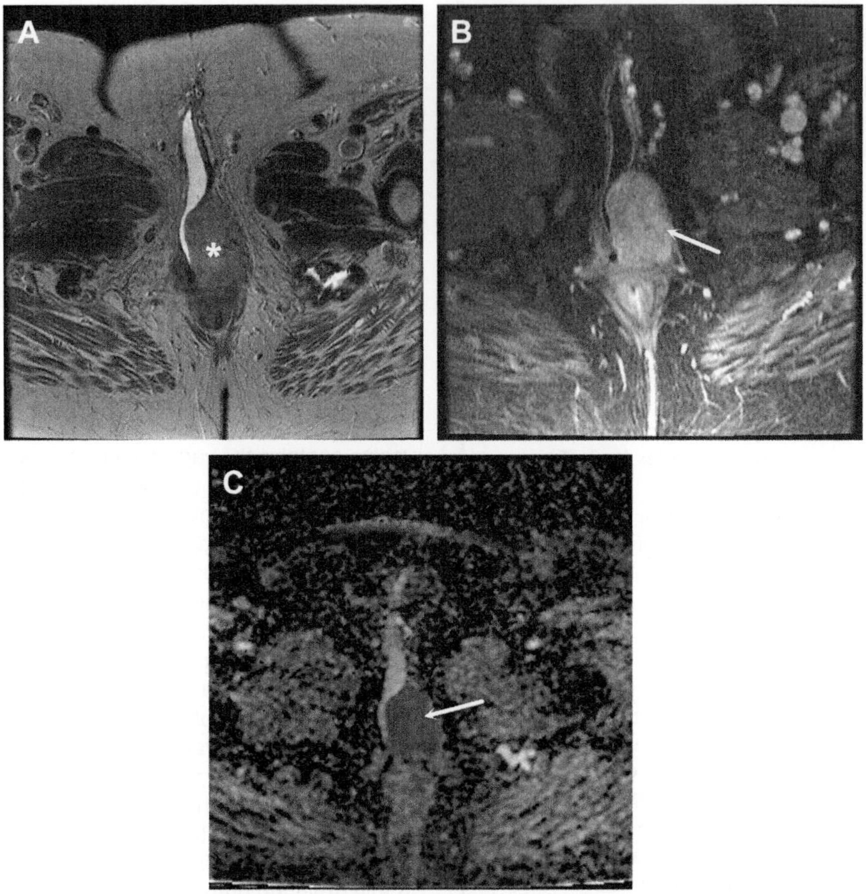

Fig. 3. Vulvar cancer. Axial TSE T2-weighted MR image (*A*) demonstrates a T2 intermediate-intensity ("evil gray") posterior left vulvar mass (*asterisk*) with extension into the ischioanal fat and involving the anterior wall of the anus, consistent with stage IV vulvar carcinoma. Axial T1-weighted FS postcontrast MR image (*B*) demonstrates avid heterogeneous enhancement of the mass, involvement of the vulvo-vaginal plexus with resultant vulvar collaterals and extension into the ischioanal fossa (*arrow*). Axial ADC map from diffusion-weighted MR image (*C*) demonstrates marked diffusion restriction of the mass (*arrow*).

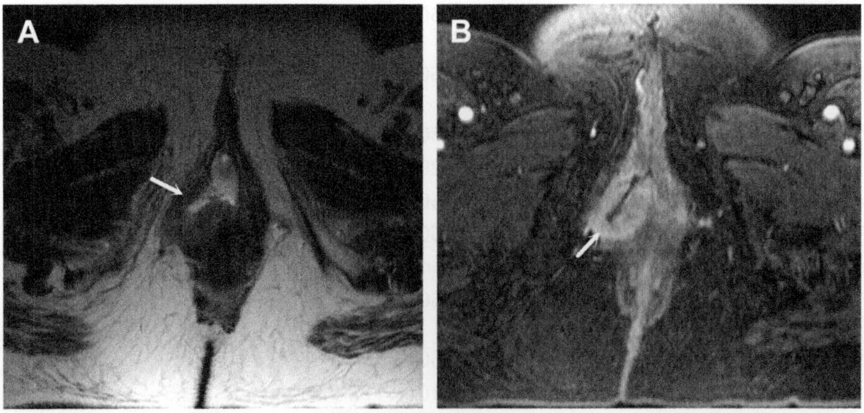

Fig. 4. Stage IB vulvar cancer. Axial TSE T2-weighted MR image (*A*) demonstrates an ulcerated right posterior vulvar mass (*arrow*). Axial T1-weighted FS postcontrast MR image (*B*) demonstrates avid enhancement of the ulcerated mass (*arrow*).

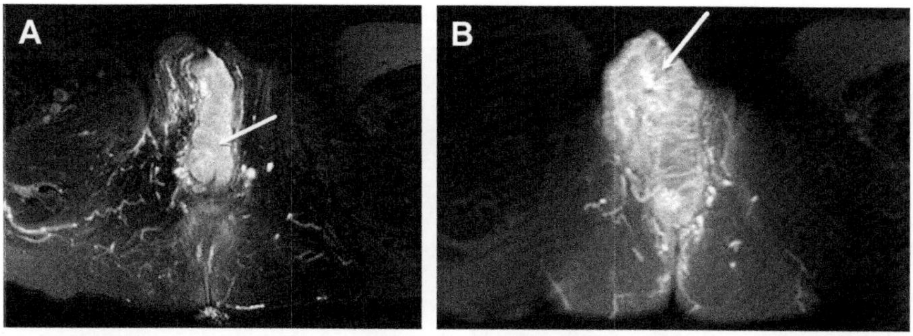

Fig. 5. Vulvar cancer. Axial T2-weighted FS MR image (*A*) demonstrates a large T2-hyperintense anterior vulvar mass (*arrow*) involving the mons pubis, labia, clitoris, vulvar-vaginal plexus, and anterior wall of the anus consistent with at least a stage II vulvar carcinoma. Axial T1-weighted FS postcontrast MR image (*B*) demonstrates avid enhancement of this mass (*arrow*).

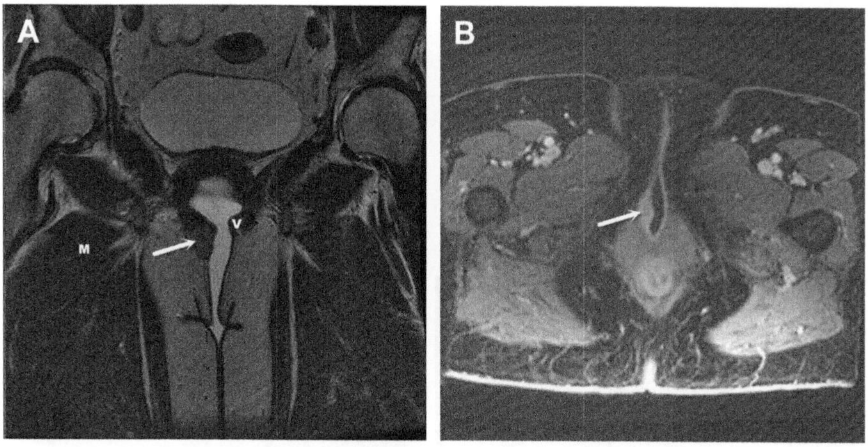

Fig. 6. Vulvar cancer. Coronal TSE T2-weighted MR image (*A*) demonstrates a small right labia minora mass (*arrow*), slightly T2 hyperintense to skeletal muscle (M) and the vaginal submucosa and muscularis layers (V) biopsy proven to be a vulvar SCC. Axial T1-weighted FS postcontrast MR image (*B*) demonstrates uniform enhancement of the mass (*arrow*).

Lymphatic drainage of the vulva is primarily through the superficial inguinal lymph nodes.[15,16] The superficial inguinal lymph nodes can be subdivided into 3 groups: a medial group, medial to the femoral vein and greater saphenous vein; an intermediate group near the femoral and saphenous vein; and a lateral group in the lateral third of the groin. The deep inguinal (also referred to as femoral) lymph nodes are located medial to the femoral vein and drain to the external iliac lymph nodes.

PATHOLOGY AND STAGING

Vulvar carcinoma is squamous cell in origin in 90% of cases.[16] Melanoma, basal cell carcinoma, Paget disease, Bartholin gland cancer, and adenocarcinoma are much rarer forms of vulvar malignancies.[1,16] Human papillomavirus (HPV)-associated vulvar squamous cell carcinoma

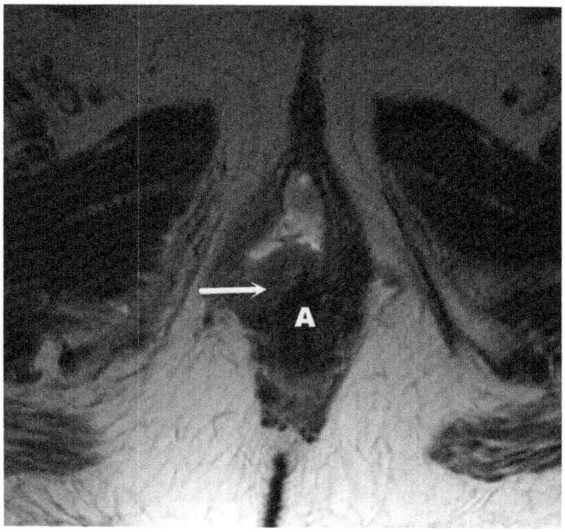

Fig. 7. Vulvar cancer. Axial TSE T2-weighted MR image demonstrates a right vulvar mass abutting the anus (A) without definite mucosal invasion (*arrow*).

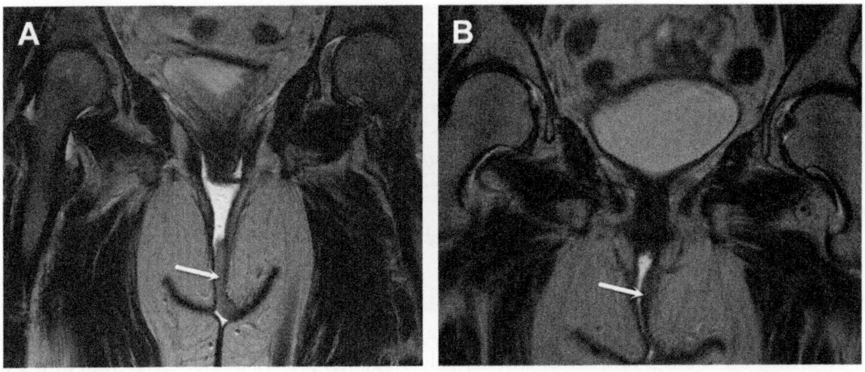

Fig. 8. Posttreatment imaging of vulvar cancer. Coronal TSE T2-weighted MR image demonstrates a superficial left vulvar mass (*A, arrow*). After chemotherapy and radiation, there is only mild residual T2-hypointense thickening of the left vulva (*B, arrow*).

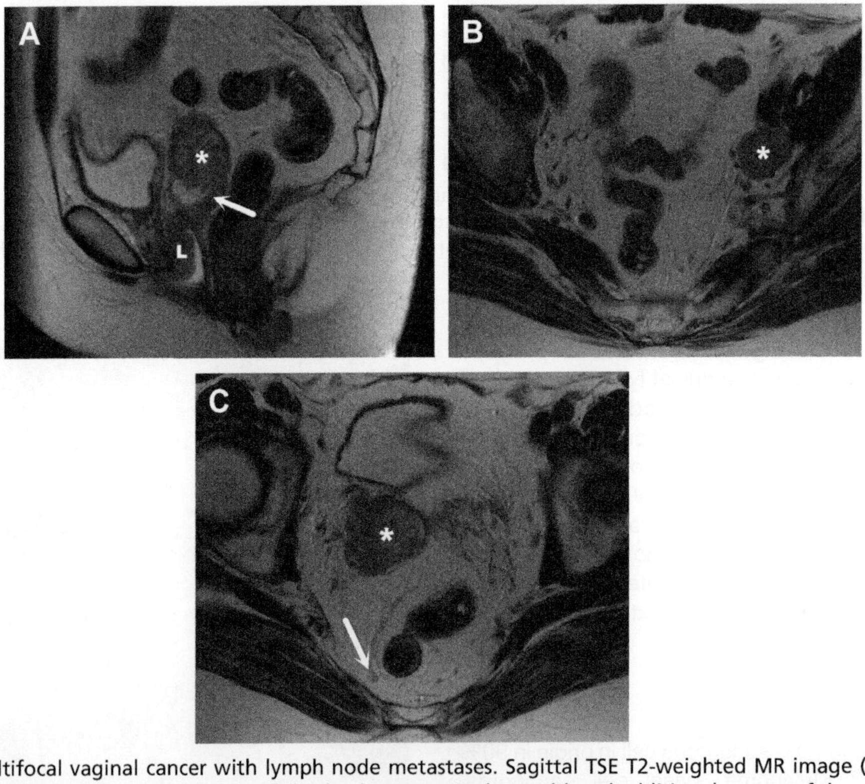

Fig. 9. Multifocal vaginal cancer with lymph node metastases. Sagittal TSE T2-weighted MR image (*A*) demonstrates multifocal vaginal carcinoma with both a lower vaginal mass (L) and additional masses of the mid (*arrow*) and upper vagina (*asterisk*). Axial TSE T2-weighted MR image (*B*) demonstrates a rounded, enlarged left external iliac lymph node consistent with lymph node metastasis (seen with upper vaginal disease) (*asterisk*). Axial TSE T2-weighted MR image (*C*) demonstrates the upper vaginal mass in the right vaginal cuff (*asterisk*) and a suspicious mesorectal lymph node (seen with lower vaginal disease, *arrow*).

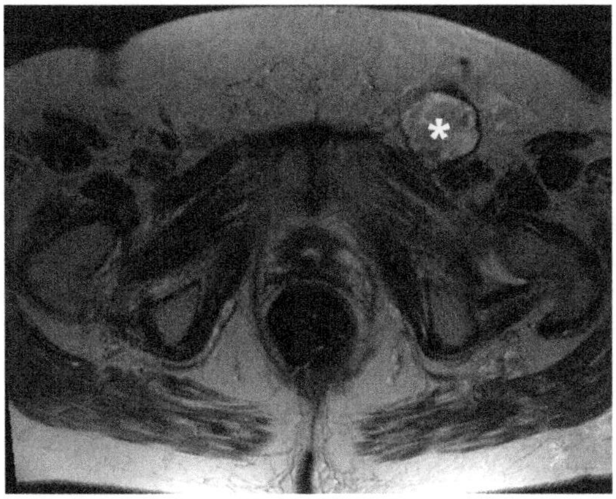

Fig. 10. Necrotic lymph node metastasis in vulvar cancer. Axial TSE T2-weighted MR image demonstrates an enlarged, necrotic left inguinal lymph node (*asterisk*) in a patient with vulvar cancer.

(SCC) presents in women younger than 60 years, is associated with vulvar intraepithelial neoplasia, and may be multifocal with associated vaginal and cervical tumors.[16,17] Non–HPV-associated vulvar SCC presents in older women, is associated with lichen sclerosis or vulvar inflammation, and is more typically unifocal.[18] The most recent revision of the International Federation of Gynecology and Obstetrics (FIGO) staging system for vulvar cancer from 2009 guides the clinicopathologic staging of vulvar cancer.[19]

Similarly, vaginal cancer is overwhelmingly squamous cell in origin, representing 80% to 90% of cases.[20] Clear-cell adenocarcinoma, resulting from in utero exposure to diethylstilbestrol (DES), is rarely seen today due to cessation of the use of DES in pregnancy, but previously represented 4% to 10% of vaginal tumors and developed in young women.[3,20] Other less frequent histologic subtypes of vaginal malignancies include melanoma, sarcoma, carcinoid, and small-cell neuroendocrine. Like vulvar cancer, HPV has been implicated in the development of vaginal SCC.[21] Vaginal cancer is staged clinically according to the 2009 FIGO staging system, as many patients will not undergo surgical management.[3]

MR Imaging Protocol

Pelvic MR protocols used for staging and surveillance in vulvar or vaginal tumors may vary from

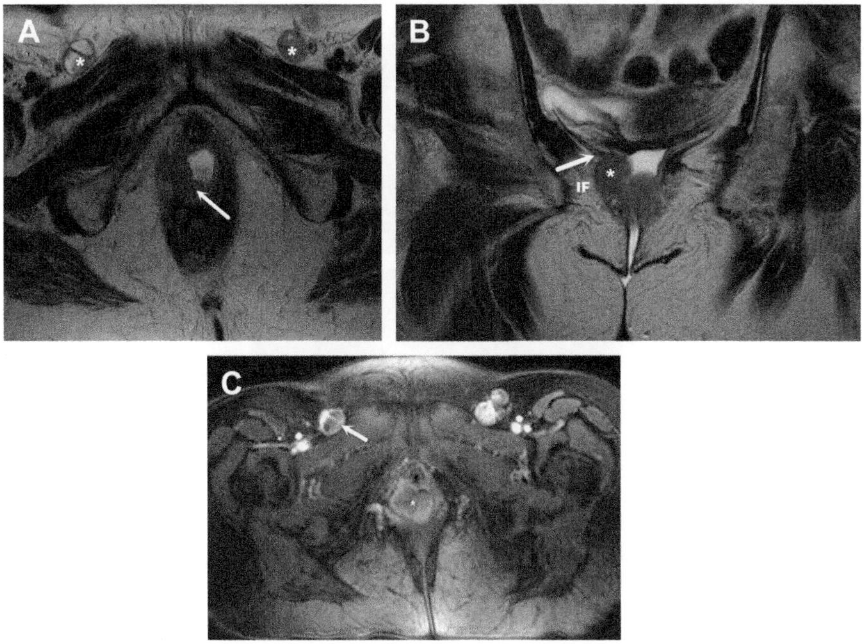

Fig. 11. Vaginal cancer. Axial TSE T2-weighted MR image (*A*) demonstrates a T2 intermediate-intensity lobular vaginal mass with well-defined nodular soft tissue margins that extends into the adjacent paravaginal fat laterally and abuts the anterior wall of the anus posteriorly (*arrow*) and associated with necrotic inguinal lymph nodes bilaterally (*asterisks*). Coronal TSE T2-weighted MR image (*B*) demonstrates invasion of the puborectalis muscle (*arrow*) and ischioanal fossa (IF) by the lobulated vaginal mass (*asterisk*). Axial T1-weighted FS postcontrast MR image (*C*) demonstrates enhancement of the primary vaginal mass (*asterisk*) and necrotic inguinal lymphadenopathy (*arrow*).

one institution to the next. At the Mallinckrodt Institute of Radiology, the patient is asked to void before entering the MR imaging suite. The patient is then asked to self-administer 20 mL of a water-soluble gel into the vaginal vault before beginning the MR examination.[22,23] A pelvic or torso phased array coil is used for the study. The examination begins with acquisition of localizer imaging and a coronal breath-hold T2-weighted single-shot turbo spin-echo sequence (SSTSE) covering the entire pelvic cavity, with sufficient cranial extent to visualize the kidneys (specifically to assess for hydronephrosis). The initial precontrast sequences include a series of multiplanar high-resolution TSE T2-weighted imaging of the entire pelvis and axial small field of view T2-weighted images of the female reproductive system, gradient-recalled echo (GRE) T1-weighted in-phase and out-of-phase axial chemical shift imaging (a routine component of our female pelvic MR protocols), echo planar diffusion-weighted axial imaging with b values of 50, 500, and 1000 (with a calculated apparent diffusion coefficient [ADC] map), and 3-dimensional (3D) spoiled gradient-echo fat-suppressed T1-weighted axial imaging of the pelvis. An extracellular gadolinium contrast agent is administered at a dose of 0.1 mmol/kg at an injection rate of 2 mL/s. After an 18-second delay, dynamic T1 spoiled gradient-echo fat-suppressed axial imaging is performed at 15-second intervals for 3 scans, to best achieve arterial, venous, and equilibrium phase images; followed by sagittal and coronal oblique post–contrast-enhanced images.

MR IMAGING FINDINGS

Vulvar Cancer

Vulvar cancer manifests on MR imaging as a T1 hypointense to isointense, T2 intermediately

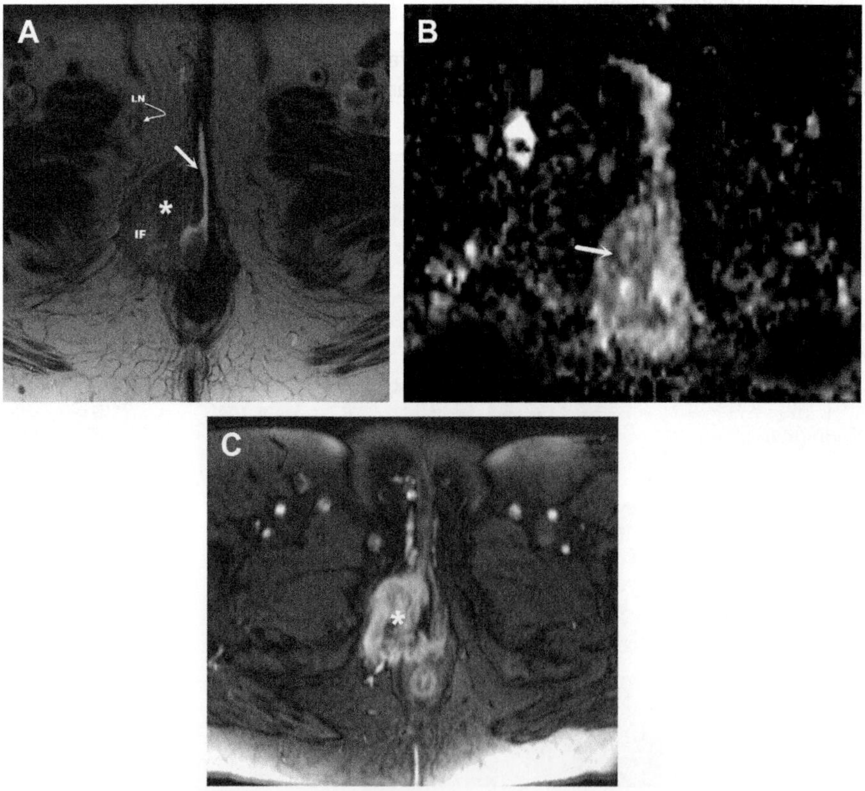

Fig. 12. Vulvo-vaginal cancer. Axial TSE T2-weighted MR image (*A*) demonstrates a large ulcerated T2 intermediate-intensity ("evil gray") right vulvo-vaginal mass (*asterisk*) extending through the vaginal submucosa and muscularis layers (*arrow*) involving the puborectalis muscle, anterior wall of the anus, and the IF, and a small centrally necrotic right inguinal lymph node (LN, *curved arrow*). Axial ADC map from diffusion-weighted MR image (*B*) demonstrates marked diffusion restriction of the vulvo-vaginal mass (*arrow*). Axial T1-weighted FS post-contrast MR image (*C*) demonstrates avid enhancement of the ulcerated vulvo-vaginal mass (*asterisk*) involving the vulvo-vaginal plexus with several vulvar collaterals, and extravaginal extension into the ischioanal fat.

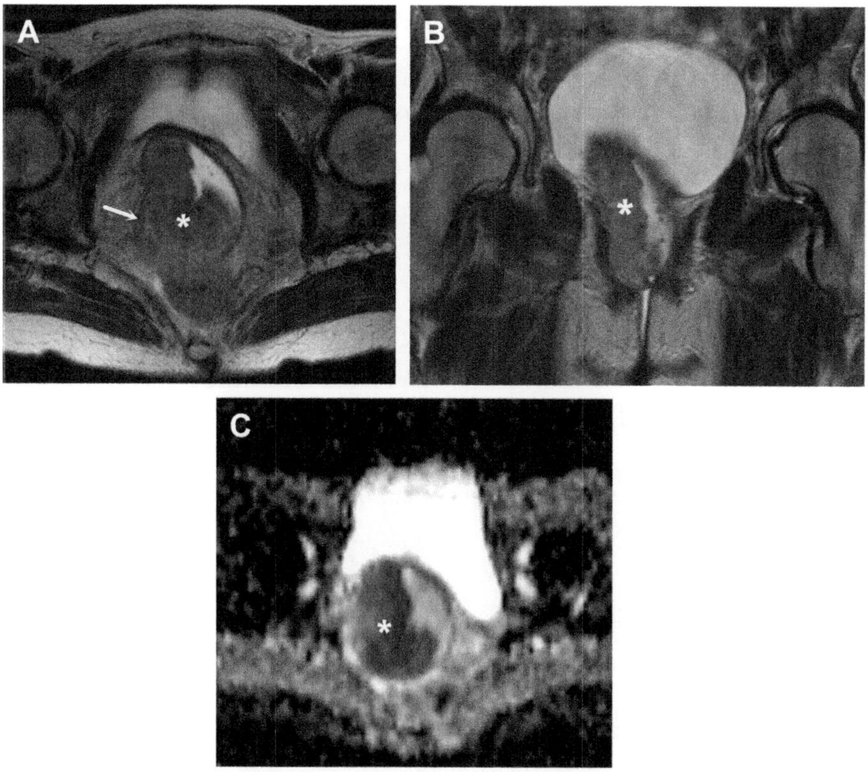

Fig. 13. Vaginal cancer. Axial TSE T2-weighted MR image (*A*) demonstrates a large lobulated vaginal mass (*asterisk*) with loss of the T2 hypointense margin of the right vaginal wall submucosa and muscularis (*arrow*), and infiltrative extravaginal extension into the parametrium. Coronal TSE T2-weighted MR image (*B*) demonstrates the extent of the vaginal mass (*asterisk*), involving the entire length of the vagina with involvement of the puborectalis muscle. Axial ADC map from diffusion-weighted MR image (*C*) demonstrates marked hypointensity of the vaginal mass (*asterisk*), in keeping with dense cellularity of the vaginal tumor.

hyperintense ("evil gray"), solidly enhancing mass with associated diffusion restriction (**Figs. 3–6**).[16,24,25] Diffusion-weighted imaging may aid in tumor detection with better tumor-to-normal tissue contrast than T2-weighted imaging.[26] The use of fat suppression with contrast-enhanced imaging improves lesion conspicuity.[27] As the presence of a vulvar mass is rarely in doubt when patients are referred for pelvic MR imaging, the emphasis is on defining the anatomic extent of the tumor. Involvement of superficial structures, such as the labia minora and majora, urethra, and clitoris, and deeper organs, such as the vagina and anus by tumor, as well as size of the tumor, should be assessed (**Fig. 7**).

MR imaging is also valuable in evaluating for tumor response, tumor recurrence and posttreatment complications, similar to vaginal cancer.[27] Unlike vaginal cancer, vulvar cancer is often treated with multiple surgeries and reconstructions, and

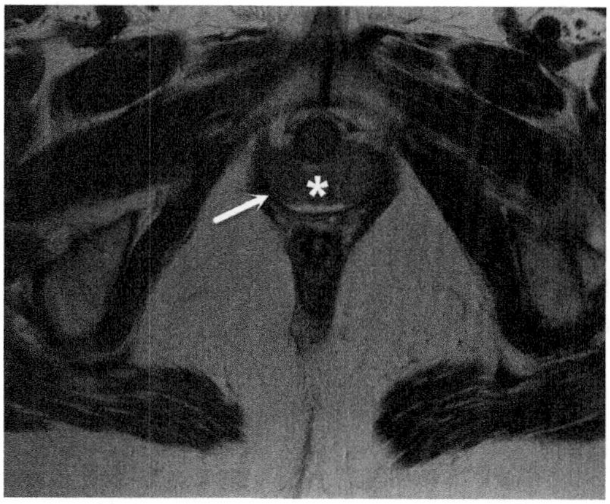

Fig. 14. Stage I vaginal cancer. Axial TSE T2-weighted MR image demonstrates a lower vaginal mass (*asterisk*) without extravaginal extension, indicated by an intact T2 hypointense rim of the vaginal submucosa and muscularis (*arrow*).

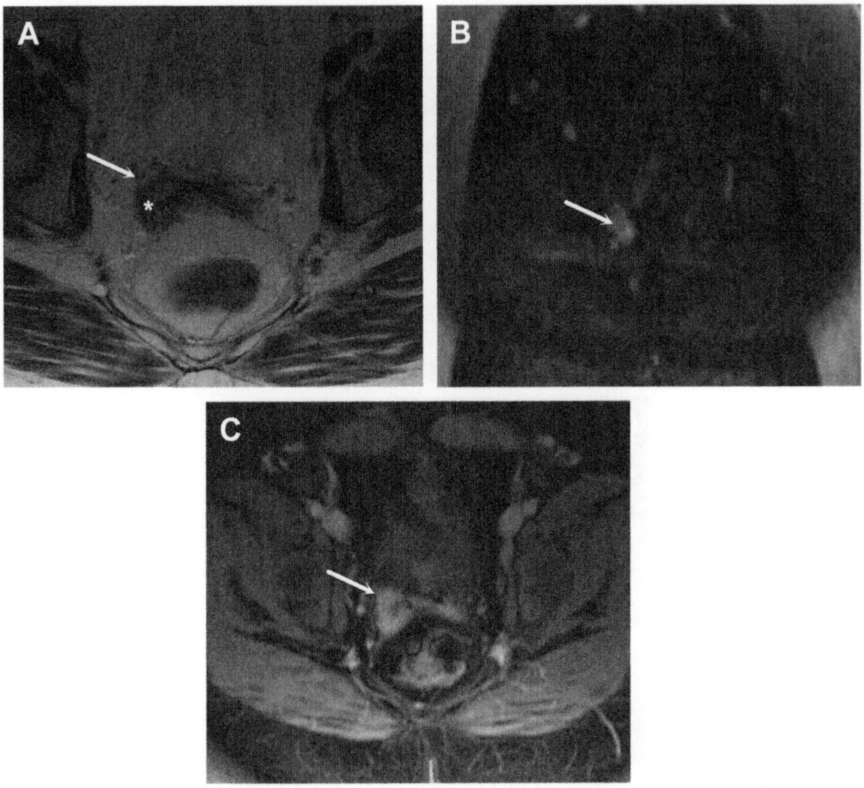

Fig. 15. Stage II vaginal cancer. Axial TSE T2-weighted MR image (*A*) demonstrates asymmetric masslike thickening of the right vaginal cuff (*asterisk*) with spiculations of tissue extending into the paravaginal fat (*arrow*). Axial diffusion-weighted MR image with b value of 1000 (*B*) demonstrates abnormal diffusion restriction of the right vaginal cuff (*arrow*). Axial T1-weighted FS postcontrast MR image (*C*) demonstrates hyperenhancement of the thickened right vaginal cuff with extension of tumor into the paravaginal fat (*arrow*).

surveillance imaging should be interpreted with an understanding of the postoperative anatomy and expected changes (**Fig. 8**). Early-stage tumors, such as stage I and smaller stage II tumors, are treated with wide local resection (stage IA) or radical local resection/modified vulvectomy (Stage IB/II).[8,28] Lymph node status (see the next section) is assessed with sentinel lymph node sampling and/or inguinofemoral lymph node dissection. Positive lymph nodes and/or the presence of bulky or locally advanced stage disease, including larger stage II and stage III/IV tumors, are most frequently treated with external-beam radiation therapy and chemotherapy.

Lymph Nodes

Lymph node staging is a critical component of determining a patient's treatment plan and prognosis. The most important determinant of overall survival with vulvar cancer is the presence of positive inguinofemoral lymph nodes, conferring FIGO stage III disease status and a 5-year survival rate of approximately 50%.[28,29] Higher-stage

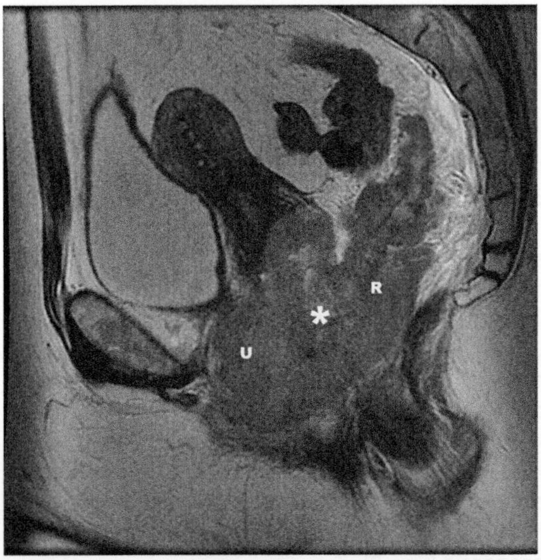

Fig. 16. Stage IV vaginal cancer. Sagittal TSE T2-weighted MR image demonstrates a large, T2 intermediate-intensity "evil gray" infiltrative vaginal mass (*asterisk*) with gross extension into the pelvic fat, urethra (U) and rectum (R), consistent with a stage IV vaginal carcinoma.

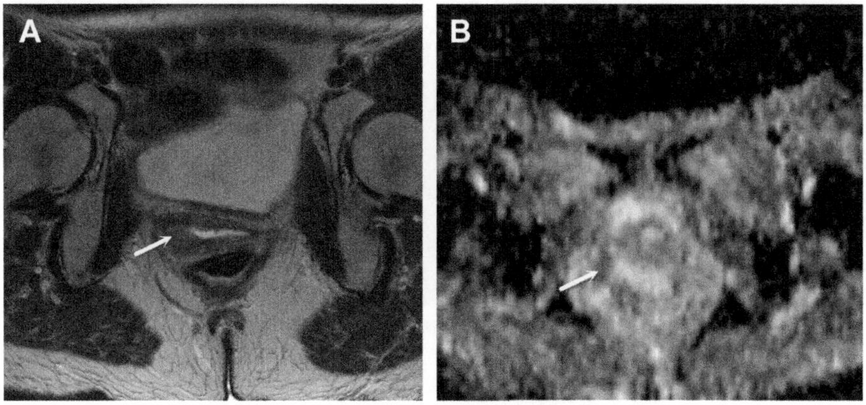

Fig. 17. Posttreatment imaging of vaginal cancer. Axial TSE T2-weighted (*A*) and ADC (*B*) MR image of the patient from **Fig. 5** after treatment with definitive chemoradiation demonstrates marked interval decrease in size of the vaginal mass (*arrow*) from the original presentation with small residual tumor with persistent extravaginal extension (*A*) and diffusion restriction (*B*).

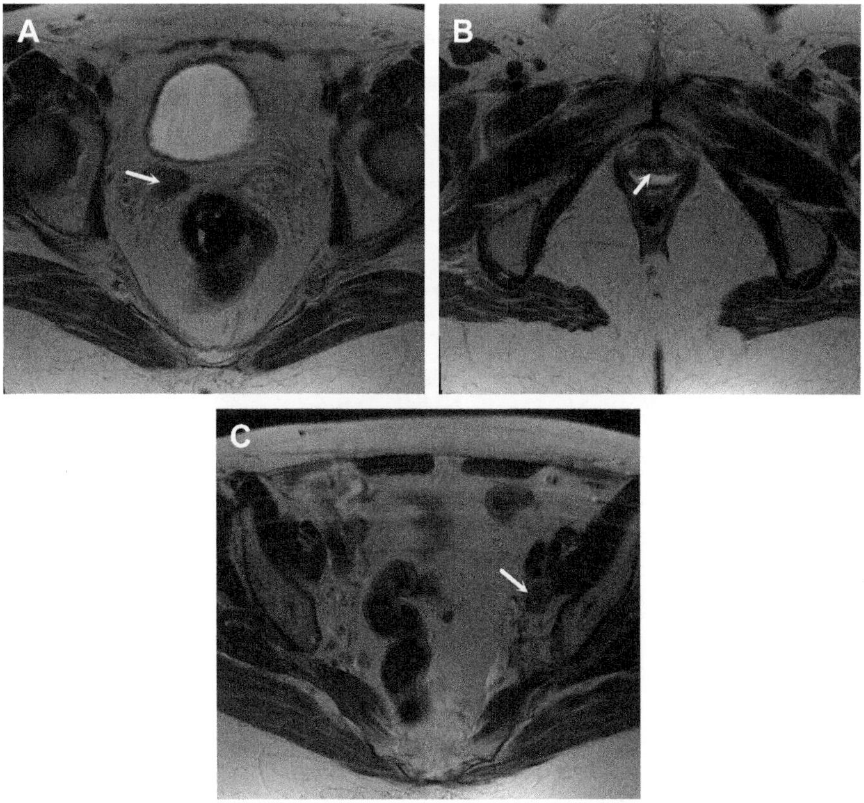

Fig. 18. Posttreatment imaging of vaginal cancer. Axial TSE T2-weighted MR image of the patient with vaginal carcinoma from **Fig. 19** after treatment with chemoradiation demonstrates marked interval reduction in size of the right vaginal cuff mass (*A, arrow*), near complete resolution of the lower vaginal mass with a mild amount of residual anterior vaginal thickening (*B, arrow*) and decreased size of left external iliac lymph nodes (*C, arrow*).

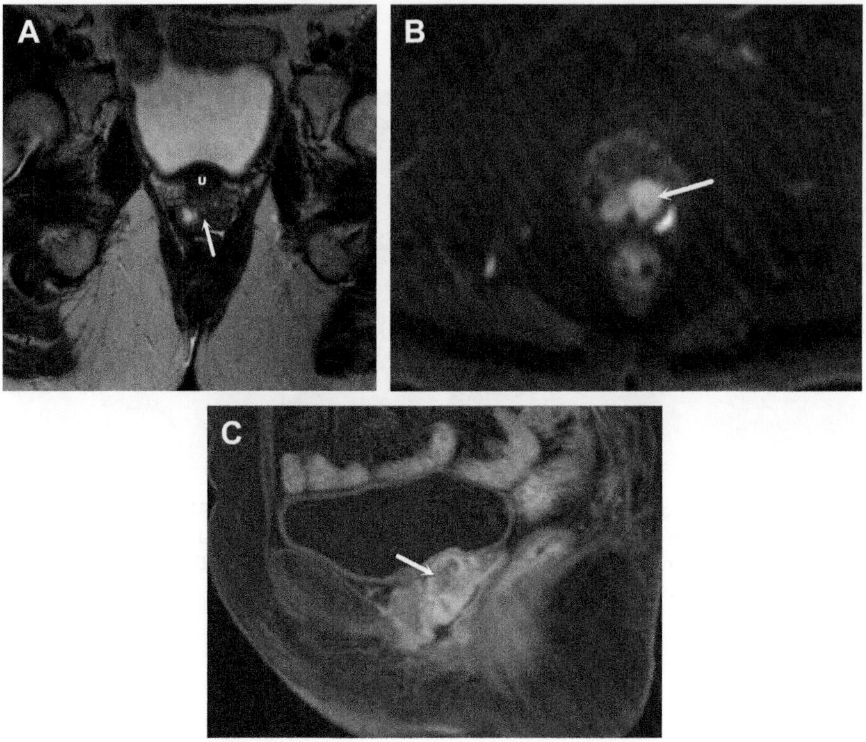

Fig. 19. Recurrent vaginal cancer. Axial TSE T2-weighted MR image (*A*) in a patient posttreatment demonstrates a recurrent anterior vaginal carcinoma (*arrow*) with foci of T2 hyperintensity abutting the urethra (U). Axial diffusion-weighted MR image with a b value of 500 (*B*) demonstrates diffusion restriction of the anterior vaginal recurrence (*arrow*), aiding in distinction from posttreatment fibrosis. Sagittal T1 FS postcontrast MR image (*C*) demonstrates peripheral enhancement of the recurrent anterior vaginal carcinoma (*arrow*).

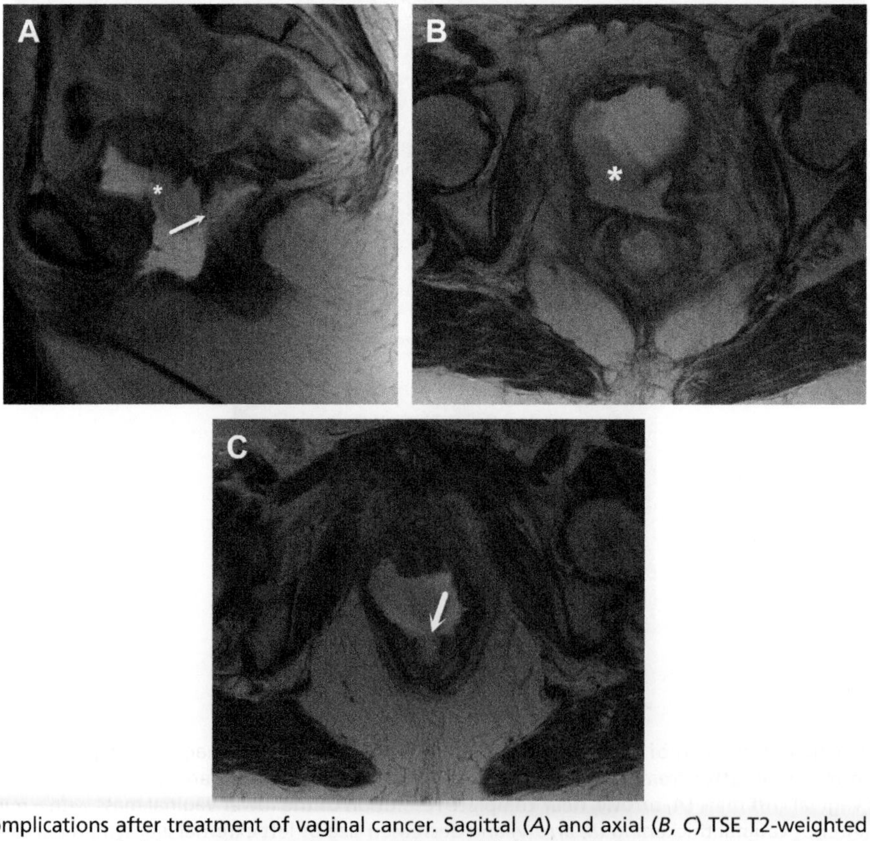

Fig. 20. Complications after treatment of vaginal cancer. Sagittal (*A*) and axial (*B*, *C*) TSE T2-weighted MR image demonstrates rectovaginal (*arrows*) and vesicovaginal (*asterisks*) fistulas that developed after definitive radiation therapy of a vaginal carcinoma.

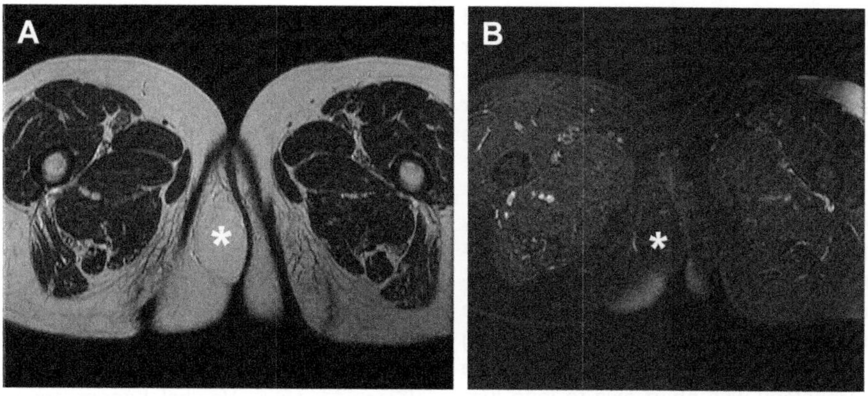

Fig. 21. Vulvar lipoma. Axial TSE T2-weighted MR image (*A*) demonstrates a well-demarcated, smooth T2 hyperintense right vulvar mass (*asterisk*), with similar signal intensity to subcutaneous fat, with signal loss of the mass (*asterisk*) on FS TSE T2-weighted MR image (*B*), confirming the internal fat content within a vulvar lipoma.

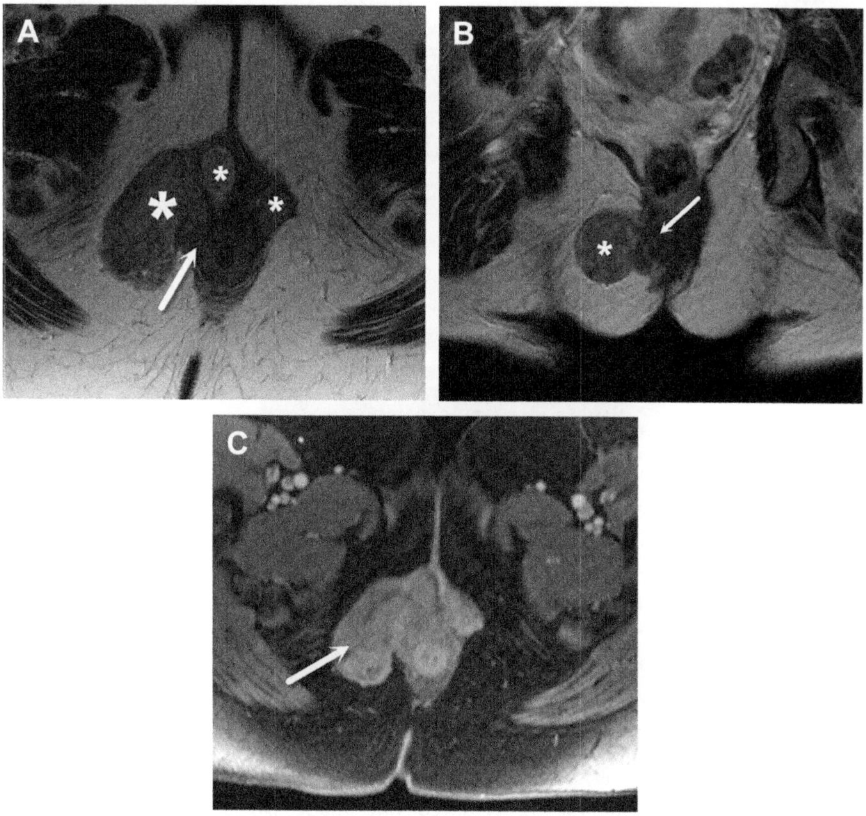

Fig. 22. Vulvar leiomyoma. Axial TSE T2-weighted MR image (*A*) demonstrates a multilobulated T2 hypointense vulvar mass (*asterisks*) abutting the anus (*arrow*). Coronal T2-weighted MR image (*B*) demonstrates that the right-sided component of the vulvar mass (*asterisk*) closely abuts the anal sphincter (*arrow*). Axial T1-weighted FS post-contrast MR image (*C*) demonstrates avid uniform enhancement of the mass (*arrow*).

vaginal cancers are more likely to be associated with pathologic node involvement and lower 5-year survival rates even with adjuvant radiotherapy treatment, in the 40% to 70% range for stage II disease compared with 100% for stage I disease.[30]

Lymph node staging of vulvar and vaginal carcinoma by MR imaging can be complicated by false-positive inguinal lymph nodes due to inflammation from ulcerated lesions and coexisting pelvic infection. A variety of lymph node features are suggestive of malignant involvement, including short axis diameter greater than 10 mm, a more rounded morphology with short axis to long axis (S to L) ratio >0.75, cystic changes within the lymph node, and irregular lymph node contour (**Fig. 9**).[24,31] Of these imaging features when imaging vulvar cancer lymph node metastases, S to L ratio greater than 0.75 yields the greatest overall accuracy (85%), the presence of necrosis is the most specific (93%) (**Fig. 10**), and readers' confidence in lymph node metastasis is most sensitive (87%).

Vaginal Cancer

Morphologically, vaginal tumors may present as an ulcerated mass with ill-defined margins or a lobulated soft tissue component, or as an annular constricting mass with circumferential thickening (**Figs. 11–13**).[32] Vaginal tumors are typically T1 isointense to skeletal muscle and of intermediate T2 hyperintensity (greater than muscle, less than water) ("the evil gray").[32,33] Fat-suppressed (FS)

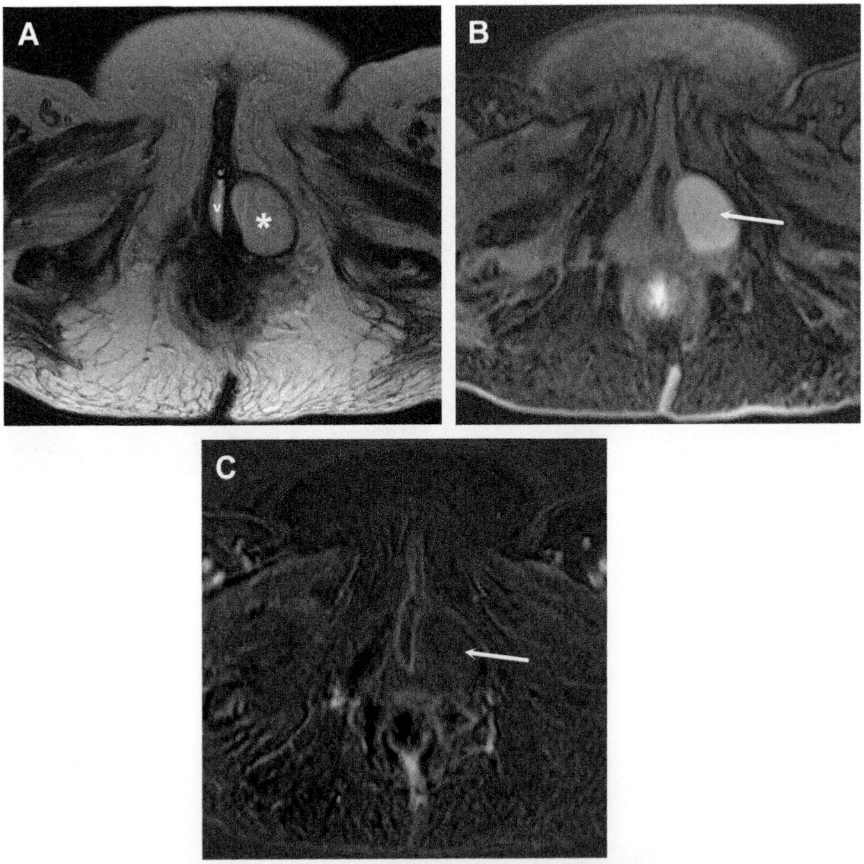

Fig. 23. Bartholin gland cyst. Axial TSE T2-weighted MR image (*A*) demonstrates a left paravaginal T2-hyperintense lesion (*asterisk*) at the level of the vaginal introitus (V). Axial T1-weighted fat precontrast MR image (*B*) demonstrates that the lesion is T1 hyperintense (*arrow*) with no internal enhancement after contrast administration on subtraction imaging (*C*), consistent with a hemorrhagic or proteinaceous Bartholin gland cyst.

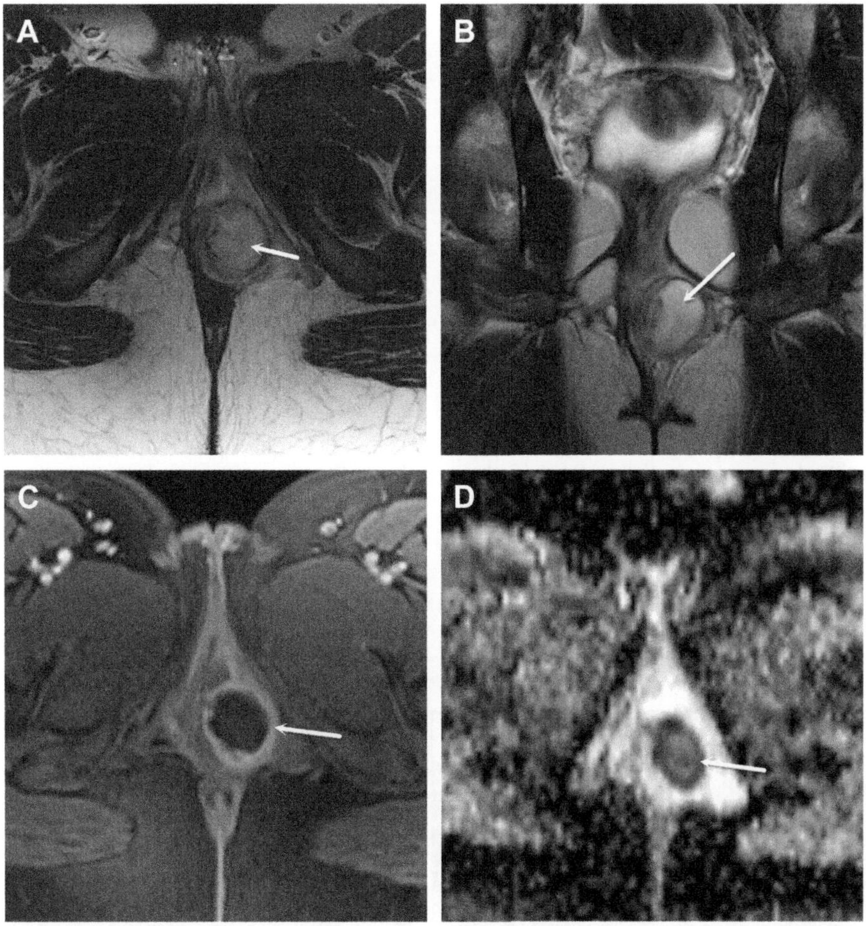

Fig. 24. Bartholin gland abscess. Axial (*A*) and coronal (*B*) TSE T2-weighted MR image demonstrates a left labial T2 hyperintense lesion with thickened, irregular borders and internal debris (*arrow*). Axial T1-weighted FS post-contrast MR image (*C*) demonstrates enhancement of the irregular thickened rim of the lesion and central non-enhancement (*arrow*). Axial ADC map from diffusion-weighted MR image (*D*) demonstrates marked diffusion restriction of the contents of the lesion (*arrow*), consistent with pus within a Bartholin gland abscess.

T1-weighted dynamic contrast-enhanced imaging depicts early tumoral enhancement in the first 45 to 90 seconds after contrast administration,[34] which may helpful in the setting of evaluation for recurrent disease or after radiation therapy.[14] Diffusion-weighted imaging has demonstrated promise with other gynecologic cancers, such as cervical cancer, in more accurately quantifying tumor volume and predicting treatment response and survival.[35]

MR imaging staging of vaginal cancer has been proposed in alignment with the FIGO clinical staging system.[14,33] For stage I tumors, the tumor should be confined to the mucosa, demonstrated on MR imaging with preservation of the T2-hypointense submucosal and muscularis layers (**Fig. 14**). Stage II tumors extend beyond the muscularis into the paravaginal fat (**Fig. 15**), disrupting the T2-hypointense submucosal and muscularis layers. Coronal and sagittal TSE T2-weighted imaging are crucial adjuncts to

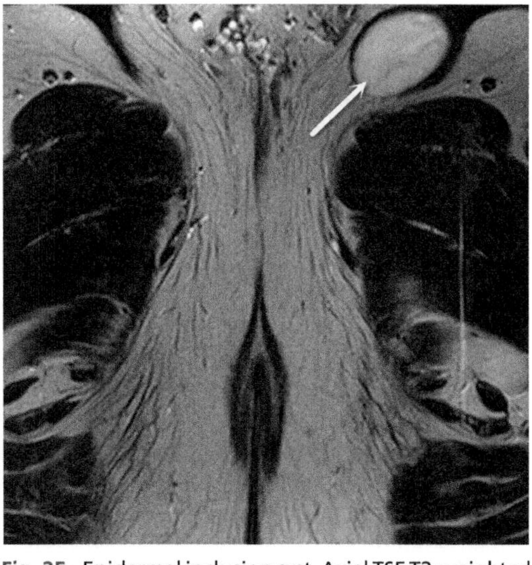

Fig. 25. Epidermal inclusion cyst. Axial TSE T2-weighted MR image demonstrates a T2-hyperintense subcutaneous lesion extending to the skin surface (*arrow*).

axial images in assessing for subtle loss of T2 hypointensity of the vaginal stroma. Stage III tumors extend to the pelvic side wall, with involvement of the obturator internus, levator ani, or piriformis, external or internal iliac vessels, or bony structures (see **Fig. 11**C). Involved musculature may have abnormally high T2 signal and be tethered, and assessment of hydronephrosis is helpful in tumors with extravaginal extension. Stage IVA disease indicates involvement of adjacent organs, involving the mucosal layer of the bladder, rectum, or urethra, or extension beyond the true pelvis (**Fig. 16**). The presence of distant metastases places the patient in the Stage IVB category, including disease in the lungs or liver.

The relative location and stage of the vaginal tumor dictates the treatment paradigm.[30] Small early-stage upper vaginal tumors can be treated with upper vaginectomy, radical hysterectomy, and pelvic lymph node dissection. Rarely, small distal vaginal tumors may be amenable to treatment with total vaginectomy or vulvovaginectomy and inguinofemoral lymph node dissection. However, in most patients with vaginal cancer, especially those with locally advanced disease, primary treatment is with definitive radiation therapy (external-beam radiation therapy and/or intracavitary/interstitial brachytherapy) and concurrent chemotherapy.

Imaging of the posttreatment patient serves to assess for residual or recurrent tumor, or

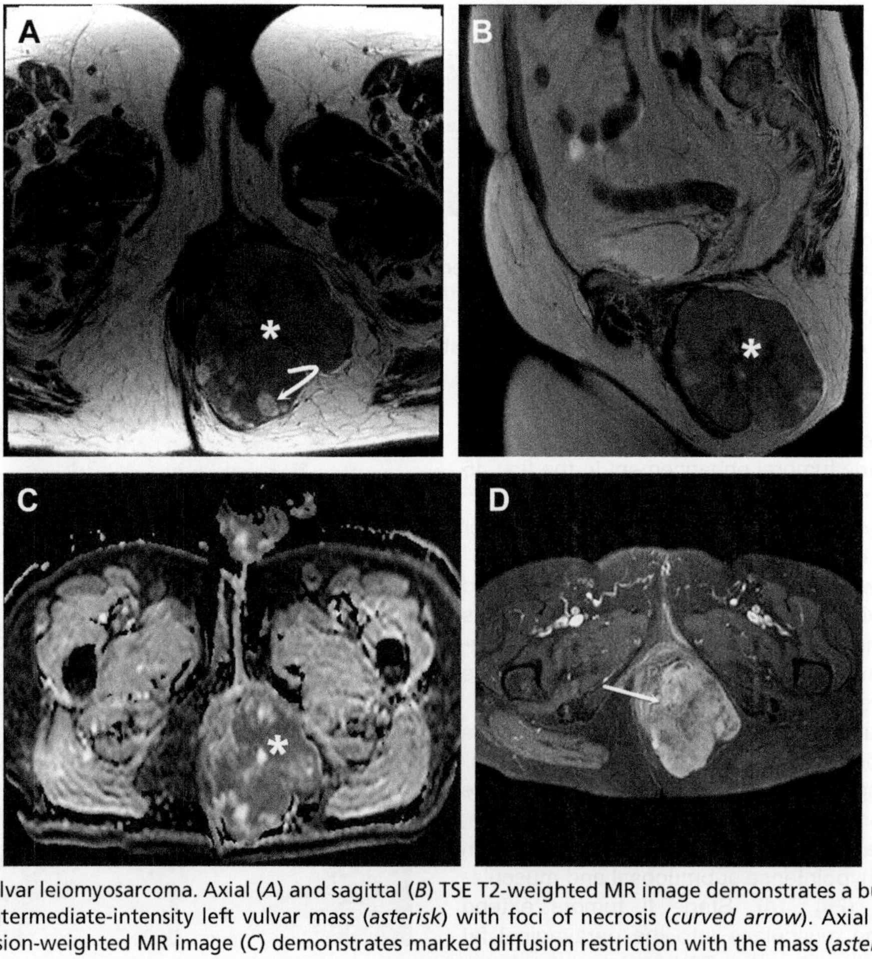

Fig. 26. Vulvar leiomyosarcoma. Axial (*A*) and sagittal (*B*) TSE T2-weighted MR image demonstrates a bulky, lobulated T2 intermediate-intensity left vulvar mass (*asterisk*) with foci of necrosis (*curved arrow*). Axial ADC map from diffusion-weighted MR image (*C*) demonstrates marked diffusion restriction with the mass (*asterisk*). Axial T1-weighted FS postcontrast MR image (*D*) demonstrates avid heterogeneous enhancement (*straight arrow*) of the mass. The presence of necrosis and hemorrhage may aid in distinguishing leiomyosarcoma from epithelial vulvar cancer, but ultimately tissue sampling is required to establish the diagnosis.

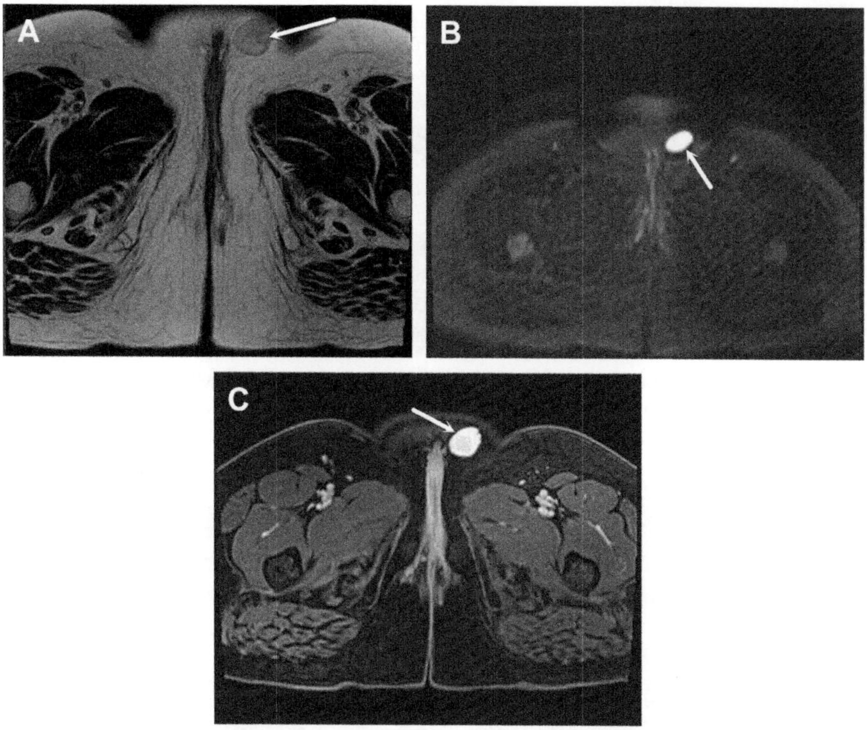

Fig. 27. Vulvar dermatofibrosarcoma protuberans, a rare sarcoma of dermal origin. Axial T2-weighted MR image (*A*) demonstrates a rounded intermediate T2-intensity subcutaneous left labia majora mass (*arrow*). Axial diffusion-weighted MR image with a b value of 1000 (*B*) demonstrates marked diffusion restriction of the mass (*arrow*). Axial T1-weighted FS postcontrast MR image (*C*) demonstrates avid homogeneous enhancement of the mass (*arrow*). The dermal location of this mass may provide a clue as to the diagnosis, and the presence of diffusion restriction and enhancement confirm the solid nature of the mass as compared with an epidermal inclusion cyst, but due to the rarity of this entity and its nonspecific MR imaging features, tissue sampling is required to establish the diagnosis.

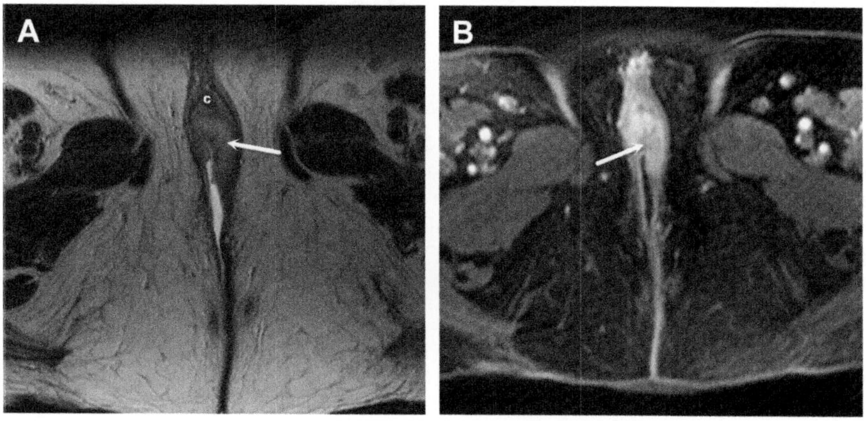

Fig. 28. Vulvar melanoma. Axial TSE T2-weighted MR image (*A*) demonstrates an anterior vulvar mass (*arrow*) abutting the clitoris (C). Axial T1-weighted FS postcontrast MR image (*B*) demonstrates avid enhancement of the mass (*arrow*). Pathology demonstrated vulvar melanoma, although by imaging the mass is indistinguishable from an SCC.

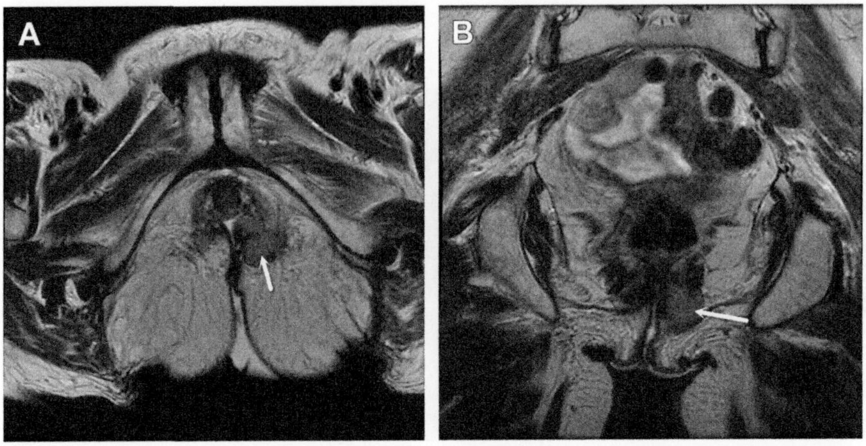

Fig. 29. Bartholin gland carcinoma. Axial (*A*) and coronal (*B*) TSE T2-weighted MR image demonstrates a vulvar mass (*arrow*) in the expected region of the left Bartholin gland that involved the lower vagina, surgically staged and pathologically proven to be stage II Bartholin gland vulvar carcinoma.

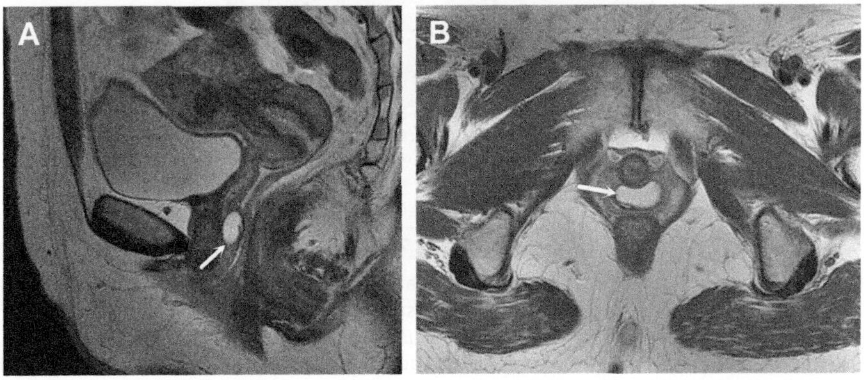

Fig. 30. Gardner duct cyst. Sagittal (*A*) and axial (*B*) TSE T2-weighted MR image demonstrates a T2 hyperintense lesion within the lower third anterior vaginal wall (*arrow*).

posttreatment complications. Locoregional recurrence is common in vaginal cancer, developing in up to a quarter of patients at 5 years and accounting for up to 80% of relapsed disease in higher stages.[14] Local recurrence occurs relatively quickly, with up to 90% seen by 5 years posttreatment. Staging and tumor location predict recurrence, with higher-stage disease and lower/posterior vaginal disease more likely to recur. MR imaging can be helpful in distinguishing between posttreatment fibrosis and tumor recurrence, using a combination of high T2 signal to differentiate from T2 hypointense fibrosis and masslike enhancement and diffusion restriction (**Figs. 17–19**).[32,36] Complications including vesicovaginal and rectovaginal fistulae are relatively common and well depicted by MR imaging, particularly on T2-weighted imaging (**Fig. 20**).[14] Other pelvic complications, such as radiation cystitis or proctitis, are also readily demonstrated on MR imaging. PET with fludeoxyglucose (FDG-PET)/CT may serve as a complementary role in both the initial evaluation of vaginal and vulvar

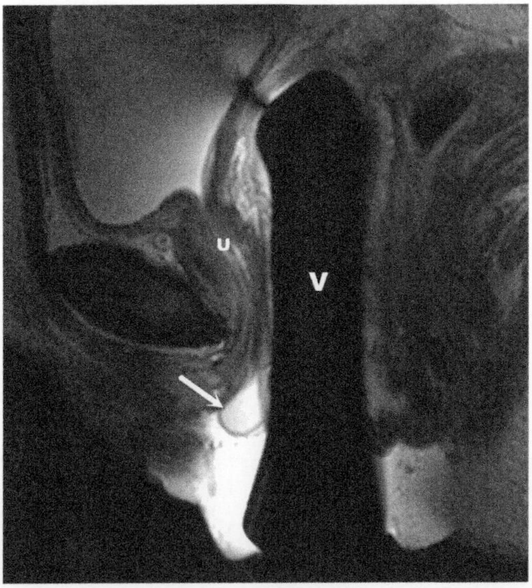

Fig. 31. Skene gland cyst. Sagittal TSE T2-weighted MR image with an endovaginal coil (V) demonstrates a teardrop-shaped cyst (*arrow*) anterior the vagina near the external meatus of the urethra (U).

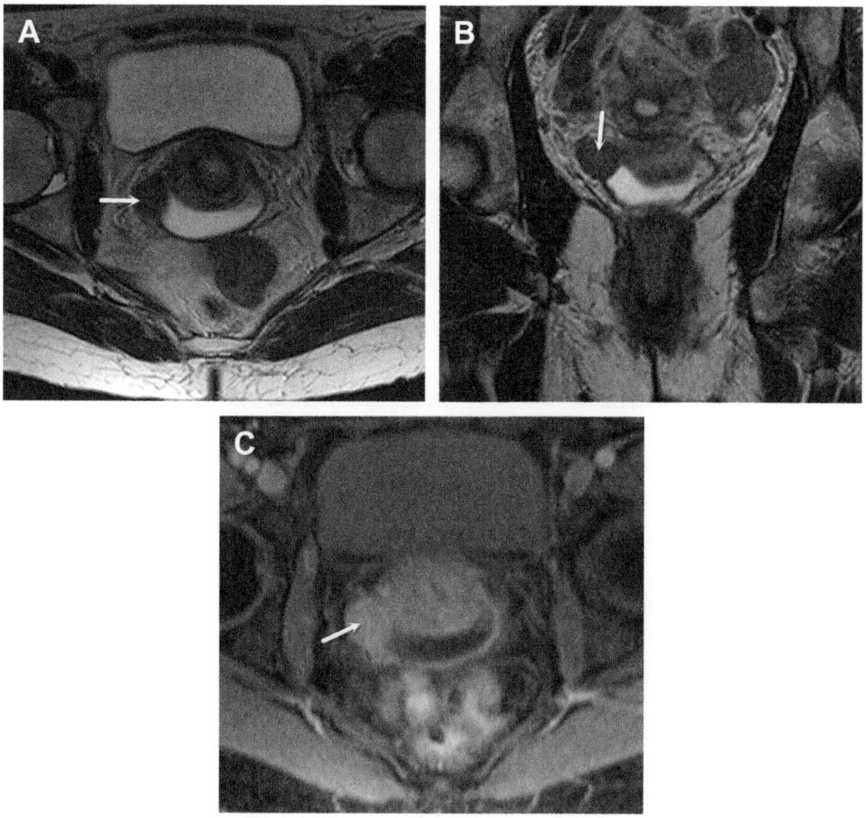

Fig. 32. Vaginal leiomyoma. Axial (*A*) and coronal (*B*) TSE T2-weighted MR image demonstrates a T2 hypointense, rounded, well-defined submucosal mass arising from the right vaginal cuff (*arrows*). Axial T1-weighed FS postcontrast MR image (*C*) demonstrates homogeneous enhancement of the mass (*arrow*). Although the diagnosis can be suggested based on imaging features, tissue sampling is required to establish the diagnosis.

tumors and also in the surveillance on follow-up evaluation for local recurrence and distant metastases. PET/MR imaging offers similar capabilities as PET/CT in detection of gynecologic malignancies but may offer better tumor delineation in staging, particularly identification of parametrial/paravaginal invasion and invasion of adjacent structures.[10,11]

DIFFERENTIAL DIAGNOSIS

Other vulvar disease processes that should be considered when assessing for vulvar malignancy with MR imaging include benign lesions such as lipomas (**Fig. 21**), leiomyomas (**Fig. 22**), Bartholin gland cysts (**Fig. 23**) and abscesses (**Fig. 24**), epidermal inclusion cysts (**Fig. 25**), and hematomas, along with malignant processes such as sarcoma (**Figs. 26** and **27**), lymphoma, melanoma (**Fig. 28**), and Bartholin gland carcinoma (**Fig. 29**).

The differential diagnosis for vaginal masses includes Gardner duct cysts (**Fig. 30**), Skene gland cysts (**Fig. 31**), leiomyomas (**Fig. 32**), hematocolpos (**Fig. 33**), sarcomas (**Fig. 34**), and metastatic disease, particularly from endometrial cancer (**Fig. 35**).

SUMMARY

Vulvar and vaginal cancers are uncommon lesions accounting for fewer than 10% of gynecologic malignancies. Radiologists should be familiar with pelvic imaging anatomy, using an optimal MR protocol, accurately staging the primary tumor and involved lymph nodes using key MR imaging features, and keeping a differential diagnosis for vaginal and vulvar masses in mind to provide maximal value in the care of these patients.

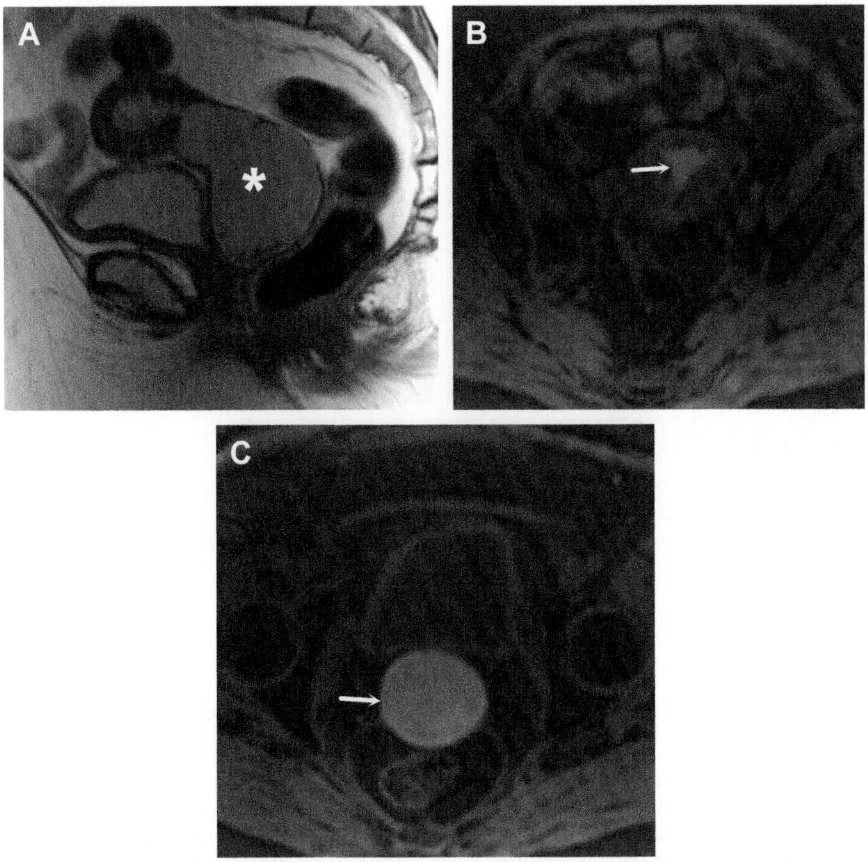

Fig. 33. Hematometrocolpos. Sagittal TSE T2-weighted MR image (*A*) demonstrates marked dilation of the vagina with T2 moderately hyperintense material (*asterisk*). Axial T1-weighted FS MR image demonstrates marked pre-contrast T1 hyperintensity of material (*arrows*) filling the endometrial canal (*B*) and vagina (*C*), indicative of blood products in this patient with hematometrocolpos secondary to vaginal stenosis resulting from radiation therapy for cervical cancer.

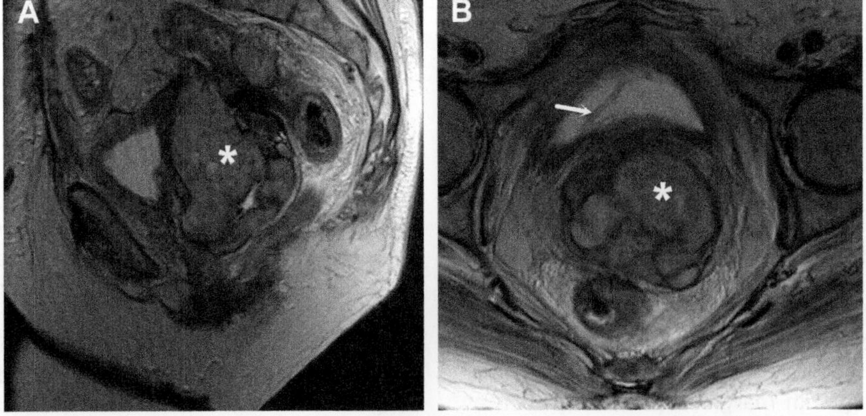

Fig. 34. Vaginal leiomyosarcoma. Sagittal (*A*) and axial (*B*) TSE T2-weighted MR image demonstrates a bulky mass filling the entire vagina (*asterisk*). A right nephroureteral stent is in place (*arrow*).

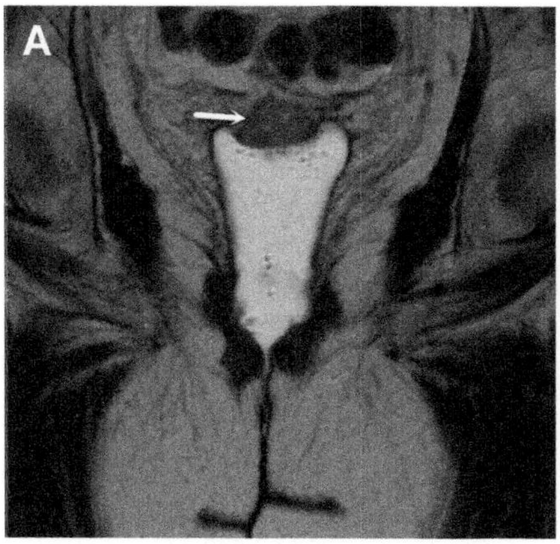

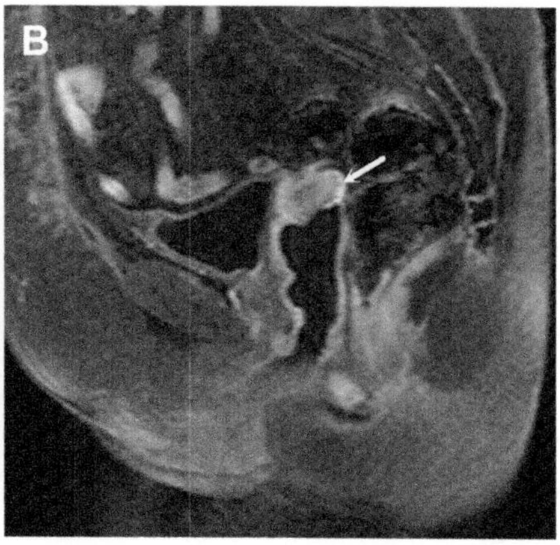

Fig. 35. Recurrent endometrial cancer. Coronal TSE T2-weighted MR image (*A*) demonstrates a vaginal cuff mass (*arrow*) in a patient status post total abdominal hysterectomy for endometrial cancer, consistent with recurrent endometrial carcinoma. Sagittal T1-weighted FS postcontrast MR image (*B*) demonstrates enhancement of the vaginal cuff mass (*arrow*).

REFERENCES

1. Stehman FB, Look KY. Carcinoma of the vulva. Obstet Gynecol 2006;107:719–33.
2. Hiniker SM, Roux A, Murphy JD, et al. Primary squamous cell carcinoma of the vagina: prognostic factors, treatment patterns, and outcomes. Gynecol Oncol 2013;131:380–5.
3. Rajaram S, Maheshwari A, Srivastava A. Staging for vaginal cancer. Best Pract Res Clin Obstet Gynaecol 2015;29:822–32.
4. Siegler E, Segev Y, Mackuli L, et al. Vulvar and vaginal cancer, vulvar intraepithelial neoplasia 3 and vaginal intraepithelial neoplasia 3: experience of a referral institute. Isr Med Assoc J 2016;18:286–9.
5. Viens LJ, Henley SJ, Watson M, et al. Human papillomavirus-associated cancers – United States, 2008-2012. MMWR Morb Mortal Wkly Rep 2016;65:661–6.
6. What are the key statistics about vulvar cancer? Available at: http://www.cancer.org/cancer/vulvarcancer/detailedguide/vulvar-cancer-key-statistics. Accessed September 18, 2016.
7. What are the key statistics about vaginal cancer. Available at: http://www.cancer.org/cancer/vaginalcancer/detailedguide/vaginal-cancer-key-statistics. Accessed September 18, 2016.
8. Zweizig S, Korets S, Cain JM. Key concepts in management of vulvar cancer. Best Pract Res Clin Obstet Gynaecol 2014;28:959–66.
9. Hacker NF, Eifel PJ, van der Velden J. Cancer of the vagina. Int J Gynaecol Obstet 2012;119(Suppl 2):S97–9.
10. Queiroz MA, Kubik-Huch RA, Hauser N, et al. PET/MRI and PET/CT in advanced gynaecological tumours: initial experience and comparison. Eur Radiol 2015;25:2222–30.
11. Bagade S, Fowler KJ, Schwarz JK, et al. PET/MRI evaluation of gynecologic malignancies and prostate cancer. Semin Nucl Med 2015;45:293–303.
12. Ssi-Yan-Kai G, Thubert T, Rivain AL, et al. Female perineal diseases: spectrum of imaging findings. Abdom Imaging 2015;40:2690–709.
13. Lee SI, Oliva E, Hahn PF, et al. Malignant tumors of the female pelvic floor: imaging features that determine therapy. AJR Am J Roentgenol 2011;196:S15–23.
14. Gardner CS, Sunil J, Klopp AH, et al. Primary vaginal cancer: role of MRI in diagnosis, staging and treatment. Br J Radiol 2015;88:20150033.
15. Bipat S, Fransen GA, Spikjerboer AM, et al. Is there a role for magnetic resonance imaging in the evaluation of inguinal lymph node metastases in patients with vulva carcinoma? Gynecol Oncol 2006;103:1001–6.
16. Kim KW, Shinagare AB, Krajewski KM, et al. Update on imaging of vulvar squamous cell carcinoma. Am J Radiol 2013;201:W147–57.
17. Hampl M, Deckers-Figiel S, Hampl JA, et al. New aspects of vulvar cancer: changes in localization and age of onset. Gynecol Oncol 2008;109:340–5.
18. Gadducci A, Tana R, Barsotti C, et al. Clinico-pathological and biological prognostic variables in squamous cell carcinoma of the vulva. Crit Rev Oncol Hematol 2012;83:71–83.
19. Mutch DG. The new FIGO staging system for cancers of the vulva, cervix, endometrium and sarcomas. Gynecol Oncol 2009;115:325–8.
20. Gadducci A, Fabrini MG, Lanfredini N, et al. Sqaumous cell carcinoma of the vagina: natural history, treatment modalities and prognostic factors. Crit Rev Oncol Hematol 2015;93:211–24.
21. Daling JR, Madeleine MM, Schwartz SM. A population-based study of squamous cell vaginal cancer: HPV and cofactors. Gynecol Oncol 2002;84:263–70.

22. Young P, Daniel B, Sommer G, et al. Intravaginal gel for staging of female pelvic cancers—preliminary report of safety, distension, and gel-mucosal contrast during magnetic resonance examination. J Comput Assist Tomogr 2012;35:253–6.
23. Brown MA, Mattrey RF, Stamato S, et al. MRI of the female pelvis using vaginal gel. Am J Radiol 2005; 185:1221–7.
24. Viswanathan C, Kirschner K, Truong M, et al. Multimodality imaging of vulvar cancer: staging, therapeutic response, and complications. Am J Radiol 2013;200:1387–400.
25. Griffin N, Grant LA, Sala E. Magnetic resonance imaging of vaginal and vulval pathology. Eur Radiol 2008;18:1269–80.
26. Wakefield JC, Downey K, Kyriazi S, et al. New MR techniques in gynecologic cancer. Am J Radiol 2013;200:249–60.
27. Lin G, Chen CY, Liu FY, et al. Computed tomography, magnetic resonance imaging and FDG positron emission tomography in the management of vulvar malignancies. Eur Radiol 2015;25:1267–78.
28. NCCN Guidelines Version 1. 2017 vulvar cancer (squamous cell carcinoma). Available at: https://www.nccn.org/professionals/physician_gls/pdf/vulvar.pdf. Accessed October 9, 2016.
29. Bosquet JG, Magrina JF, Gaffey TA, et al. Long-term survival and disease recurrence in patients with primary squamous cell carcinoma of the vulva. Gynecol Oncol 2005;97:828–33.
30. Lee LJ, Jhingran A, Kidd E, et al. American College of Radiology ACR appropriateness criteria: management of vaginal cancer. Oncology 2013;27:1166–73.
31. Kataoka MY, Sala E, Baldwin P, et al. The accuracy of magnetic resonance imaging in staging of vulvar cancer: a retrospective multi-centre study. Gynecol Oncol 2010;117:82–7.
32. Parikh JH, Barton DP, Ind TE, et al. MR imaging features of vaginal malignancies. Radiographics 2008; 28:49–63.
33. Taylor MB, Dugar N, Davidson SE, et al. Magnetic resonance imaging of primary vaginal carcinoma. Clin Radiol 2007;62:549–55.
34. Kinkel K, Ariche M, Tardivon A, et al. Differentiation between recurrent tumor and benign conditions after treatment of gynecologic pelvic carcinoma: value of dynamic contrast-enhanced subtraction MR imaging. Radiology 1997;204:55–63.
35. Hameeduddin A, Sahdev A. Diffusion-weighted imaging and dynamic contrast-enhanced MRI in assessing response and recurrent disease in gynaecological malignancies. Cancer Imaging 2015;15:3.
36. Testa AC, Di Legge A, Virgilio B, et al. Which imaging technique should we use in the follow up of gynaecological cancer? Best Pract Res Clin Obstet Gynaecol 2014;28:769–91.

MR Imaging of Pelvic Emergencies in Women

Ursula S. Knoepp, MD[a,*,1], Michael B. Mazza, MD[a,2], Suzanne T. Chong, MD, MS[a,3], Ashish P. Wasnik, MD[b,4]

KEYWORDS

• Female pelvis • Adnexa • Pelvic emergencies • Pregnancy • Pelvic pain • MR imaging • Appendicitis

KEY POINTS

- Lower abdominal/pelvic pain is one of the commonest presenting complaints for emergency department visits in women of all ages.
- Imaging plays a key role in diagnosis, triage, and management of these patients with appropriate clinical and laboratory correlation.
- Although pelvic sonography remains the imaging modality of choice in initial assessment of these women, MR imaging has proven to be an excellent adjunct modality in evaluation of indeterminate or equivocal sonographic findings, especially in pregnant women.
- Radiologists should be familiar with commonly encountered pelvic emergencies in pregnant and nonpregnant women, including the spectrum of MR imaging features, to make correct and timely diagnoses and facilitate appropriate patient management.

INTRODUCTION

Lower abdominal/pelvic pain is one of the most common presenting symptoms for emergency department (ED) visit among women of all ages.[1,2] These symptoms can be attributed to gynecologic, urologic, gastrointestinal, or other causes. Several of these entities may have nonspecific clinical and laboratory findings, presenting a dilemma for clinical decision making and patient care. Imaging remains an integral component in patient evaluation, directing the diagnosis and management in many cases. Ultrasonography is an established first-line imaging modality in evaluation of female pelvic symptoms in the emergent and nonemergent setting due to its wide accessibility, cost-effectiveness, and lack of ionizing radiation with acceptable sensitivity and specificity in diagnosing most pelvic pathologies.[3] Although computed tomography (CT) is the imaging test of choice for many diseases in the ED, it is rarely the first choice when acute gynecologic pathologies are suspected, due to poor soft tissue contrast of the pelvic reproductive organs and the use of ionizing radiation.[4] Over the past few decades, MRI has emerged as an excellent second-line imaging option in patients with inconclusive sonographic findings and/or contraindication to CT (mostly pregnancy), due to its

Disclosure Statement: The authors have nothing to disclose.

[a] Emergency Radiology Division, Department of Radiology, University of Michigan Health System, Ann Arbor, MI 48105, USA; [b] Abdominal Imaging Division, Department of Radiology, University of Michigan Health System, Ann Arbor, MI 48105, USA
[1] Present address: Taubman Center Floor B1 140 A, 1500 East Medical Center Drive, SPC 5302, Ann Arbor, MI 48109.
[2] Present address: Taubman Center Floor B1 140 B, 1500 East Medical Center Drive, SPC 5302, Ann Arbor, MI 48109.
[3] Present address: Taubman Center Floor B1 141, 1500 East Medical Center Drive, SPC 5302, Ann Arbor, MI 48109.
[4] Present address: 1500 East Medical Center Drive, B1 D502, Ann Arbor, MI 48109.
* Corresponding author. 139 Laurin Drive, Ann Arbor, MI.
E-mail addresses: ursulakn@med.umich.edu; ursulaw10@gmail.com

Magn Reson Imaging Clin N Am 25 (2017) 503–519
http://dx.doi.org/10.1016/j.mric.2017.03.009

lack of ionizing radiation, superior soft tissue resolution, and technological advancements allowing for isotropic, multiplanar imaging.[5–7]

This article presents a comprehensive review of the role of MR imaging in pelvic emergencies in pregnant and nonpregnant patients. Although the major emphasis is on gynecologic pathologies, commonly encountered gastrointestinal pathologies are also presented.

IMAGING PROTOCOLS

Although MR imaging of the pelvis may be performed at 1.0, 1.5, or 3.0 T, 3.0 T is preferred because of superior signal to noise ratio, spatial resolution, and shorter acquisition time afforded by the higher magnetic field strength. A multichannel phased array surface coil is used, which allows for parallel imaging to speed up acquisition time while increasing spatial resolution.[8] An intramuscular injection of glucagon (an antiperistaltic agent) may be administered to suppress bowel motion, improving visualization of the adnexal and peritoneal surfaces. The patient's pregnancy status must be ascertained before administration of gadolinium-based contrast agents, which are contraindicated in pregnancy.[9]

At our institution, we obtain the following sequences on our routine MRI pelvis studies in nonpregnant patients on either a 1.5-T or preferably 3.0-T magnet (depending on magnet availability), summarized in **Tables 1** and **2**. The first sequence is a rapidly acquired, heavily T2-weighted (T2W) sequence (single-shot fast spin echo [SSFSE]) in the coronal plane. The sagittal T2W fast spin echo (FSE) is performed with smaller field of view and higher spatial resolution, and is especially useful for assessing the orientation of the uterus ("uterine lie"), to demonstrate the uterine zonal anatomy, and evaluate anatomic landmarks for subsequent sequences. Based on the uterine lie, short and long axis, T2W images (FSE) are then obtained. T1-weighted (T1W) sequences with in-phase and opposed-phase imaging and with fat suppression are obtained to aid in the detection of lipid-rich lesions and distinguish them from hemorrhagic and/or proteinaceous cysts. Depending on the clinical indication and the patient's pregnancy status, contrast-enhanced images may be acquired after the intravenous administration of gadolinium by using fat-saturated T1W sequence (spoiled gradient recalled echo). **Table 3** summarizes the protocol used in pregnant patients suspected of having acute appendicitis.

PREGNANCY-RELATED EMERGENCIES

Ectopic Pregnancy

Ectopic pregnancy refers to implantation of the fertilized ovum outside the endometrial cavity. It constitutes approximately 2% of total pregnancies and is a leading cause of maternal death in the first trimester of pregnancy.[10,11] Most ectopic pregnancies occur in the ampullary and isthmic portions of the fallopian tube, with other rare sites being interstitial, adnexal, cervical, and ovarian.[12] Risk factors for ectopic pregnancy include prior

Table 1
MR protocol female pelvis (nonpregnant) at 1.5 T or 3.0 T

	Coronal T2	Sagittal T2	Oblique Long Axis T2	Oblique Short-Axis T2	Axial T1 In/ Out-Phase	Axial DWI	Axial T1-FS Pre and Postcontrast
Pulse sequence	SSFSE	FSE	FSE	FSE	SPGR	EPI	SPGR
Repetition time, ms	4000	3000–5000	3000–5000	3000–5000	185	Shortest	Shortest
Echo time, ms	100	90	120	120	2.3/4.6	Shortest	Shortest
Matrix, frequency × phase	256 × 128	512 × 224	512 × 224	512 × 224	256 × 160	128 × 128	320 × 160
Slice thickness, mm	5	5	4	4	5	5	4
Flip angle	90	90	90	90	70	90	7
FOV	40	24–32	20–24 (to fit)	20–24 (to fit)	28–34	40	20–24 (to fit)

Abbreviations: DWI, diffusion-weighted imaging; EPI, echo planar imaging; FOV, field of view; FS, fat saturation; FSE, fast spin echo; SPGR, spoiled gradient recalled echo; SSFSE, single-shot fast spin echo; TSE, turbo spin echo.

Table 2
MR protocol female pelvis at 3.0 T

	Coronal T2	Sagittal T2	Oblique Long Axis T2	Oblique Short-Axis T2	Axial T1 In/Out-phase	Axial DWI	Axial T1-FS Pre and Postcontrast
Pulse sequence	SSFSE	FSE	FSE	FSE	SPGR	EPI	SPGR
Repetition time, ms	4000	3000–5000	3000–5000	3000–5000	185	Shortest	Shortest
Echo time, ms	100	90	120	120	2.3/4.6	Shortest	Shortest
Matrix, frequency × phase	256 × 128	512 × 224	512 × 224	512 × 224	256 × 160	128 × 128	320 × 160
Slice thickness, mm	5	5	4	4	5	5	4
Flip angle	90	90	90	90	70	90	7
FOV	40	24–32	20–24 (to fit)	20–24 (to fit)	28–34	40	20–24 (to fit)

Abbreviations: DWI, diffusion-weighted imaging; EPI, echo planar imaging; FOV, field of view; FS, fat saturation; FSE, fast spin echo; SPGR, spoiled gradient recalled echo; SSFSE, single-shot fast spin echo; TSE, turbo spin echo.

ectopic pregnancy, pelvic inflammatory disease, endometriosis, use of an intrauterine device, congenital uterine anomalies, and prior gynecologic surgery.[10] When a patient with a positive pregnancy test lacks a sonographically apparent intrauterine pregnancy, an ectopic pregnancy should be considered.[13]

The role of MR in ectopic pregnancy is limited when sonographic diagnosis is clear, because clinically stable patients are followed with serial serum human chorionic gonadotropin (βhCG) level and/or ultrasound, and unstable patients with suspected ectopic pregnancy undergo exploratory laparotomy. However, MR imaging is often helpful when the diagnosis or location of ectopic pregnancy is unclear, or to evaluate myometrial thickness in sonographically suspected interstitial pregnancy before intervention.[12,14] Further, ectopic pregnancy on MR imaging may be identified as an incidental finding in evaluation of suspected pelvic/adnexal mass, appendicitis, or bowel pathology in the pregnant patient.

The most specific finding of a tubal ectopic pregnancy is an extrauterine gestational sac in the adnexa, often separate from the ovary, which follows the signal characteristics of a cyst: low internal signal intensity on T1W imaging (T1WI) and high signal intensity on T2W imaging (T2WI), often surrounded by a T2 high signal intensity edematous wall. A hematosalpinx also may be present.[14] Additional and less specific imaging features of tubal ectopic pregnancy on MR imaging include heterogeneous or hemorrhagic extraovarian mass and hemoperitoneum.[15] Tubal ectopic

Table 3
MR protocol pregnant appendicitis 1.5 T

	Coronal T2	Axial T2	Axial T2 FS	Axial T1 In/Out-Phase
Pulse sequence	SSFSE	SSFSE	FSE	SPGR
Repetition time, ms	Min	Min	Min	Min
Echo time, ms	110	80	80	80
Matrix, frequency × phase	256 × 128	256 × 128	256 × 128	256 × 160
Slice thickness, mm	3	3	3	3
FOV, cm	40	36	36	36

Adult contrast dosage (nonpregnant), 0.2 mL/kg body weight gadolinium; method of administration, intravenous power injection @ 2 mL/s.

Abbreviations: FOV, field of view; FS, fat saturation; FSE, fast spin echo; SPGR, spoiled gradient recalled echo; SSFSE, single-shot fast spin echo; TSE, turbo spin echo.

pregnancy must be distinguished from a common and clinically benign diagnosis: corpus luteum cyst. Corpus luteum cysts are intraovarian (intraovarian ectopic pregnancy is extremely rare) and appear as a thick-walled cystic structure that may demonstrate internal hemorrhage, with high T1 and low T2 signal intensity.[13]

Very rarely, ectopic pregnancies may occur within a cesarean delivery scar. Although most can be diagnosed with sonography, in equivocal cases MR imaging may aid in diagnosis. These ectopic pregnancies are surrounded by myometrium and fibrous tissue within the anterior wall of the lower uterine segment. Complications include uterine rupture and hemorrhage; thus, timely diagnosis is crucial[13] (**Fig. 1**). MR imaging also is helpful in evaluation of interstitial ectopic pregnancy. Interstitial pregnancies are located within the interstitial or myometrial segment of the fallopian tube, surrounded by a thin rim of myometrial tissue (less than 5 mm) with potential to rupture with advancing gestational age. Interstitial ectopic pregnancies characteristically present later than tubal ectopic pregnancies, as they slowly grow and distend the portion of the fallopian tube that is surrounded by the muscular myometrium. Therefore, interstitial ectopic may result in significant maternal morbidity and mortality with inaccurate and untimely diagnosis. Although the ultrasound finding of an eccentrically located intrauterine gestation sac near the cornua with surrounding thin myometrium is suggestive of the diagnosis, MR imaging may contribute to diagnosis of equivocal cases by means of multiplanar imaging and high soft tissue resolution. The gestational sac with a yolk sac and/or fetal tissue is identified eccentrically with thin rind of myometrium measuring less than 5 mm (**Fig. 2**).[14] An intact junctional zone on MR imaging separating the gestational sac from the endometrium helps distinguish an interstitial pregnancy from a normally located but eccentric pregnancy.[15]

A potential pitfall to consider is a cornual pregnancy, which is defined as a pregnancy located within one horn of a bicornuate or septate uterus. Cornual pregnancies also are eccentric in location and may demonstrate less than 5 mm of preserved surrounding myometrium. MR imaging helps identify uterine morphology in this case.[10,15]

Subchorionic Hemorrhage and Abruption

Placental abruption is the premature separation of a normally implanted placenta from the uterine wall.[16] Abruption is the leading cause of third trimester vaginal bleeding, affects approximately 1% of pregnancies, and is associated with up to 25% of perinatal deaths.[17,18] MR imaging is superior to ultrasound for the detection of placental abruption because MR imaging has greater accuracy for characterizing intrauterine blood products.[19] The placenta demonstrates homogeneous signal intensity in the early second trimester and gradually becomes heterogeneous with maturation in late pregnancy on MR imaging. The normal thickness of the placenta ranges from 2 to 4 cm.[17] On T2WI, the placenta demonstrates low or isointense signal and is isointense on the T1WI to the surrounding myometrium. The placental-myometrial interface may be visualized as a fine line of low signal on T2WI.[20] Normal placental septae appear as a regular pattern of

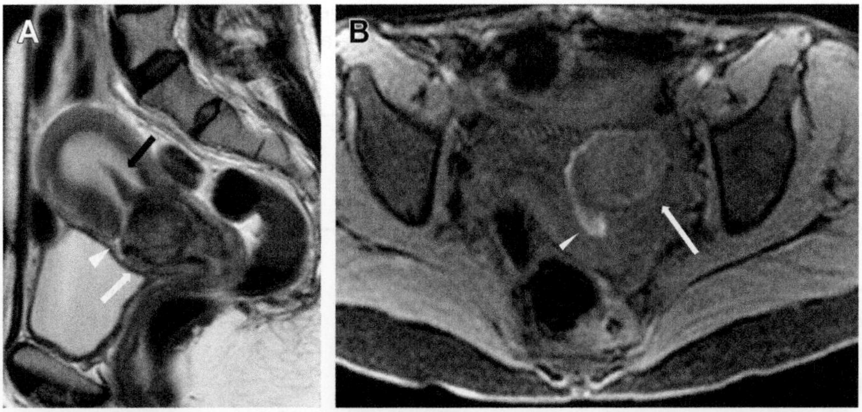

Fig. 1. Cesarean delivery scar in ectopic pregnancy. (*A*) Sagittal T2WI in a patient with positive pregnancy test demonstrates a heterogeneous lesion (*arrow*) associated with the cesarean delivery scar (*arrowhead*) and low-signal blood products in the endometrial canal on T2WI (*black arrow*). (*B*) Axial noncontrast T1WI with fat saturation demonstrates the heterogeneous lesion with internal foci of high signal intensity (*arrow*) and high signal fluid within the canal (*arrowhead*) consistent with blood products.

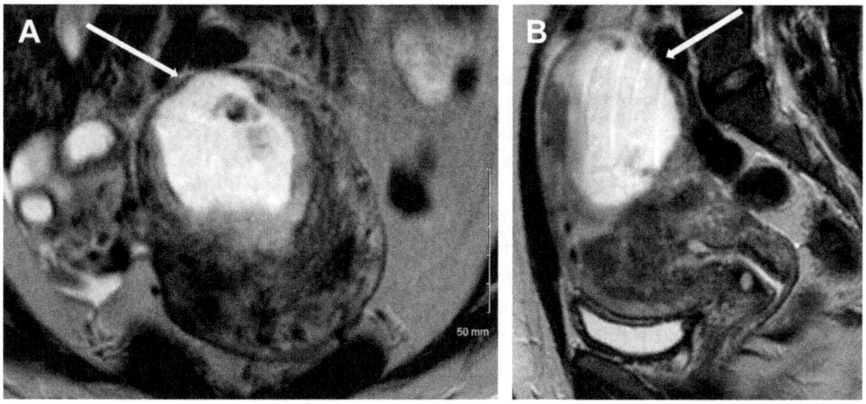

Fig. 2. Interstitial ectopic pregnancy. (*A*) Coronal T2WI demonstrates a heterogeneous predominantly high-signal lesion (*arrow*) located eccentrically to the right within the uterine fundus, with 1 to 2 mm of surrounding myometrium. (*B*) Corresponding sagittal T2WI depicts the abnormally located gestational sac with marked myometrial thinning (*arrow*) consistent with an interstitial ectopic pregnancy.

thin lines that are low signal on T2WI. Normal subplacental vascularity and the umbilical cord insertion site in the placenta appear as flow voids.[17]

T1WI and diffusion-weighted imaging (DWI) have been shown to be more sensitive than sonography in detecting intrauterine hemorrhagic lesions secondary to better soft tissue contrast and wider anatomic coverage.[21] On MR, placental abruption demonstrates signal characteristics related to the age of blood products, with high-signal or low-signal blood products clearly distinguished from the placenta, which is isointense to the surrounding myometrium[19,20,22] (**Fig. 3**). Comparing various MR sequences, Masselli and colleagues[21] found that DWI and T1WI have improved detection of placental abruption (sensitivity of 100%, specificity of 94%, diagnostic accuracy 100% and 97%, respectively) over T2W half Fourier rapid acquisition with relaxation enhancement (RARE) (sensitivity 94%, diagnostic accuracy 87%) and true Fast Imaging with Steady state Precession (FISP) sequences (sensitivity 79%, diagnostic accuracy 90%).

Retained Products of Conception

Histologically, retained products of conception (RPOC) refers to intrauterine tissue composed of trophoblasts and numerous chorionic villi that invade the decidua basalis of the endometrium and persist after delivery or termination of pregnancy.[23] RPOC may be seen in approximately 1% of all term pregnancies, but occurs at a higher frequency after second trimester delivery or termination of pregnancy.[24] Ultrasound findings of thickened endometrium with vascularized soft tissue favor RPOC in the postpartum patient with bleeding. Potential pitfalls and related differential diagnosis may include uterine arteriovenous malformation and gestational trophoblastic disease.[23] Most RPOCs may be diagnosed with sonography.[25] MR imaging is helpful to further evaluate equivocal sonographic findings.[17,23] On MR

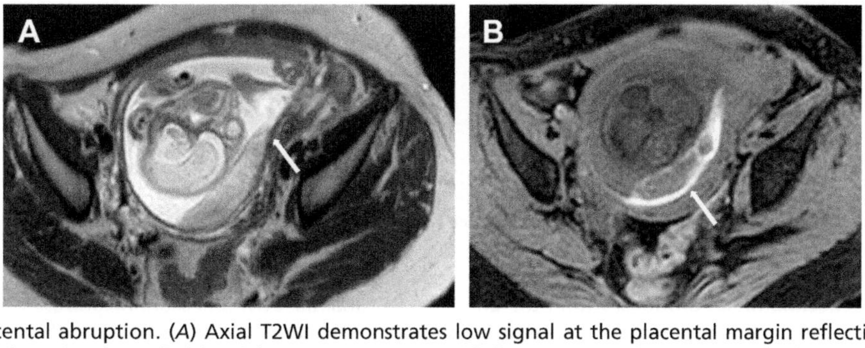

Fig. 3. Placental abruption. (*A*) Axial T2WI demonstrates low signal at the placental margin reflecting hemorrhage and abruption (*arrow*). (*B*) Axial noncontrast T1WI with fat saturation demonstrates high signal in the retroplacental region consistent with hemorrhage and abruption (*arrow*).

imaging, RPOCs are seen as heterogeneous soft tissue within the endometrial cavity, with variable signal intensity and enhancement depending on the degree of necrosis and hemorrhage (**Fig. 4**). In contrast to uterine arteriovenous malformations (UAVMs), which are myometrial based, RPOCs are endometrial/intracavitary in location.[23]

Gestational trophoblastic disease (GTD) may have similar imaging appearance to RPOC. However, laboratory parameters are helpful in differentiating the two, with significantly elevated serum β-hCG levels in GTD versus low β-hCG, or even within normal nonpregnant limits, in RPOC.[26]

Uterine Arteriovenous Malformation

UAVM should be a diagnostic consideration in patients presenting with excessive vaginal bleeding postpartum, or after uterine instrumentation including dilation and curettage.[27] Rarely, the patient may present with high-output cardiac failure secondary to vascular steal phenomenon.[28]

UAVMs are composed of a tangle of different-sized arteries and veins without an intervening capillary network,[29] and can be acquired or congenital, the former being more common. Congenital UAVMs result from abnormal embryologic development of vasculature with multiple abnormal arterial-venous communications including a central nidus; acquired UAVMs have arterial-venous fistulous communications lacking a nidus.[30] Acquired UAVMs have been associated with trauma, infection, cancer, endometriosis, GTD, and fibromas.[31] Pregnancy has been associated in the pathogenesis of acquired arteriovenous malformations (AVMs). Venous sinuses formed after chorionic villi necrosis can scar the myometrium and lead to AVM formation.[30]

Gray-scale sonographic findings are nonspecific and may include heterogeneity of the myometrium, intramural mass, tubular anechoic or hypoechoic channels within the myometrium possibly protruding into the endometrium. Color Doppler is valuable in demonstrating vascular flow within these channels. Doppler spectral evaluation shows characteristic features of high velocity and low resistance flow.[29] MR provides confirmation in cases with non-diagnostic or equivocal sonographic features. AVMs demonstrate serpiginous flow voids which disrupt the junctional zone on T1 and T2-weighted images, and may be associated with prominent parametrial

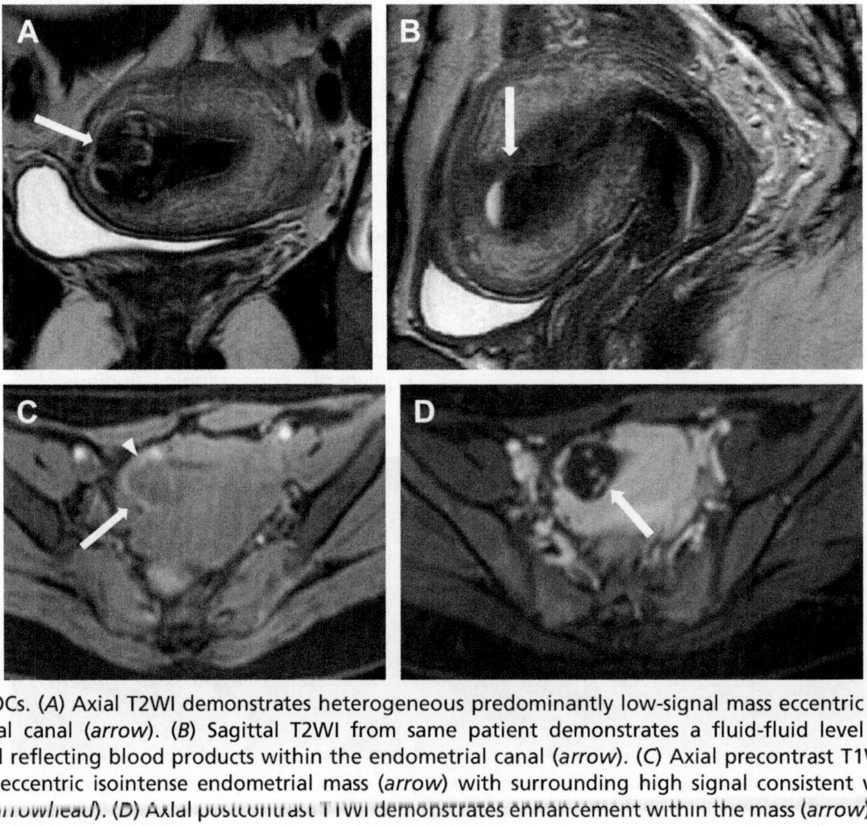

Fig. 4. RPOCs. (*A*) Axial T2WI demonstrates heterogeneous predominantly low-signal mass eccentric within the endometrial canal (*arrow*). (*B*) Sagittal T2WI from same patient demonstrates a fluid-fluid level with low-signal fluid reflecting blood products within the endometrial canal (*arrow*). (*C*) Axial precontrast T1WI demonstrates an eccentric isointense endometrial mass (*arrow*) with surrounding high signal consistent with blood products (*arrowhead*). (*D*) Axial postcontrast T1WI demonstrates enhancement within the mass (*arrow*) consistent with surgically proven RPOC.

flow voids as well. If a myometrial soft tissue mass is present, it demonstrates heterogeneous signal intensity on T1 and T2-weighted images with enhancing vascular channels on post contrast images along with an early draining vein[23,32] (**Fig. 5**).

NONOBSTETRIC GYNECOLOGIC EMERGENCIES

Hemorrhagic Cysts and Endometriomas

Dominant functional follicles are routinely identified on imaging (ultrasound, CT, MRI) as simple fluid-containing cysts measuring up to 3 cm in premenopausal women. At times the functional follicle may continue to enlarge, measuring up to 5 cm, and still is considered benign in premenopausal women.[33] Hemorrhage can occur within these cysts, sometimes manifesting as acute pelvic pain. The pain associated with these cysts is thought to be due to stretching of the ovarian capsule, mass effect, or leakage of fluid or blood from the cyst. Some patients may present to the ED with hypotension and/or syncope if large enough volumes of blood are lost.[34] By contrast, endometriomas are rarely acutely symptomatic.

Sonographically, a simple functional cyst is seen as a well-defined anechoic unilocular lesion with thin imperceptible wall. Those up to 5 cm can be ignored, as these are almost always benign in premenopausal women. Simple cysts measuring more than 7 cm, although often benign, may warrant evaluation with MR to assess internal morphology for any subtle mural nodule or soft tissue component. Hemorrhagic cysts classically demonstrate low-level internal echoes and avascular reticulations (due to fibrin mesh) on ultrasound. When a hemorrhagic cyst measures more than 5 cm, follow-up imaging in 6 to 12 weeks helps differentiate it from a persisting endometrioma.[33] At times, MR may be used to visualize the full extent of large or inaccessible cysts, confirm the diagnosis of endometrioma, and/or look for additional endometriotic implants.[35]

On MR imaging, functional cysts are unilocular with low signal on T1WI, high signal on T2WI, and no internal postcontrast enhancement. Hemorrhagic cysts can demonstrate variable signal depending on age of blood products. Subacute blood (deoxyhemoglobin) demonstrates intermediate signal on T1WI and low signal on T2WI. As

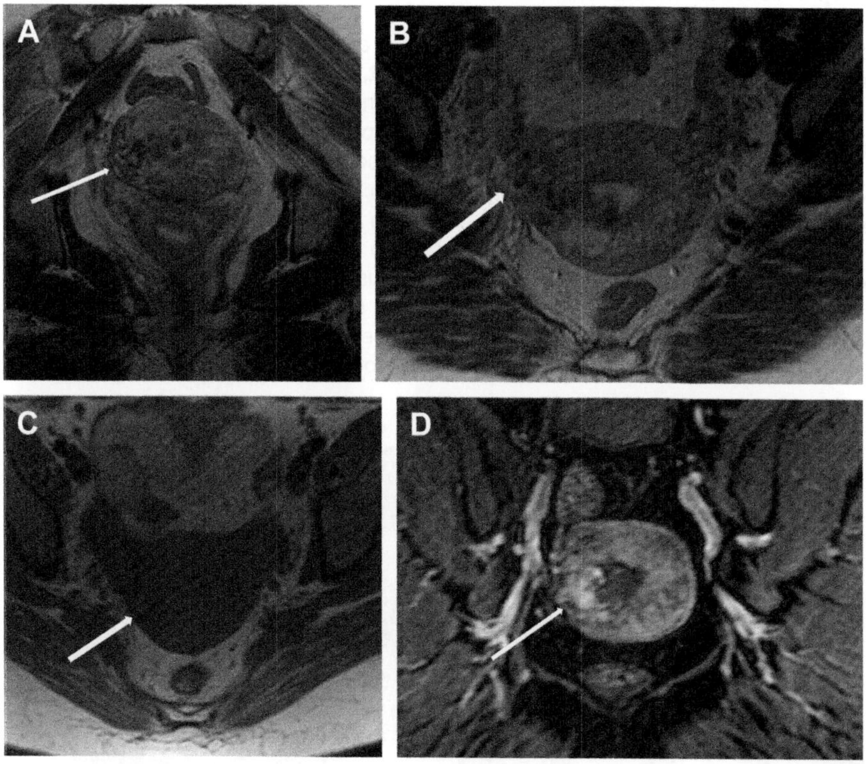

Fig. 5. UAVM. (*A*) Axial oblique T2WI demonstrates intramural flow voids (*arrow*). (*B*) Axial T2WI demonstrates nonspecific parametrial flow voids (*arrow*) associated with myometrial flow voids consistent with UAVM. (*C*) Axial T1WI demonstrates intramural flow void (*arrow*). (*D*) Axial oblique postcontrast T1WI demonstrates enhancement within the intramural flow voids (*arrow*) seen on the precontrast images consistent with UAVM.

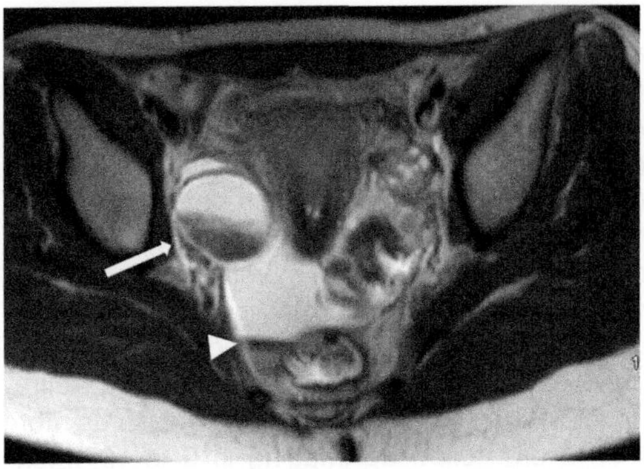

Fig. 6. Ruptured hemorrhagic cyst. Axial T2WI demonstrates a fluid-fluid level within a right adnexal lesion (*arrow*) consistent with hemorrhagic cyst. Low signal reflects layering blood products. There are also layering blood products with the same imaging characteristics layering in the pelvis consistent with a hematocrit level (*arrowhead*) from hemorrhagic cyst rupture.

the blood products age, gradually increasing signal intensity is seen on T1WI due to the presence of intracellular methemoglobin. At times a fluid-blood level or hematocrit level may be seen[36] (**Fig. 6**). In contrast, endometrioma shows high signal on T1WI with intermediate low signal intensity on T2WI ("T2-shading") from varying age of subacute to chronic blood products.[37]

Adnexal Torsion

Adnexal/ovarian torsion occurs due to twisting of an enlarged ovary/adnexa (with or without mass) and fallopian tube along its vascular pedicle, causing vascular compromise leading to ischemia and infarction. It is a surgical emergency accounting for approximately 2% to 3% of all gynecologic emergencies.[38] Accurate and timely diagnosis and intervention is crucial in salvaging the ovary, and imaging remains integral in evaluation of suspected torsion. Although most patients present with acute pelvic or lower quadrant pain, rarely it may be asymptomatic with nonspecific clinical presentation.[37,39] The degree of pain may vary, and pain may be intermittent in the case of torsion-detorsion.[40] Usually adnexal torsion involves the ovary and the fallopian tube and rarely the tube alone. In isolated fallopian tube torsion, the ipsilateral ovary can be normal in size.[41] Torsion also may occur in pregnant patients and should be considered in the differential diagnosis in pregnant women presenting with right lower quadrant pain.[36] Undiagnosed and untreated adnexal torsion can lead to significant morbidity and even mortality, and the longer the delay to diagnosis, the lower the chance of ovarian salvage.[40,42] Imaging plays a critical role in helping to ensure timely diagnosis and treatment to preserve fertility in women of child-bearing age. Sonography is the first-line imaging modality in patients suspected of adnexal torsion and MR imaging is used as a second-line examination.[37,40]

On sonography, the most common finding in torsion is ovarian enlargement, whereas the most specific finding is the "whirlpool" sign, describing the twisted vascular pedicle, although this may not always be depicted.[43] If Doppler flow is absent, a diagnosis of torsion may be made with confidence.[44] However, given dual ovarian blood supply from the ovarian and uterine arteries, the presence of flow does not entirely exclude torsion.[43–45] The MR imaging findings of adnexal torsion most commonly include ovarian enlargement with the early sign of stromal edema depicted as diffuse high signal on T2WI within the ovary.[44,46,47] The stromal edema displaces follicles to the periphery, creating the characteristic appearance of a torsed ovary (**Fig. 7**). The presence of an

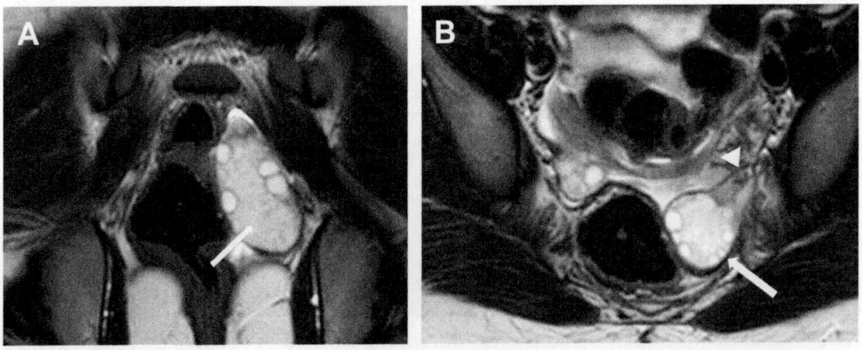

Fig. 7. Ovarian torsion. (*A*) Axial long-axis oblique T2WI demonstrates stromal edema (*arrow*). (*B*) Axial T2WI in the same patient demonstrates peripheral displacement of the follicles due to stromal edema (*arrow*) and beaking of the fallopian tube (*arrowhead*) consistent with surgically proven ovarian torsion.

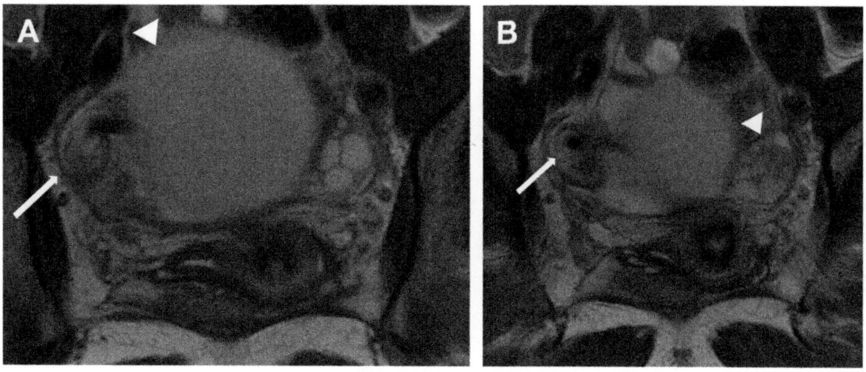

Fig. 8. Whirlpool sign. (*A*) Coronal T2WI demonstrates swirling of the vascular pedicle (*arrow*) of the right ovary (not pictured). Partially visualized right ovarian cystic lesion, which was the cause of torsion (*arrowhead*). (*B*) Swirling of the vascular pedicle (*arrow*) and normal contralateral left ovary (*arrowhead*).

underlying ovarian lesion may obscure the ovary and limit evaluation for stromal edema.[46] High signal on T1WI and T2WI within the ovary indicates hemorrhagic infarction and necrosis and is best appreciated on fat-saturated sequences.[37,44,48] The multiplanar capabilities of MR imaging aid in identifying the twisted vascular pedicle ("Whirlpool sign")[44] (**Fig. 8**). Dynamic postcontrast subtraction imaging should be used to best detect decreased or absent ovarian enhancement.[32] A torsed ovary will demonstrate varying degrees of diminished enhancement, which correlates with the severity of devascularization.[36,46,48] Comparison with the other ovary may be helpful to appreciate enhancement differences.[49] Additional MR imaging findings have been described and include infiltration of the pelvic fat, associated mass, tubal thickening, tubal edema (increased signal on T2WI), and uterine deviation.[46,47,49]

Pelvic Inflammatory Disease

Pelvic inflammatory disease (PID) accounts for approximately a quarter of all ED visits for pelvic pain, and is one of the most common causes of pelvic pain in sexually active women.[4,7] PID is caused by ascending infection, usually polymicrobial, that begins as cervicitis and can progress to endometritis, salpingitis, tubo-ovarian complex, and if untreated to tubo-ovarian abscess (TOA). Patients typically present with fever, lower abdominal pain, vaginal discharge, elevated inflammatory serum markers, leukocytosis, and cervical motion tenderness.[4,32] PID that ascends to the perihepatic region to cause right upper quadrant pain is known as Fitz-Hugh-Curtis syndrome. PID remains a leading cause of infertility, increases the risk of ectopic pregnancy, and may cause chronic pelvic pain.[32,50]

Pelvic sonography can usually identify inflammatory changes within the pelvis, hydro or pyosalpinx, or a fluid collection, but MR imaging may contribute additional information in advanced PID or disease refractory to initial treatment.[50,51] The sensitivity, specificity, and accuracy of MR imaging for PID are 95%, 89%, and 93%, respectively.[52] Pelvic inflammation manifests on fat-suppressed T2WI as an ill-defined area of

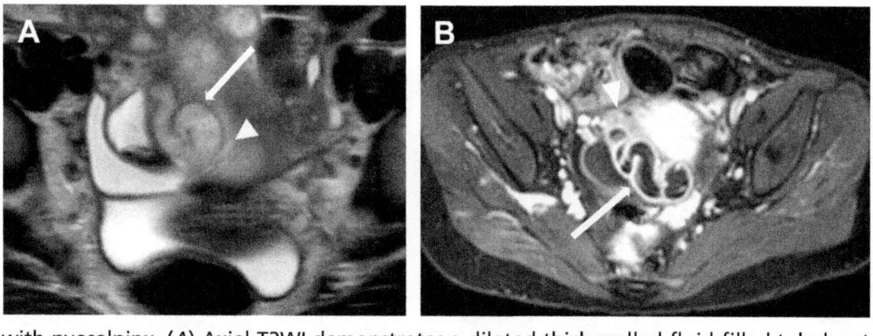

Fig. 9. PID with pyosalpinx. (*A*) Axial T2WI demonstrates a dilated thick-walled fluid-filled tubular structure (*arrow*) with surrounding edema (*arrowhead*). (*B*) Axial postcontrast T1WI demonstrates enhancement of the thick-walled fluid-filled tubular structure (*arrow*) and enhancement of the surrounding tissues (*arrowhead*) consistent with pyosalpinx and surrounding inflammation.

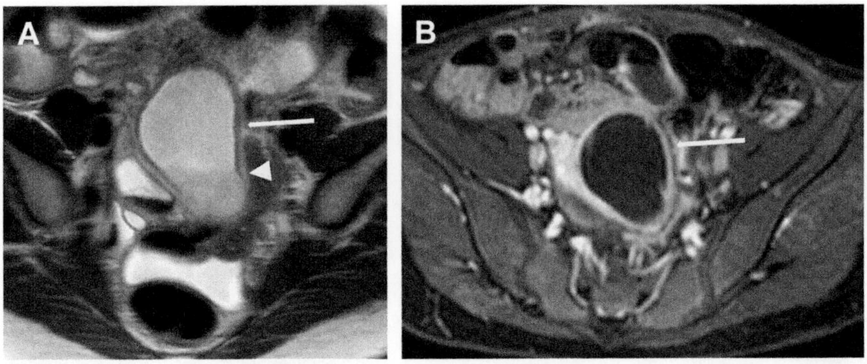

Fig. 10. Pelvic inflammatory disease with TOA. (*A*) Axial T2WI demonstrates a thick-walled high signal intensity lesion (*arrow*) with a fluid-pus level (*arrowhead*). (*B*) Axial postcontrast fat-saturated T1WI demonstrates rim enhancement of the lesion (*arrow*) consistent with TOA.

heterogeneous high signal intensity that can be either localized in the adnexa or can be extensive throughout the pelvis, with corresponding hyperenhancement on postcontrast fat-saturated T1WI.[32,47] Pyosalpinx manifests as a dilated fluid-filled tubular structure with thickened enhancing walls on fat-saturated postcontrast T1WI (**Fig. 9**). The appearance of pyosalpinx on T1WI and T2WI may be heterogeneous depending on the amount of protein and blood mixed with the fluid.[4,52] Multiplanar images can be helpful in distinguishing pyosalpinx from bowel or multilocular cystic adnexal lesion.[52]

Tubo-ovarian complex refers to an inflammatory mass in which the tube and the ovary are still distinguishable structures, whereas the term TOA reflects extensive inflammation with loss of distinction between the tube and ovary. The MR imaging appearance of a TOA is an irregular, multiloculated, fluid-filled structure with thick walls. The contents may be mildly high in signal on T1WI due to high protein content,[7,52] demonstrating marked postcontrast enhancement of the wall and surrounding soft tissue (**Fig. 10**).[7,32]

Degenerating Leiomyomas (Fibroids)

Leiomyomas (fibroids) are benign smooth muscle tumors and the most common gynecologic tumor in reproductive-age women.[51,53] Their growth is hormone dependent; therefore, they can grow during pregnancy and with oral contraceptive use.[47,54] Based on the location, fibroids are classified as intramural (in the myometrium/wall), subserosal (projecting outside the wall), and submucosal (protruding into the endometrial cavity). As fibroids enlarge, they may outgrow their blood supply causing hyaline (cystic), myxoid, or red (hemorrhagic infarct) degeneration.[4,51,54] Conversion to sarcoma has been reported, but is extremely rare.[55] Acute pain may occur secondary to mass effect, hemorrhage, degeneration, torsion of a pedunculated fibroid, or prolapse of a submucosal fibroid.[4,54] Patients with degenerating fibroids may present with fever, leukocytosis, and physical examination findings that overlap or mimic other disease processes, such as such as acute appendicitis, adnexal torsion, and PID. Red degeneration of a fibroid

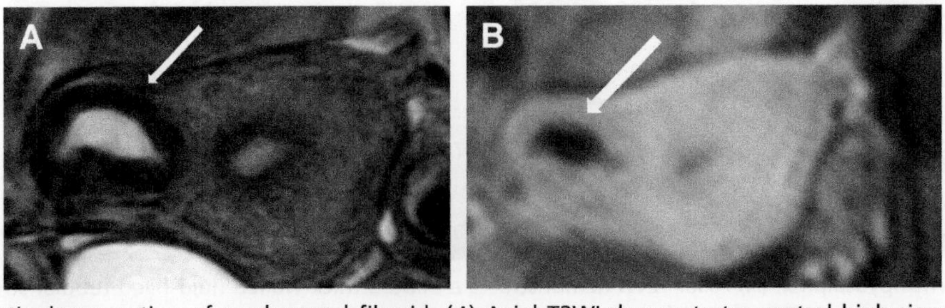

Fig. 11. Cystic degeneration of a subserosal fibroid. (*A*) Axial T2WI demonstrates central high signal with the fibroid (*arrow*). (*B*) Axial postcontrast T1WI demonstrates a lack of enhancement of the central portion of the fibroid (*arrow*), which has undergone cystic degeneration.

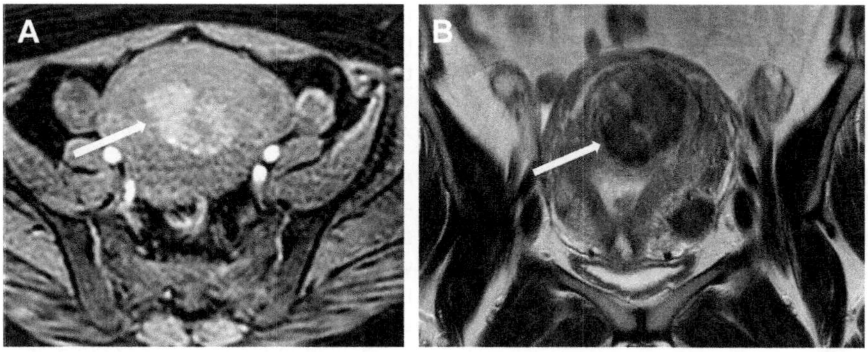

Fig. 12. Hemorrhagic or red degeneration of fibroid. (*A*) Axial fat-saturated T1WI demonstrates high signal within the intramural fibroid (*arrow*). (*B*) Corresponding low signal within the fibroid on coronal T2WI (*arrow*) consistent with hemorrhagic degeneration.

most often occurs in pregnancy and has also been described in association with oral contraceptive use. It is caused by thrombosis and occlusion of the venous outflow, resulting in venous congestion and marked increase in tumor size.[4,54]

Transabdominal and transvaginal sonography can visualize fibroids,[56] but MR imaging is more accurate at depicting the number, location, and internal tissue characteristics of uterine fibroids. It is a useful adjunct examination for indeterminate pelvic masses incidentally seen on CT, or for cases in which sonography is inconclusive.[54] The multiplanar capabilities and superior contrast resolution are helpful for determining whether a pelvic mass is ovarian or uterine in origin; for example, pedunculated fibroids or hose arising from the broad ligament may mimic ovarian masses. Fibroids typically are isointense to muscle on T1WI and homogeneously hypointense on T2WI. Degenerating fibroids are heterogeneous due to cystic or hemorrhagic changes. An early finding of degeneration is heterogeneous hyperintensity on T2WI due to interstitial edema[47,54] (**Fig. 11**). Red degeneration shows diffuse or peripheral increased signal intensity on T1WI with variable signal intensity on T2WI[32,54] (**Fig. 12**). Postcontrast images are helpful in identifying degenerating fibroids as poorly or nonenhancing areas of heterogeneity.[7,47,51,54]

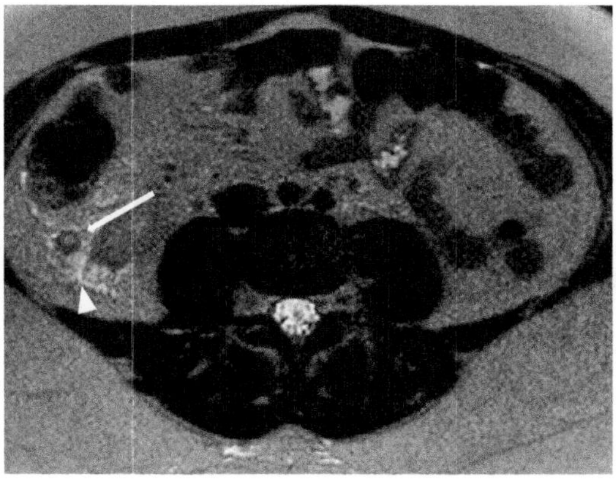

Fig. 13. Acute appendicitis. Axial T2WI demonstrates a dilated, thick-walled, fluid-filled tubular structure (*arrow*) in the right lower quadrant with surrounding fluid (*arrowhead*) consistent with acute appendicitis.

GASTROINTESTINAL EMERGENCIES

Acute Appendicitis

Acute appendicitis is one of the most common surgical emergencies presenting to the ED. The classic presentation is a patient with fever, elevated white blood cells, and periumbilical pain that migrates to the right lower quadrant (McBurney point). The most appropriate initial imaging test for suspected acute appendicitis is patient dependent: graded compression sonography is recommended for pregnant or pediatric patients and CT is recommended for all other patients.[57] The diagnostic performance of MR imaging for uncomplicated and complicated acute appendicitis is similar to CT.[58] However, CT confers ionizing radiation and should be avoided in certain populations. Therefore, if sonographic findings are equivocal and the patient is a child, pregnant, or allergic to iodinated contrast, MR imaging is recommended.[36,47,59,60]

The normal appendix measures up 6 mm in diameter and is low signal on T1WI and T2WI due to intraluminal air.[61] The abnormal appendix is dilated ($\geq$7 mm) and fluid filled with wall thickening measuring greater than 2 mm and surrounding inflammatory fat stranding, best depicted on T2WI[36] (**Fig. 13**). A normal appendix may not always be visualized, but a lack of secondary findings of inflammation makes the diagnosis of

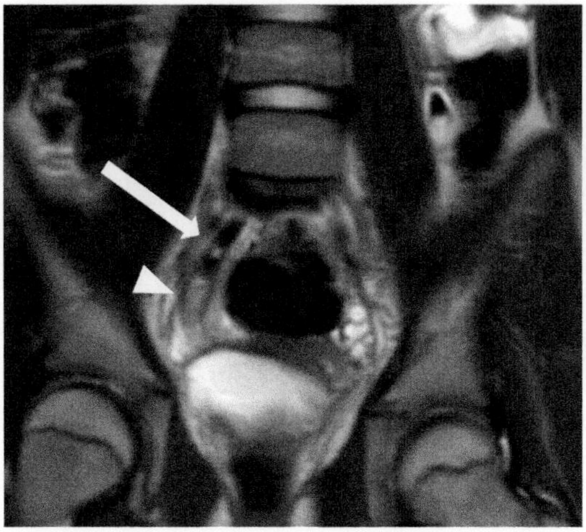

Fig. 14. Acute appendicitis, appendicoliths. Coronal T2WI demonstrates 2 low-signal appendicoliths (*arrow*) within a dilated, fluid-filled appendix (*arrowhead*) consistent with acute appendicitis.

acute appendicitis highly unlikely.[59,60] Short tau inversion recovery (STIR) and other fat-saturated T2WI sequences increase the conspicuity of edema and fluid by suppressing the high signal of fat. Appendicoliths demonstrate low signal intensity on all sequences[36] (**Fig. 14**). If protocols include diffusion-weighted sequences or contrast, the inflamed appendix demonstrates linear restricted diffusion and enhancement within the abnormal wall.[5,47]

Perforated appendicitis is diagnosed if extraluminal air or an abscess is identified. Extraluminal air is low signal intensity on all sequences.[62] An abscess may be suggested without intravenous (IV) contrast if an extraluminal fluid collection is identified, but IV contrast is useful to illustrate the rim enhancement of an abscess and distinguish it from phlegmon.[5] MR imaging is more sensitive for the diagnosis of ruptured appendicitis than ultrasound and CT performed in the setting of negative or inconclusive sonography.[63]

Appendicitis in Pregnancy

Acute appendicitis is the most common cause for emergent surgery in pregnant patients.[64] The symptoms of acute appendicitis in pregnant women are often nonspecific, because the location of the appendix is affected by the growing uterus. By the third trimester, the appendix may be located in the right upper quadrant.[61,65] Laboratory values also may be equivocal because mild leukocytosis is a normal finding in pregnancy.[66]

Sonography is the most appropriate initial imaging modality in the evaluation of a pregnant woman presenting with abdominal pain and concern for acute appendicitis, according to the American College of Radiology Appropriateness Criteria.[57] Sonography, however, is limited by body habitus and gas, and the appendix is often difficult to localize in pregnant women. Over the past 2 decades, many groups have demonstrated the high diagnostic accuracy of MR imaging in pregnant patients suspected of having acute appendicitis. The imaging findings mirror those found in nonpregnant patients: a dilated, thick-walled fluid-filled tubular structure with surrounding inflammatory changes (**Fig. 15**).[36,61,65,67]

We use a focused noncontrast MR protocol for this indication (see **Table 3**). In the emergency setting, Petkovska and colleagues[60] used a rapid noncontrast MR protocol by using mostly SSFSE images in patients suspected of having acute appendicitis showing a sensitivity and specificity of 97.0% and 99.4%, respectively, with a mean total room time of 14 minutes. In 2016, Duke and colleagues[68] performed a meta-analysis of 30 studies

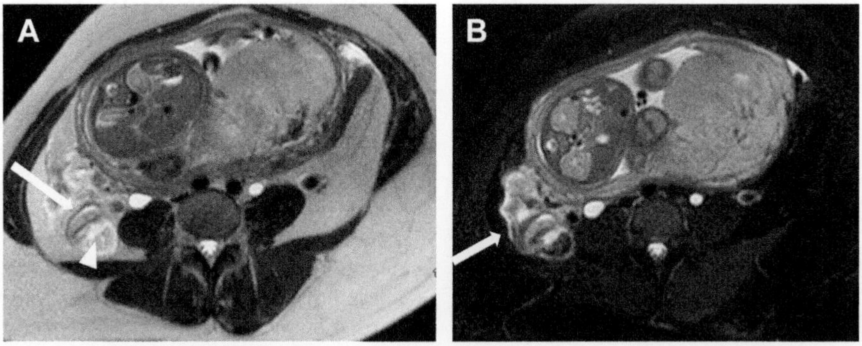

Fig. 15. Acute appendicitis in pregnancy. (*A*) Axial T2WI demonstrates a dilated thick-walled fluid-filled tubular structure in the right lower quadrant (*arrow*) with surrounding edema (*arrowhead*). (*B*) Axial STIR image rendering edema and surrounding inflammatory changes more conspicuous than in (*A*) due to fat saturation (*arrow*).

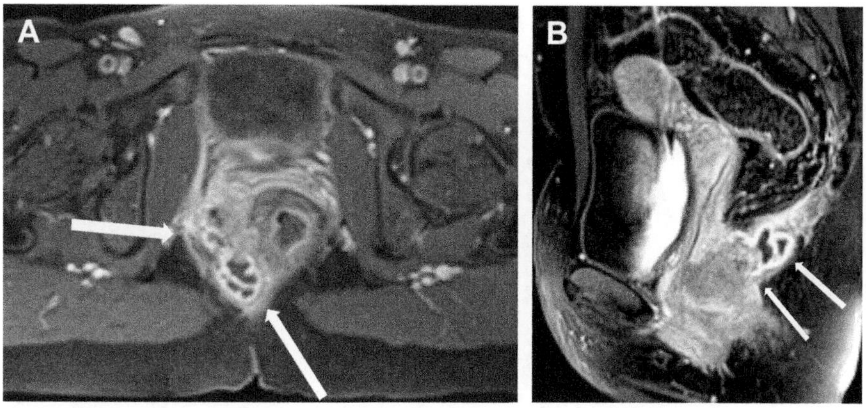

Fig. 16. IBD complications. (*A*) Axial and (*B*) sagittal postcontrast fat-saturated T1WI through pelvis shows a complex perirectal and perianal fistula and abscesses (*arrows*).

on the performance of MR imaging, which demonstrated pooled sensitivity and specificity were both 96% for the diagnosis of acute appendicitis. This analysis also showed that within the subset of pregnant patients, the sensitivity and specificity of MR imaging were 94% and 97%, respectively, whereas in the pediatric subset the sensitivity and specificity were 95% and 96%, respectively.

Inflammatory Bowel Disease

Inflammatory bowel disease (IBD) (Crohn disease and ulcerative colitis) is one of the most common bowel diseases affecting women, and is usually initially diagnosed in adolescence or early adulthood.[69] Due to its propensity to involve the terminal ileum, Crohn disease can present with pelvic or right lower quadrant pain mimicking appendicitis. In a patient with known history of IBD, such symptoms would raise suspicion for an active disease flare. Broadly speaking, ulcerative colitis is a mucosal process that is well evaluated endoscopically, whereas Crohn disease is a transmural process with a higher frequency of complications, including penetrating disease (fistula, abscess) and fibrostenosing disease (causing bowel obstruction), frequently requiring imaging evaluation for complete assessment.[70]

MR imaging is an excellent modality for initial diagnosis or follow-up in patients with known IBD to assess disease activity, severity, and complication, augmented by its lack of ionizing radiation and high soft tissue resolution for better evaluation of pelvic/perianal fistulas.[70] A dedicated MR enterography protocol should be used whenever IBD is suspected, usually including negative oral contrast for distension, IV or intramuscular spasmolytic, multiplanar T2WI, a short

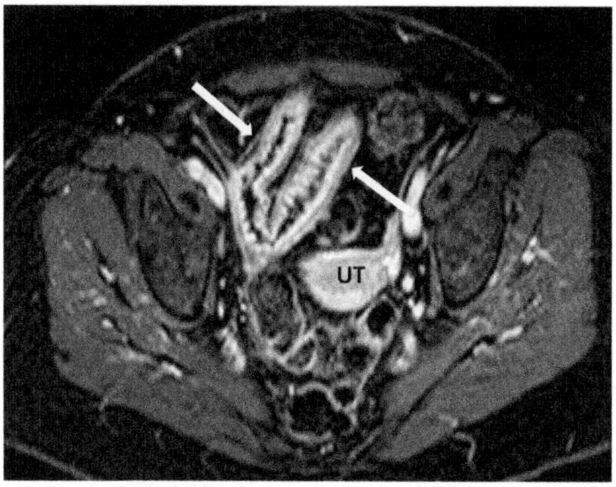

Fig. 17. IBD. Axial fat-saturated postcontrast T1WI through the pelvis in a young woman with history of Crohn disease presenting with acute right lower quadrant pain shows active inflammation in distal ileum (*arrows*). UT, uterus.

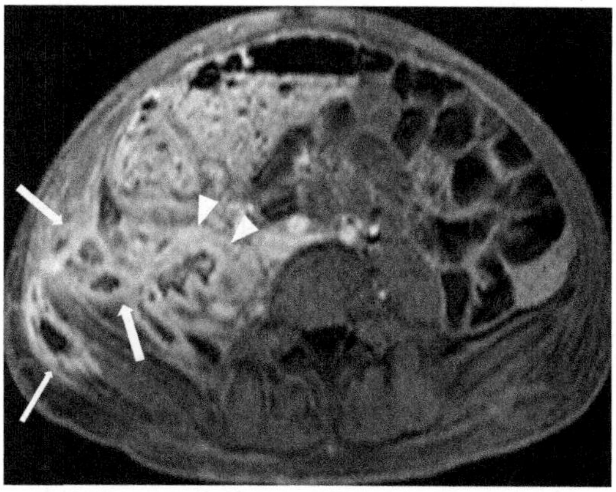

Fig. 18. IBD complications. Axial fat-saturated postcontrast T1WI through the pelvis in a woman with history of Crohn disease shows active inflammation of the bowel (*arrowheads*) with penetrating disease and right abdominal wall abscesses (*arrows*).

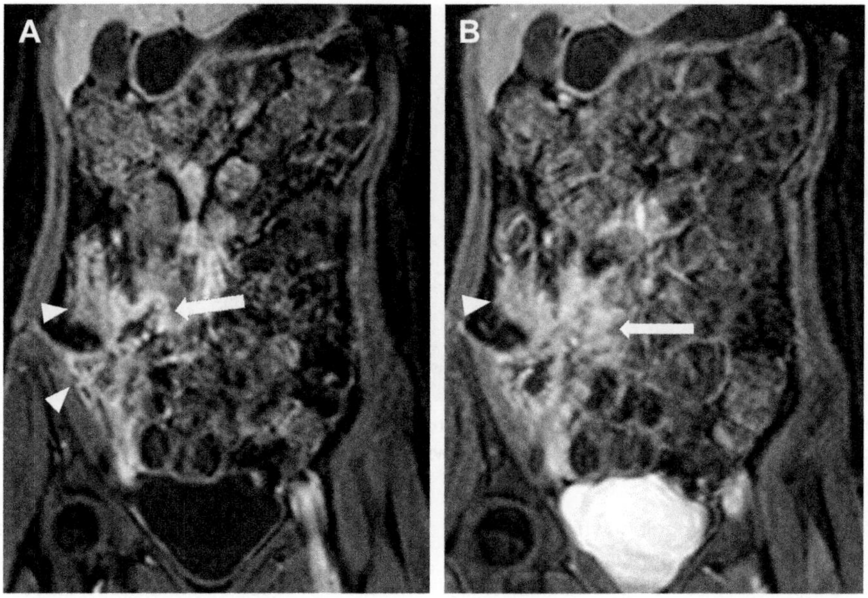

Fig. 19. IBD complications. (*A, B*) Coronal postcontrast fat-saturated T1WI in a patient with known Crohn disease shows active penetrating bowel disease (*arrowheads*) with fistualizing/tethered bowel loops (*arrows*).

repetition time (TR) sequence such as a balanced gradient echo sequence or true FISP, and precontrast and postcontrast fat-saturated T1WI in 1 or more planes.

The sensitivity and specificity of MR imaging for Crohn disease from the jejunum to the anorectal region are 94.5% and 97.0%, respectively.[71] Imaging findings in active IBD include bowel wall thickening and edema, stratified mural hyperenhancement, mesenteric hypervascularity, and lymph node enlargement.[48] Although ulcerative colitis typically shows contiguous involvement of colon starting from the rectum, Crohn disease shows skip segments of active disease with or without associated complication of bowel obstruction from stricture, enteric fistula, or abscess formation. Careful attention to perianal soft tissue and ischiorectal fossae is needed (**Fig. 16**). Short TR sequences "freeze" peristalsis and are helpful in assessing the geography of the segments involved, whereas T2WI has particular utility for fibrostenosing disease, because the thickened bowel wall usually shows intermediate signal intensity in active inflammation and low signal in fibrosis.[36] Dynamic contrast fat-saturated T1WIs are most useful in assessing the disease activity, with active disease showing stratified (or targetoid) mural hyperenhancement due to the contrast between mucosal enhancement and submucosal edema, whereas fibrostenosing disease exhibits less edema and a transmural enhancement pattern[70,71] (**Fig. 17**). A phlegmon without an abscess is seen as an ill-defined inflammatory area adjacent to actively inflamed bowel, with intermediate signal on T1WI and mild increased signal on T2WI. Abscess is diagnosed when a rim-enhancing complex fluid collection is visualized (**Fig. 18**). These are often seen with an associated fistula, which is a rim-enhancing linear fluid-filled track intervening between inflamed bowel loops or between bowel and other structures[36,72] (**Fig. 19**).

SUMMARY

MR imaging is a useful adjunct imaging modality for evaluating women presenting with acute lower abdominal/pelvic pain who have negative or inconclusive sonographic findings. Pregnancy status of the patient does alter the clinical and imaging differential diagnosis and choice of imaging modality. In pregnant women, although obstetric complications, including ectopic gestation, placental abruption, RPOCs, adnexal torsion, and degenerated fibroids are of prime concern, gastrointestinal pathologies, like acute appendicitis or acute flare of IBD, also warrant careful attention, and MR imaging is often useful in refining the diagnosis. In nonpregnant women, gynecologic pathologies, like PID, TOA, ovarian torsion, degenerated fibroids, and gastrointestinal pathologies, are of major concern, and may necessitate evaluation with MR imaging. Knowledge of imaging features in the appropriate clinical setting helps in early and accurate diagnosis, enabling timely management for better clinical outcomes.

REFERENCES

1. Curtis KM, Hillis SD, Kieke BA Jr, et al. Visits to emergency departments for gynecologic disorders in the United States, 1992-1994. Obstet Gynecol 1998; 91(6):1007–12.
2. Fawole A, Awonuga D. Gynaecological emergencies in the tropics: recent advances in management. Ann Ib Postgrad Med 2007;5(1):12–20.
3. Bhosale PR, Javitt MC, Atri M, et al. ACR appropriateness criteria® acute pelvic pain in the reproductive age group. Ultrasound Q 2016;32(2):108–15.
4. Roche O, Chavan N, Aquilina J. Radiological appearances of gynaecological emergencies. Insights Imaging 2012;3:265–75.
5. Heverhagen JT, Klose KJ. MR imaging for acute lower abdominal and pelvic pain. Radiographics 2009;29:1781–96.
6. Patel SJ, Reede DL, Katz DS, et al. Imaging the pregnant patient for nonobstetric conditions: algorithms and radiation dose considerations. Radiographics 2007;27(6):1705–22.
7. El Maati AAA, Ibrahim EAG, Mokhtar FZ. A two stage imaging protocol for evaluating women presenting with acute pelvic pain. Egypt J Radiol Nucl Med 2013;44:923–36.
8. Glockner JF, Hu HH, Stanley DW, et al. Parallel MR imaging: a user's guide. Radiographics 2005;25(5): 1279–97.
9. Kanal E, Barkovich AJ, Bell C, et al. ACR guidance document for safe MR practices: 2007. AJR Am J Roentgenol 2007;188:1447–74.
10. Lin EP, Bhatt S, Dogra VS. Diagnostic clues to ectopic pregnancy. Radiographics 2008;28(6): 1661–71.
11. Lozeau AM, Potter B. Diagnosis and management of ectopic pregnancy. Am Fam Physician 2005;72(9): 1707–14.
12. Chukus A, Tirada N, Restrepo R, et al. Uncommon implantation sites of ectopic pregnancy: thinking beyond the complex adnexal mass. Radiographics 2015;35(3):946–59.
13. Tamai K, Koyama T, Togashi K. MR features of ectopic pregnancy. Eur Radiol 2007;17(12): 3236–46.
14. Parker RA 3rd, Yano M, Tai AW, et al. MR imaging findings of ectopic pregnancy: a pictorial review. RadioGraphics 2012;32(5):1445–60.
15. Kao LY, Scheinfeld MH, Chernyak V, et al. Beyond ultrasound: CT and MRI of ectopic pregnancy. AJR Am J Roentgenol 2014;202(4):904–11.
16. Sinh P, Kuruba N. Ante-partum haemorrhage: an update. J Obstet Gynaecol 2008;28(4):377–81.
17. Masselli G, Gualdi G. MR imaging of the placenta: what a radiologist should know. Abdom Imaging 2013;38(3):573–87.
18. Sakornbut E, Leeman L, Fontaine P. Late pregnancy bleeding. Am Fam Physician 2007;75(8):1199–206.
19. Elsayes KM, Trout AT, Freidken AM, et al. Imaging of the placenta: a multimodality pictorial review. Radiographics 2009;29(5):1371–91.
20. Leyendecker JR, DuBose M, Hosseinzadeh K, et al. MRI of pregnancy-related issues: abnormal placentation. AJR Am J Roentgenol 2012;198(2):311–20.
21. Masselli G, Brunelli R, Di Tola M, et al. MR imaging in the evaluation of placental abruption: correlation with sonographic findings. Radiology 2011;259(1): 222–30.
22. Trop I, Levine D. Hemorrhage during pregnancy: sonography and MR imaging. AJR Am J Roentgenol 2001;176:607–15.
23. Sellmyer MA, Desser TS, Maturen KE, et al. Physiologic, histologic, and imaging features of retained products of conception. Radiographics 2013;33(3):781–96.
24. Wolman I, Altman E, Faith G, et al. Combined clinical and ultrasonographic work-up for the diagnosis of retained products of conception. Fertil Steril 2009; 92(3):1162–4.
25. Matijevic R, Knezevic M, Grgic O, et al. Diagnostic accuracy of sonographic and clinical parameters in the prediction of retained products of conception. J Ultrasound Med 2009;28(3):295–9.
26. Noonan JB, Coakley FV, Qayyum A, et al. MR imaging of retained products of conception. AJR Amer J Roentgenol 2003;181:435–9.
27. Manolitsas T, Hurley V, Gilford E. Uterine arteriovenous malformation–a rare cause of uterine haemorrhage. Aust N Z J Obstet Gynaecol 1994;34(2):197–9.
28. Hickey M, Fraser IS. Clinical implications of disturbances of uterine vascular morphology and function. Baillieres Best Pract Res Clin Obstet Gynaecol 2000;14(6):937–51.
29. Huang MW, Muradali D, Thurston WA, et al. Uterine arteriovenous malformations: gray-scale and Doppler US features with MR imaging correlation. Radiology 1998;206(1):115–23.
30. Hoffman MK, Meilstrup JW, Shackelford DP, et al. Arteriovenous malformations of the uterus: an uncommon cause of vaginal bleeding. Obstet Gynecol Surv 1997;52(12):736–40.
31. Laifer-Narin SL, Kwak E, Kim H, et al. Multimodality imaging of the postpartum or posttermination uterus: evaluation using ultrasound, computed tomography, and magnetic resonance imaging. Curr Probl Diagn Radiol 2014;43(6):374–85.
32. Dohke M, Watanabe Y, Okumura A, et al. Comprehensive MR imaging of acute gynecologic diseases. Radiographics 2000;20(6):1551–66.
33. Levine D, Brown DL, Andreotti RF, et al. Management of asymptomatic ovarian and other adnexal

cysts imaged at US: Society of Radiologists in Ultrasound consensus conference statement. Radiology 2010;256(3):843–54.
34. Lemonick DM. Evaluation of syncope in the emergency department. Am J Clin Med 2010;7:11–9.
35. Chamié LP, Blasbalg R, Pereira RM, et al. Findings of pelvic endometriosis at transvaginal US, MR imaging, and laparoscopy. Radiographics 2011;31: E77–100.
36. Pedrosa I, Zeikus EA, Levine D, et al. MR imaging of acute right lower quadrant pain in pregnant and nonpregnant patients. Radiographics 2007;27(3): 721–43.
37. Chiou SY, Lev-Toaff AS, Masuda E, et al. Adnexal torsion: new clinical and imaging observations by sonography, computed tomography, and magnetic resonance imaging. J Ultrasound Med 2007; 26(10):1289–301.
38. Hibbard LT. Adnexal torsion. Am J Obstet Gynecol 1985;152:456–61.
39. Hourt D, Abbott JT. Ovarian torsion: a fifteen year review. Ann Emerg Med 2001;38(2):156–9.
40. Béranger-Gibert S, Sakly H, Ballester M, et al. Diagnostic value of MR imaging in the diagnosis of adnexal torsion. Radiology 2016;279(2):461–70.
41. Gross M, Blumstein SL, Chow LC. Isolated fallopian tube torsion: a rare twist on a common theme. AJR Am J Roentgenol 2005;185(6):1590–2.
42. Bayer AI, Wiskind AK. Adnexal torsion: can the adnexa be saved? Am J Obstet Gynecol 1994; 171(6):1506–10.
43. Vijayaraghavan SB. Sonographic whirlpool sign in ovarian torsion. J Ultrasound Med 2004;23(12): 1643–9.
44. Duigenan S, Oliva E, Lee SI. Ovarian torsion: diagnostic features on CT and MRI with pathologic correlation. AJR Am J Roentgenol 2012;198(2):W122–31.
45. Peña JE, Ufberg D, Cooney N, et al. Usefulness of Doppler sonography in the diagnosis of ovarian torsion. Fertil Steril 2000;73(5):1047–50.
46. Ghossain MA, Hachem K, Buy JN, et al. Adnexal torsion: magnetic resonance findings in the viable adnexa with emphasis on stromal ovarian appearance. J Magn Reson Imaging 2004;20(3):451–62.
47. Singh AK, Desai H, Novelline RA. Emergency MRI of acute pelvic pain: MR protocol with no oral contrast. Emerg Radiol 2009;16(2):133–41.
48. Ditkofsky NG, Singh A, Avery L, et al. The role of emergency MRI in the setting of acute abdominal pain. Emerg Radiol 2014;21(6):615–24.
49. Kimura I, Togashi K, Kawakami S, et al. Ovarian torsion: CT and MR imaging appearances. Radiology 1994;190(2):337–41.
50. Chen P, Sickler K, Maklad N. Acute obstetric and gynecologic emergencies. Emerg Radiol 1998;5:306.
51. Potter AW, Chandrasekhar CA. US and CT evaluation of acute pelvic pain of gynecologic origin in nonpregnant premenopausal patients. Radiographics 2008;28:1645–59.
52. Tukeva TA, Aronen HJ, Karjalainen PT, et al. MR imaging in pelvic inflammatory disease: comparison with laparoscopy and US. Radiology 1999;210:209–16.
53. Bennett GL, Slywotzky CM, Giovanniello G. Gynecologic causes of acute pelvic pain: spectrum of CT findings. Radiographics 2002;22(4):785–801.
54. Murase E, Siegelman ES, Outwater EK, et al. Uterine leiomyomas: histopathologic features, MR imaging findings, differential diagnosis, and treatment. Radiographics 1999;19(5):1179–97.
55. Di Salvo DN. Sonographic imaging of maternal complications of pregnancy. J Ultrasound Med 2003; 22(1):69–89.
56. Amirbekian S, Hooley RJ. Ultrasound evaluation of pelvic pain. Radiol Clin North Am 2014;52(6): 1215–35.
57. Smith MP, Katz DS, Lalani T, et al. ACR Appropriateness Criteria right lower quadrant pain—suspected appendicitis. Ultrasound Q 2015;31(2):85–91.
58. Zhang H, Liao M, Chen J, et al. Ultrasound, computed tomography or magnetic resonance imaging—which is preferred for acute appendicitis in children? A Meta-analysis. Pediatr Radiol 2017;47(2):186–96.
59. Dillman JR, Gadepalli S, Sroufe NS, et al. Equivocal pediatric appendicitis: unenhanced MR imaging protocol for nonsedated children—a clinical effectiveness study. Radiology 2016;279(1):216–25.
60. Petkovska I, Martin DR, Covington MF, et al. Accuracy of unenhanced MR imaging in the detection of acute appendicitis: single-institution clinical performance review. Radiology 2016;279(2):451–60.
61. Pedrosa I, Levine D, Eyvazzadeh AD, et al. MR imaging evaluation of acute appendicitis in pregnancy. Radiology 2006;238:891–9.
62. Lam M, Singh A, Kaewlai R, et al. Magnetic resonance of acute appendicitis: pearls and pitfalls. Curr Probl Diagn Radiol 2008;37(2):57–66.
63. Leeuwenburgh MM, Wiezer MJ, Wiarda BM, et al. Accuracy of MRI compared with ultrasound imaging and selective use of CT to discriminate simple from perforated appendicitis. Br J Surg 2014;101(1):e147–155.
64. Tamir IL, Bongard FS, Klein SR. Acute appendicitis in the pregnant patient. Am J Surg 1990;160(6):571.
65. Oto A, Ernst RD, Shah R, et al. Right-lower-quadrant pain and suspected appendicitis in pregnant women: evaluation with MR imaging—initial experience. Radiology 2005;234(2):445–51.
66. Gilo NB, Amini D, Landy HJ. Appendicitis and cholecystitis in pregnancy. Clin Obstet Gynecol 2009; 52(4):586–96.
67. Cobben LP, Groot I, Haans L, et al. MRI for clinically suspected appendicitis during pregnancy. AJR Am J Roentgenol 2004;183(3):671–5.
68. Duke E, Kalb B, Arif-Tiwari H, et al. A systematic review and meta-analysis of diagnostic performance

of MRI for evaluation of acute appendicitis. AJR Am J Roentgenol 2016;206(3):508–17.
69. Loftus EV Jr. Clinical epidemiology of inflammatory bowel disease: incidence, prevalence, and environmental influences. Gastroenterology 2004;126(6):1504–17.
70. Tolan DJ, Greenhalgh R, Zealley IA, et al. MR enterographic manifestations of small bowel Crohn disease. Radiographics 2010;30(2):367–84.
71. Maccioni F, Al Ansari N, Mazzamurro F, et al. Detection of Crohn disease lesions of the small and large bowel in pediatric patients: diagnostic value of MR enterography versus reference examinations. AJR Am J Roentgenol 2014;203(5):W533–42.
72. Haggett PJ, Moore NR, Shearman JD, et al. Pelvic and perineal complications of Crohn's disease: assessment using magnetic resonance imaging. Gut 1995;36(3):407–10.

MR Imaging for Incidental Adnexal Mass Characterization

William R. Masch, MD[a,*], Dania Daye, MD, PhD[b],
Susanna I. Lee, MD, PhD[b]

KEYWORDS

• Pelvic MR imaging • Diffusion-weighted imaging • Endometrioma • Borderline tumor
• Ovarian cancer • Adnexal mass

KEY POINTS

- Incidental adnexal masses considered indeterminate for malignancy are commonly seen on computed tomography (CT) scan and ultrasound (US). Most of these prove to be benign.
- Ovarian cancer grows rapidly; thus, adnexal masses that cannot be definitively characterized as benign on imaging are resected to avoid a clinically significant delay in cancer diagnosis.
- Pelvic MR imaging increases the specificity of the imaging evaluation and enables confident diagnosis of many benign lesions.
- Incorporation of MR imaging into imaging evaluation of adnexal masses allows for decreased resection rates of benign lesions and aids in treatment planning for minimally invasive interventions.

INTRODUCTION

Incidentally detected adnexal lesions are common, identified in approximately 4% to 5% of women undergoing computed tomography (CT) scan[1,2] and in 9% to 10% of women undergoing ultrasound (US).[3] Although a source of anxiety for patients, referring clinicians, and radiologists alike, these lesions, or the overwhelming majority, are benign. Nevertheless, concern over incidentally detected adnexal lesions results in high rates of benign oophorectomies. The frequency of malignancy in premenopausal women undergoing surgical resection of an adnexal mass is well below 10%,[4,5] and that for postmenopausal women is less than 15%.[6] In the United States, between 5% and 10% of women will undergo oophorectomy for a benign adnexal lesion.[7] These numbers are not trivial given the associated surgical morbidity and downstream health consequences of early surgical menopause, which include infertility and increased prevalence of coronary artery disease, cardiovascular death, dementia, and Parkinsons disease.[8]

The incidence of ovarian cancer is known to increase with age, and the lifetime risk is approximately 1.3%.[9] Despite this, most adnexal masses identified even in elderly women are benign. One case series examining the postmortem adnexa of women who had died of nongynecologic causes found 15.4% (36/234) had adnexal cysts, only 1 of which was found to be malignant (serous borderline cancer).[10] Rapid growth rate of high-grade ovarian cancers means that the choice to defer definitive diagnosis to follow-up imaging may result in a clinically significant spread of

The authors have nothing to disclose.

[a] Department of Radiology, University of Michigan Health System, UH B2A205G, 1500 East Medical Center Drive, SPC 5030, Ann Arbor, MI 48109, USA; [b] Department of Radiology, Massachusetts General Hospital, Harvard Medical School, 55 Fruit Street, Boston, MA 02114, USA
* Corresponding author.
E-mail address: mascwill@med.umich.edu

Magn Reson Imaging Clin N Am 25 (2017) 521–543
http://dx.doi.org/10.1016/j.mric.2017.03.001
1064-9689/17/

cancer. Screening trials have shown that most ovarian cancers show rapid progression from early-stage sonographically detectable lesion to extraovarian spread with short lag times of weeks to months. In 1 trial, all 10 of the ovarian cancers detected were at stage III or IV, having developed within the 6-month interval between screening examinations.[11] A recent study examining 118 incidentally detected adnexal lesions in 2869 women consecutively screened with CT colonography found that all incidentally detected lesions were benign.[1] Ironically, during the follow-up period, 4 cases of ovarian cancer were diagnosed in the 2751 women not found to have adnexal lesions at screening CT colonography.

The differential diagnosis of adnexal masses is broad (**Box 1**) and includes ovarian and extraovarian abnormalities, which are both benign and malignant.[12] MR imaging has been shown to be the most accurate modality in adnexal mass characterization,[13] and many of the benign adnexal lesions considered indeterminate at CT and US (eg, physiologic cysts, hemorrhagic cysts, cystadenomas, mature cystic teratomas, endometriomas, hydrosalpinges, and paratubal cysts) may be confidently diagnosed as benign with MR imaging. This accuracy is due to superior soft tissue assessment and lesion localization. The diagnostic accuracy of MR imaging versus CT for diagnosis of malignancy after US detection of an indeterminate adnexal mass may be seen in **Table 1**. Confident diagnosis of adnexal lesion as benign at imaging allows for an overall decrease in resection rates for benign abnormality and appropriate triaging of patients to minimally invasive and/or fertility-sparing procedures.[14] Conversely, patients with indeterminate adnexal lesions that remain indeterminate or exhibit malignant features at MR imaging may be rapidly triaged to appropriate surgical management.

ANATOMY

The uterine adnexum (**Fig. 1**) comprises the ovary, the fallopian tube, the broad ligament, the ovarian ligament, the round ligament, and the infundibular pelvic ligament. The ovarian ligament connects the ovaries to the uterine fundus and then continues into the inguinal canal as the round ligament. The infundibular ligament, also referred to as the suspensory ligament of the ovary, is the lateral extension of the broad ligament, which anchors the ovary to the pelvic sidewall. The broad ligament is a 2-layered peritoneal fold that connects the uterus to the pelvic sidewall and the pelvic floor. Its contents include the ovary, the ovarian artery, vein, and lymphatics laterally, the uterine artery, vein, and lymphatics medially, the fallopian tube,

Box 1
Differential diagnosis of incidental adnexal masses

- Ovarian benign *(common)*
  - Epithelial
    - Physiologic cyst
    - Endometrioma
    - Cystadenoma
  - Nonepithelial
    - Mature cystic teratoma (dermoid)
    - Fibroma
- Ovarian borderline and malignant *(rare)*
  - Epithelial
    - Serous carcinoma
    - Mucinous carcinoma
    - Clear cell carcinoma
    - Endometrioid carcinoma
    - Brenner or transitional cell carcinoma
  - Nonepithelial
    - Germ cell, for example, dysgerminoma
    - Sex cord stromal, for example, granulosa cell, Seroli-Leydig cell
    - Metastases: uterine, gastrointestinal, pancreatic, & breast primaries
    - Rare histologies, for example, carcinosarcoma, primitive neuroectodermal tumor
- Extraovarian benign *(common)*
  - Uterus
    - Fibroid
    - Obstructed horn
    - Adenomyoma
  - Broad ligament
    - Fallopian tube: hydrosalpinx, hematosalpinx, pyosalpinx
    - Paratubal (paraovarian) cyst
  - Nongynecologic organs
    - Peritoneal inclusion cyst
    - Bowel: appendiceal mucocele, duplication cyst
    - Lymphatics–lymphocele, lymphangioma
    - Fibromatosis or desmoid tumor
    - Nerve sheath tumor, for example, schwannoma
- Extraovarian malignant *(very rare)*
  - Colorectal carcinoma
  - Primary peritoneal carcinoma
  - Gastrointestinal stromal tumor
  - Malignant transformation of endometriosis
  - Lymphoma
  - Mesothelioma

Note: List ordered from higher to lower incidence within each subgroup.

Table 1
Diagnostic performance for cancer detection after indeterminate ultrasound

Modality	Sensitivity %	Specificity %
CT with contrast	81 (73, 86)	87 (81–94)
MR without contrast	76 (70, 82)	97 (95, 98)
MR with contrast	81 (77, 84)	98 (97, 99)

Note: 95% CI in parentheses.

Data from Kinkel K, Lu Y, Mehdizade A, et al. Indeterminate ovarian mass at US: incremental value of second imaging test for characterization–meta-analysis and Bayesian analysis. Radiology 2005;236(1):85–94.

and the ovarian and round ligaments. Ovarian arteries originate from the abdominal aorta below the renal artery origins. The right ovarian vein generally drains into the inferior vena cava, whereas the left ovarian vein drains into the left renal vein.

The normal ovaries as well as the broad and round ligaments are typically well seen at pelvic MR imaging. Identifying these structures is a crucial component to accurate pelvic MR imaging interpretation because the identification of normal ovaries on imaging substantially informs the differential diagnosis of an adnexal mass. The ovaries are located at the junction of the broad and round ligaments, and these structures may be used as landmarks for ovarian identification. Normal ovaries in a premenopausal woman (**Fig. 2**) will have multiple nonenhancing cysts (follicles) containing homogeneously hyperintense fluid within a stroma that is intermediate in signal on T2-weighted imaging. In a postmenopausal woman, follicles may be less apparent or absent. On postcontrast T1-weighted imaging, the follicular fluid is nonenhancing, and the normal ovarian stroma is relatively hypoenhancing with respect to the myometrium. Using the ligaments as anatomic landmarks is particularly important when identifying postmenopausal ovaries that are small (usually <2 cm), lack follicles (**Fig. 3**), and can sometimes be mistaken for lymph nodes. The broad ligament may be traced laterally from the uterus, and the round ligament may be traced medially from the inguinal canal. Alternatively, on the postcontrast T1-weighted sequences, the gonadal veins may be traced inferiorly, the left from the left renal vein and the right from the inferior vena cava, to the points where they drain the ovary.

IMAGING PROTOCOL

MR imaging of the female pelvis for characterization of adnexal masses is best performed with a small field of view and a phased-array surface coil to maximize soft tissue contrast and signal-to-noise.[15] Multiplanar fast spin-echo T2 (FSE T2)-weighted imaging in sagittal, axial, and coronal planes comprises the backbone of pelvic imaging. The high soft tissue contrast afforded by these sequences allows for both anatomic localization and tissue characterization (see **Fig. 2**A, B). These sequences are typically the most helpful for localization of adnexal lesions as either ovarian or extraovarian. FSE T2-weighted imaging is also helpful in determining whether the lesion is a unilocular cyst, mixed solid and cystic, or homogeneously solid. T1-weighted imaging without and with fat saturation allows for detection of adnexal lesions containing macroscopic fat. The fat-saturated T1-weighted imaging is used to identify ovarian endometriomas, extraovarian endometriosis, and other lesions with blood degradation products, such as hemorrhagic cysts.[16]

Contrast-enhanced T1-weighted MR imaging with fat saturation is necessary to obtain optimum

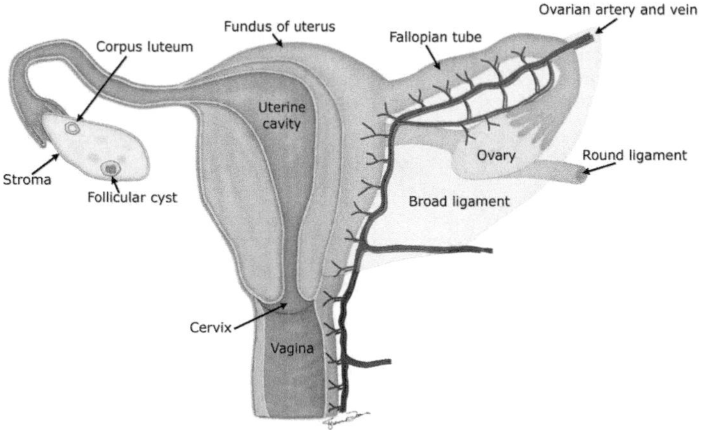

Fig. 1. Uterine adnexa containing the ovaries and fallopian tubes. Posterior view of the female ligaments and viscera shows the broad ligament draping over the uterus and extending laterally to the pelvic sidewall. The round ligament is a continuation of the ovarian ligament and courses laterally from the broad ligament to enter the internal inguinal ring before terminating in the labia majora. (*Courtesy of* Susanne Loomis, MS, FBCA, REMS Media Services, Mass General Imaging, Boston, MA.)

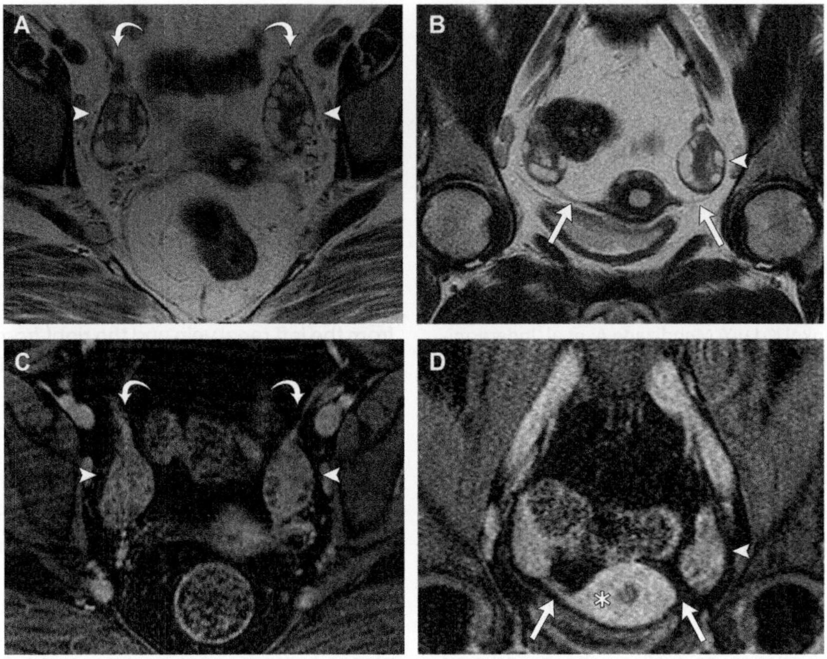

Fig. 2. Normal ovaries. T2-weighted (*A, B*) and postgadolinium fat-saturated T1-weighted (*C, D*) axial (*A, C*) and coronal (*B, D*) images of a 22-year-old woman show ovaries (*arrowheads*) with multiple cysts containing T2-weighted hyperintense nonenhancing fluid and solid stroma that is of intermediate T2-weighted signal and enhances less avidly than the uterine myometrium (*asterisk*). The ovaries are located at the intersection of the broad ligaments (*straight arrows*) originating from the uterus and the round ligaments (*curved arrows*) that extend into the inguinal canal.

sensitivity and specificity in adnexal mass characterization.[13] The authors obtain dynamic (multiphasic) postcontrast imaging in the sagittal plane, primarily for assessment of the lesion relative to the uterine myometrium versus endometrium. Subtraction imaging is helpful in confirming the presence or absence of soft tissue enhancement, particularly when assessing tissue that contains natively high T1-weighted signal such as an endometrioma.[17] Solid enhancing tissue within an ovarian lesion raises suspicion for malignancy; however, soft tissue enhancement is not pathognomonic for malignancy because benign neoplasms may have enhancing soft tissue as well.[14,18] Although some institutions obtain high-temporal-resolution true dynamic contrast-enhanced images with washin and washout curves, the benefit of this has not yet been shown. Recent studies comparing the kinetics of contrast enhancement between benign and malignant lesions have suggested that lesions exhibiting rapid, robust enhancement with washout have a higher likelihood of malignancy.[19–22]

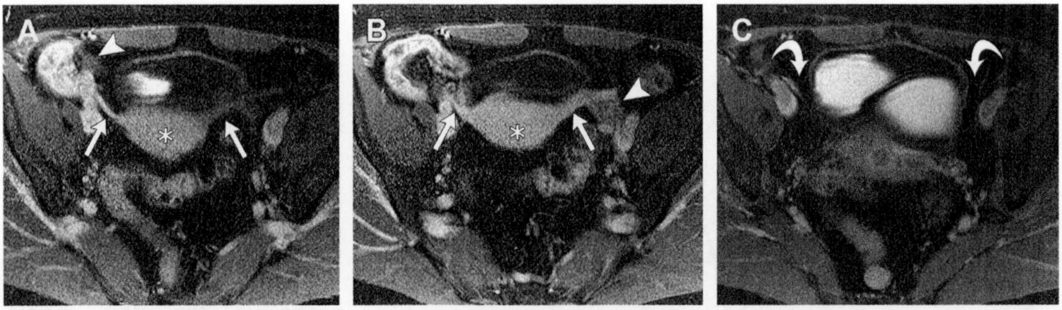

Fig. 3. Ovarian localization using anatomic landmarks. Axial postgadolinium T1-weighted images from most craniad to most caudad (*A–C*) views in a 56-year-old woman show the ovaries (*arrowheads*) at the intersections of the broad ligaments (*straight arrows*) and the round ligaments (*curved arrows*). The broad ligaments are seen extending laterally from the uterus (*asterisk*), and the round ligaments are seen extending into the inguinal canal.

Diffusion-weighted imaging (DWI) has traditionally been used for lesion detection in body imaging.[23] However, there is increasing evidence supporting its use in lesion characterization,[24–26] with qualitative assessment affording more accuracy than isolated measurement of apparent diffusion coefficient (ADC) value.[27] When evaluating an ovarian lesion for restricted diffusion, internal reference may be made to the myometrium and/or small bowel wall. Assessment for restricted diffusion requires concurrent evaluation of both DWI and ADC maps. A lesion is considered to demonstrate restricted diffusion if it is hyperintense on DWI and hypointense or isointense on the ADC map. As both benign and malignant ovarian lesions may exhibit restricted diffusion, the presence of restricted diffusion in and of itself does not definitively characterize a lesion as malignant. For instance, both mature cystic teratomas and high-grade serous carcinomas (**Fig. 4**A–D) typically show regions of diffusion restriction.[28] However, it is very rare for a malignant ovarian lesion not to exhibit restricted diffusion; therefore, lack of diffusion restriction in the solid components of an ovarian lesion may be used as a reliable marker of benignity (see **Fig. 4**E–H).[25–27] The important MR pulse sequences for adnexal mass characterization are summarized in **Table 2**.

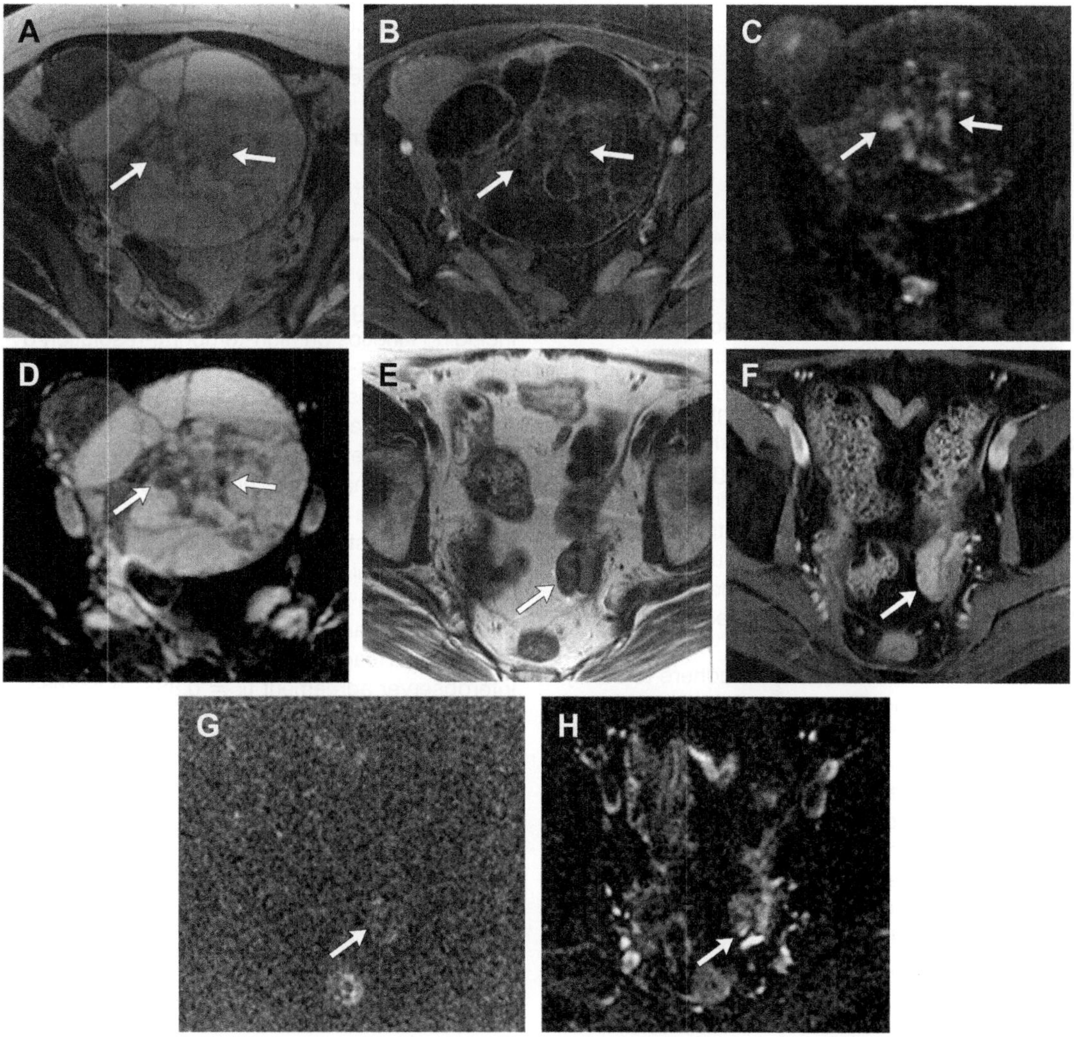

Fig. 4. DWI of ovarian masses. Axial T2-weighted images (*A, E*), postgadolinium T1-weighted images (*B, F*), DWIs (*C, G*), and ADC maps (*D, H*) of a 48- year-old woman with malignant cystadenocarcinoma (*A, D*) (*arrows*) and of a 52-year-old woman with benign fibroma (*E–H*) (*arrows*). The solid portions of the cystadenocarcinoma (*arrows, A–D*) are hyperintense on DWI and hypointense on ADC, indicating restricted diffusion. The fibroma (*arrows, E–H*) is hypointense on DWI and isointense on ADC, indicating lack of restricted diffusion. Signal intensity is internally compared with the uterine myometrium or small bowel wall. Diagnoses were confirmed on pathology.

Table 2
Key MR pulse sequences for adnexal mass characterization

MR Pulse Sequence	Relevant Diagnostic Features
Multiplanar FSE T2-weighted imaging (sagittal, axial, coronal)	• Identification of normal ovaries (if present) • Lesion localization (ie, ovarian versus extraovarian) • Lesion characterization (wide range of soft tissue contrast)
T1-weighted imaging without and with fat saturation	• Macroscopic fat of dermoid cyst • Endometrioma and endometriosis (homogeneously high signal on the fat-saturation T1-weighted sequence)
Precontrast- and dynamic contrast-enhanced (eg, 20 s, 60 s, and 3 min after bolus) T1-weighted imaging	• Soft tissue enhancement (fluid, debris, and calcifications will not enhance) • Kinetics of contrast enhancement (rapid early enhancement with washout suggests malignancy; slow continuous increase in enhancement suggests benignity; internal comparison may be made to the myometrium)
Subtraction imaging	• Enhancing tissue within structures that have natively high signal on fat-saturated T1-weighted imaging (eg, presence or absence of soft tissue enhancement in an endometrioma)
Diffusion-weighted imaging	• Presence of diffusion restriction is sensitive but not specific for malignancy • Absence of diffusion restriction is specific but not sensitive for benignity

Imaging in Pregnancy

In the setting of pregnancy, pelvic MR imaging, with its high soft tissue contrast, wide field of view, and lack of ionizing radiation, is recommended to characterize an incidentally detected adnexal mass. MR imaging has the capacity to noninvasively and accurately diagnose a lesion as benign, obviating longitudinal imaging follow-up or intervention. Although hypothetical risks of heat deposition and acoustic injury have been raised at high field strengths, no adverse fetal effects of MR have been documented in the past 3 decades of imaging in pregnancy.[29] Nevertheless, examination performance should adhere to safety guidelines published by imaging societies.[30] Some institutions prefer to limit scanning of pregnant patients to 1.5 T because experience with 3-T scanning to date is limited. Because no fetal harm has been documented, scanning can be performed any time during pregnancy as clinically indicated. However, contrast administration should be avoided because gadolinium-based contrast agents readily pass through the placental barrier into the fetal circulation.[30]

STANDARDIZED REPORTING SYSTEM: ADNEX MR

In 2013, the ADNEX MR SCORING system was created in an effort to standardize radiologists' reporting of adnexal lesions.[31] Lesions are assigned a score from 1 to 5 based on MR imaging features, which include morphologic appearance, T1 and T2 signal, and enhancement features, including kinetics on high-temporal-resolution dynamic contrast-enhanced sequences, and diffusion characteristics. An ADNEX MR score of 1 denotes no mass present; 2 denotes a benign mass; 3 denotes a probably benign mass; 4 denotes a mass that is indeterminate for malignancy; and 5 denotes a mass that is probably malignant. In the validation study, lesions assigned an ADNEX score of 4 or higher were associated with malignancy with 93.5% sensitivity and 96.6% specificity, and no malignant masses were assigned a score of 1 or 2. Readers in the study exhibited high interobserver agreement ($\kappa = 0.888$) in scoring.[31] Aside from standardizing the reporting of adnexal masses, the scoring system also provides a framework for providing recommendations to guide clinical care. Patients assigned an ADNEX MR score of 4 or 5 should be referred for oncologic evaluation, whereas patients assigned ADNEX MR scores of 1 or 2 need no further management or follow-up for their ovarian finding. Patients assigned an ADNEX MR score of 3 may be followed at the discretion of the radiologist and referring clinician.

DIAGNOSTIC CRITERIA: BENIGN OVARIAN LESIONS

Simple ovarian cysts are common in women of all ages and occur in approximately 20% of postmenopausal women.[32] The underlying histopathology of a simple ovarian cyst cannot be determined by its imaging features. In premenopausal women, most simple cysts are follicles or follicular cysts, both of which reflect normal ovarian function.[33] In premenopausal and postmenopausal women, simple cysts can also represent benign cystadenomas (**Fig. 5**).[34] Regardless of the underlying histopathology, ovarian lesions meeting all of the MR criteria for a simple cyst should be considered benign and do not require follow-up. Most cysts will spontaneously resolve, and available data from follow-up of simple cysts indicate that the risk of progression to cancer approaches zero.[32,34–36] For an ovarian cyst to be considered simple by MR imaging criteria, it must be unilocular and smooth walled, lack internal enhancement, have uniformly T1-weighted hypointense and T2-weighted hyperintense signal, and exhibit no diffusion restriction. Notably, simple cysts do not contain solid mural nodules, septations, intrinsic T1-weighted hyperintense signal indicating blood or fat, or any internal nonmural enhancement.

Endometriosis is defined as ectopic endometrial glandular tissue located outside of the uterus. It is estimated that up to 10% of premenopausal women are affected by endometriosis.[37]

There are 3 types of endometriosis with surface implants along the pelvic peritoneum and ovaries; ovarian cysts, endometriomas, comprising endometrial tissue (**Fig. 6**); and deep pelvic endometriosis where implants invade the subperitoneal tissues to involve the fibromuscular pelvic structures and organs.[38] The latter 2 forms may be detected as an indeterminate adnexal mass at CT or US. The most important MR sequence for diagnosis of endometriosis is the fat-suppressed T1-weighted sequence; lesions with marked hyperintensity on this sequence may be diagnosed as endometriosis with a high degree of specificity.[39] Hemorrhagic cysts (**Fig. 7**) can also demonstrate T1-weighted hyperintensity and are the primary differential consideration in the diagnosis of endometriomas. However, when compared with endometriomas (see **Fig. 7**A, B), hemorrhagic cysts (see **Fig. 7**C, D) tend to be inhomogeneous in internal signal and their T1-weighted hyperintense and T2-weighted hypointense signal are clearly less marked.[40] High concentrations of extracellular methemoglobin in endometriomas from repeated cycles of hemorrhage produce the pronounced T2-weighted hypointensity, known as "shading," that is not seen in hemorrhagic cysts.[41] The presence of a hematosalpinx is near-diagnostic of endometriosis and can further increase specificity.[42] Nonenhancing fluid portions of endometriomas can frequently demonstrate diffusion restriction, and this feature should not raise concern for malignancy in the absence of enhancing soft tissue components.[43]

Mature cystic teratomas of the ovary, or dermoid cysts (**Fig. 8**), are benign neoplasms comprising well-differentiated cells from at least 2 of the 3 germ cell layers.[44] They are the most common ovarian neoplasm in premenopausal patients,[5] and their incidence peaks near age 30.[45] Definitive diagnosis of mature cystic teratoma on MR is made according to specific and reproducible criteria at the molecular level by identifying the presence of macroscopic fat within the mass. Fat demonstrates high signal on T1-weighted imaging; this signal is lost when fat-suppression pulse sequences are applied. Most mature teratomas of the ovary exhibit restricted diffusion within the sebaceous fluid of the cyst component.[28] Contrast enhancement in benign mature teratomas is often seen. Malignant transformations of mature teratomas have been

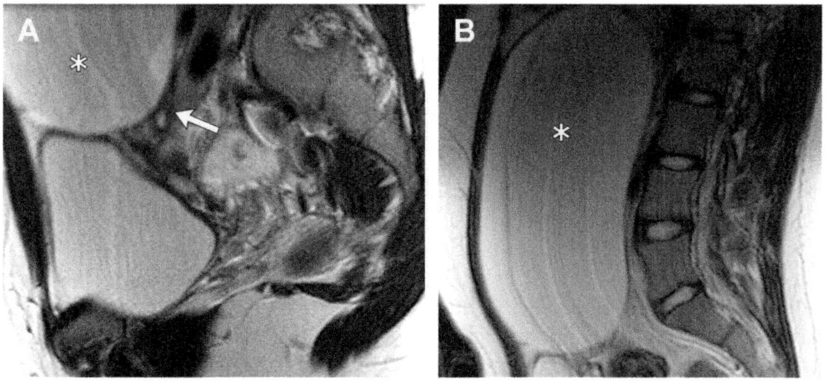

Fig. 5. Benign cystadenoma. Sagittal T2-weighted images (*A*, *B*) of a 20-year-old woman with an adnexal cyst on ultrasound show an 18-cm unilocular lesion (*asterisk*) with a thick uniform wall and homogeneously T2-weighted hyperintense fluid arising from the ovary (*arrow*). Diagnosis was confirmed on pathology.

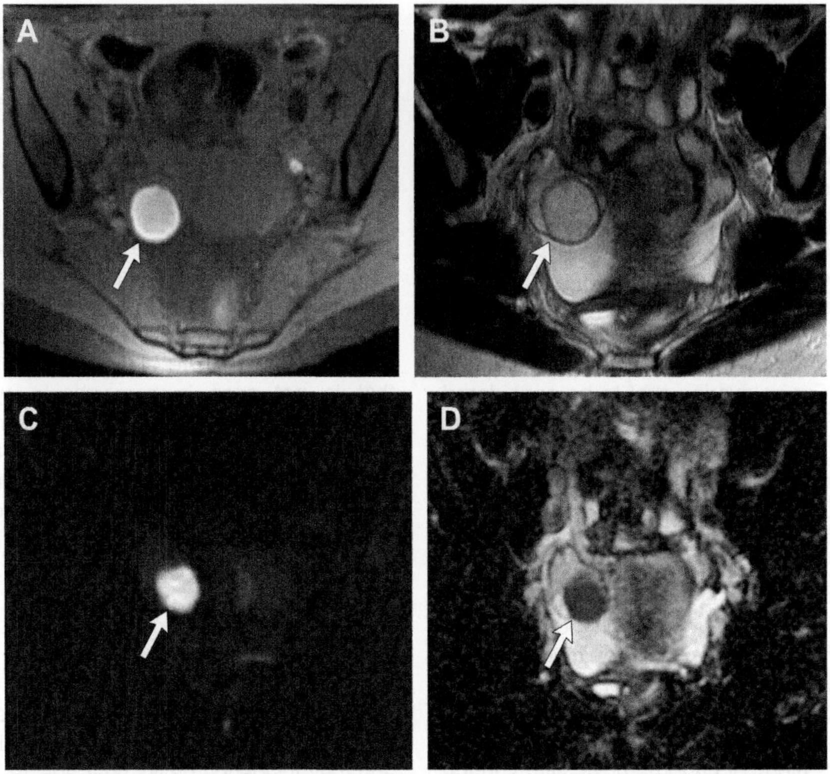

Fig. 6. Endometrioma. Axial fat-saturated T1-weighted image (*A*), T2-weighted image (*B*), DWI (*C*), and ADC map (*D*) of a 24-year-old woman with right lower quadrant pain show a 3-cm right ovarian unilocular cyst (*arrow*). The cyst fluid is homogeneously hyperintense on fat-saturated T1-weighted imaging and exhibits restricted diffusion. Note that the fluid is hyperintense on T2-weighted imaging and lacking in "shading." Diagnosis was confirmed on pathology.

described[46]; however, such events are rare, thought to occur in well less than 1% of lesions,[45] and typically occur in the seventh decade of life.[44]

Fibromas and fibrothecomas are benign tumors of the ovary comprising spindle-shaped fibroblasts and collagen. Fibrothecomas contain theca cells, which produce estrogen, and can clinically be differentiated from fibromas based on serum hormone levels. Although these tumors are the most common sex cord stromal tumors of the ovary, they are rare and account for only 4% of all ovarian neoplasms.[47,48] Fibromas (**Fig. 9**) have a characteristic MR imaging appearance. They are completely solid, homogeneously T2 and T1 hypointense (due to their high collagen content), exhibit homogenous low-level enhancement less than that of the myometrium, and do not restrict diffusion.[48–50] A lesion arising from the ovary with these features may be confidently diagnosed as fibroma or fibrothecoma. Broad ligament or pedunculated fibroids (leiomyomas) comprise the primary differential diagnosis consideration, and fibromas are often misdiagnosed as fibroids on imaging. When evaluating a fibrous pelvic tumor at MR, delineating the presence or absence of normal ovaries becomes central to image interpretation. Inability to identify a normal ovary ipsilateral to a fibrous mass, although not excluding the diagnosis of a fibroid, should promote consideration of fibroma or fibrothecoma. Enhancement characteristics should also be assessed, because fibromas and fibrothecomas are hypoenhancing relative to normal myometrium and most fibroids.[50] MR imaging diagnostic criteria for benign ovarian lesions are summarized in **Table 3**.

DIAGNOSTIC CRITERIA: BENIGN EXTRAOVARIAN LESIONS

Many incidental adnexal masses are extraovarian lesions arising from the uterus, the fallopian tube, or the surrounding pelvic organs. The overwhelming majority of extraovarian adnexal lesions are benign (see **Box 1**), and identification of an ipsilateral normal ovary (see **Fig. 8**) indicates a high likelihood of a benign diagnosis (the

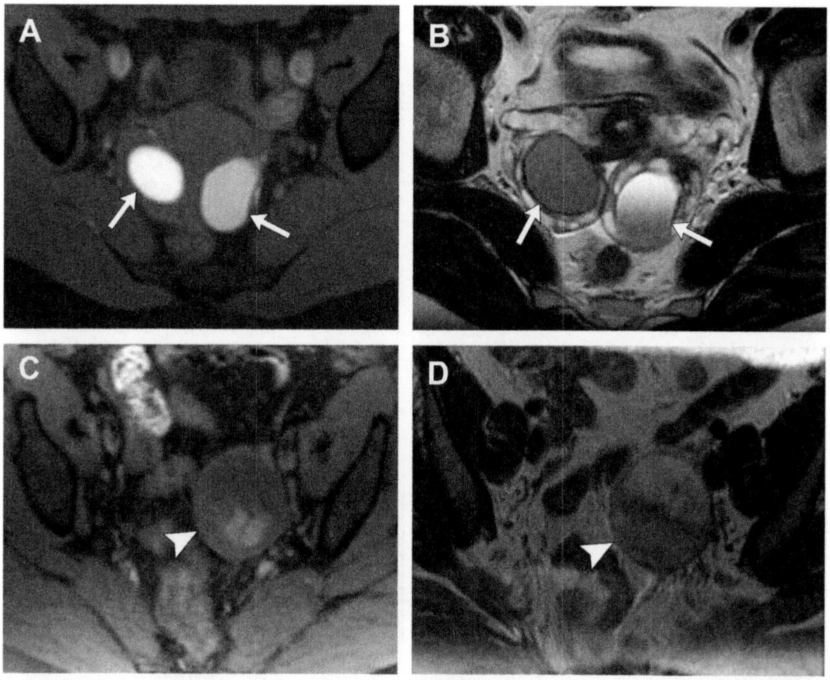

Fig. 7. Endometrioma versus hemorrhagic ovarian cyst. Axial fat-saturated T1- (*A, C*) and T2- (*B, D*) weighted images of bilateral endometriomas (*arrows, A, B*) and a left hemorrhagic cyst (*arrowhead, C, D*). Note that, on the fat-saturated T1-weighted imaging, the endometriomas and the hemorrhagic cyst all exhibit hyperintense signal; however, the former are homogenous in signal and the latter is heterogeneous in signal. Both entities exhibit T2-weighted hypointense signal seen as "shading" in endometriomas (*arrows, B*) and within the fluid-fluid level in the hemorrhagic cyst (*arrowhead, D*). Diagnosis of endometrioma was confirmed with laparoscopy. The hemorrhagic cyst was noted to resolve on follow-up ultrasound.

occasional malignant extraovarian adnexal mass typically presents as a metastasis in the setting of disseminated cancer, rarely a diagnostic dilemma). Once a mass is identified as extraovarian, a thorough search for another organ of origin should be performed to render a specific diagnosis. Attachment to the uterus suggests that the lesion could reflect a subserosal or pedunculated fibroid (**Fig. 10**) or adenomyoma (**Fig. 11**). Both lesions are characteristically low in T2-weighted signal[51]; however, foci of hyperintense signal on fat-saturated T1-weighted imaging suggest the presence of ectopic endometrial tissue and punctate hemorrhage within an adenomyoma.[52] Because fibroids are common and protean, an extraovarian mass originating from the uterine myometrium should be considered a fibroid, even when imaging features are atypical (eg, cystic, hemorrhagic, diffusion restricted). However, MR imaging cannot exclude the possibility of the rare underlying leiomyosarcoma in such a setting.[53] If the adnexal mass is on the right, effort should be made to identify the normal appendix, because appendiceal mucoceles (**Fig. 12**) can present as incidental adnexal masses. MR may miss the presence of characteristic calcifications, but communication with the cecum is diagnostic.[54] Nerve sheath tumors (**Fig. 13**), when large, may contain cystic components and may mimic adnexal lesions.[55] These lesions may be confidently diagnosed based on their location along the known course of nerve roots, their high T2-weighted signal, and their avid contrast enhancement.

Not all extraovarian adnexal lesions may be diagnosed by localizing their attachment to adjacent pelvic organs. Most of these arise from the fallopian tube or from pelvic adhesions. Here, morphologic features (unilocular or septated cysts) and localization separate from a normal ipsilateral ovary, allowing for a benign diagnosis. Peritoneal inclusion cysts (**Fig. 14**) typically arise in premenopausal women with pelvic adhesions that trap fluid released from ovarian cysts,[56] resulting in collections of fluid around an ovary. These lesions carry no malignant potential. They typically contain thin uniform septations, are located lateral to the broad ligament, conform to

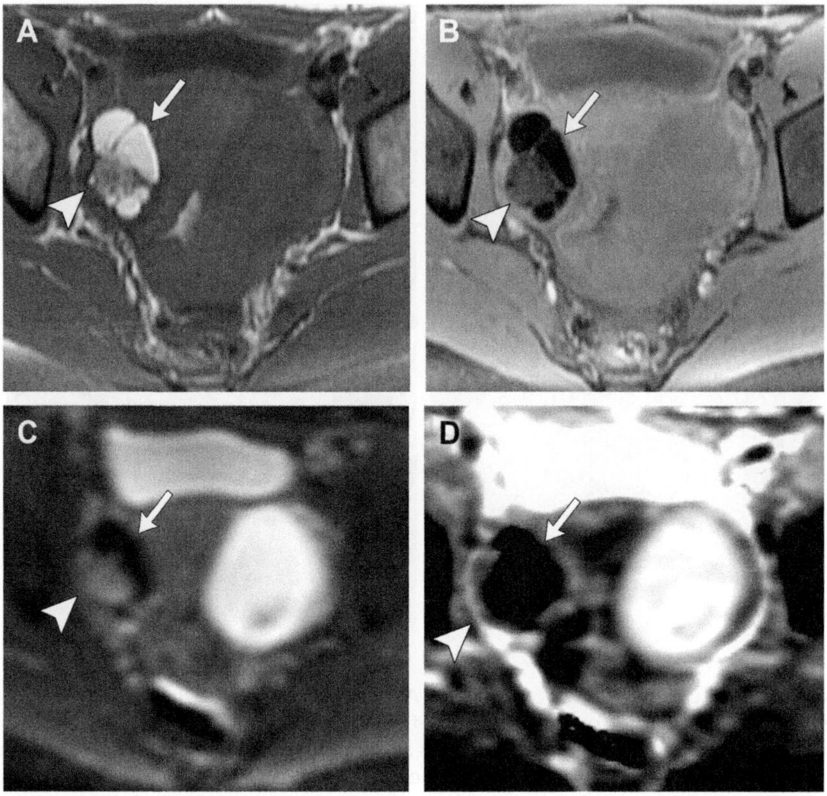

Fig. 8. Mature cystic teratoma or dermoid cyst. Axial T1-weighted images without (*A*) and with (*B*) fat saturation, DWI (*C*), and ADC map (*D*) of a 4.5-cm right ovarian mass (*arrow*) in a 34-year-old woman. The mass was noted to be an enlarging complex cyst at ultrasound. There is loss of signal within the mass on the fat-saturated T1-weighted image confirming the presence of macroscopic fat (*B*). The solid nodule (*arrowhead*) demonstrates diffusion restriction. Diagnosis was confirmed on pathology.

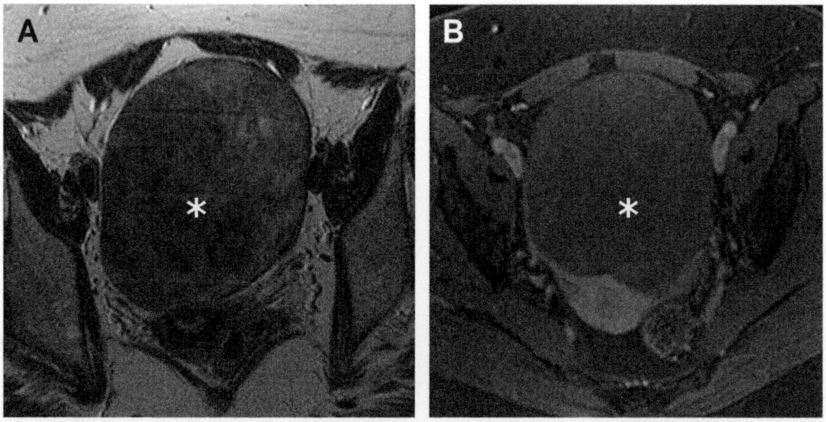

Fig. 9. Fibroma. Axial T2-weighted (*A*) and postgadolinium fat-saturated T1-weighted (*B*) images of a 10-cm well-circumscribed solid adnexal lesion (*asterisk*) in a 55-year-old woman with a history of fibroids. The right adnexal lesion exhibits relatively uniform T2-weighted hypointense signal and low-level contrast enhancement. A normal left ovary is identified; however, a normal right ovary is not seen. A right ovarian fibroma was included in the differential diagnosis and confirmed on pathology.

Table 3
MR imaging features for diagnosing an ovarian lesion as benign

Pathology	Morphology	T1[a]	T2[a]	DWI[a]	Contrast Enhancement[a]
Mature cystic teratoma (dermoid cyst)	Mixed solid and cystic (possible)	Hyperintense signal that suppresses with fat saturation (required)	NA	Portions of lesion with restricted diffusion (possible)	Portions enhance (possible)
Endometrioma	Unilocular cyst with uniformly smooth wall (required)	Homogeneous internal fluid "lightbulb-bright" hyperintensity (required)	Homogeneous internal fluid hyperintensity, isointensity, or hypointensity (required)	Restricted diffusion of internal fluid (possible)	No internal enhancement (required)
Fibroma	Completely solid (required)	Homogeneously isointense or hypointense (required)	Homogeneously hypointense (required)	No restricted diffusion (required)	Homogeneous enhancement less than myometrium (required)
Physiologic cyst or cystadenoma	Unilocular cyst with uniformly smooth wall (required)	Homogenous internal fluid hypointensity (required)	Homogeneous internal fluid hyperintensity (required)	No restricted diffusion (required)	No internal enhancement (required)

Abbreviation: NA, not applicable, that is, no typical imaging feature.
[a] Relative to uterine myometrium or small bowel wall.

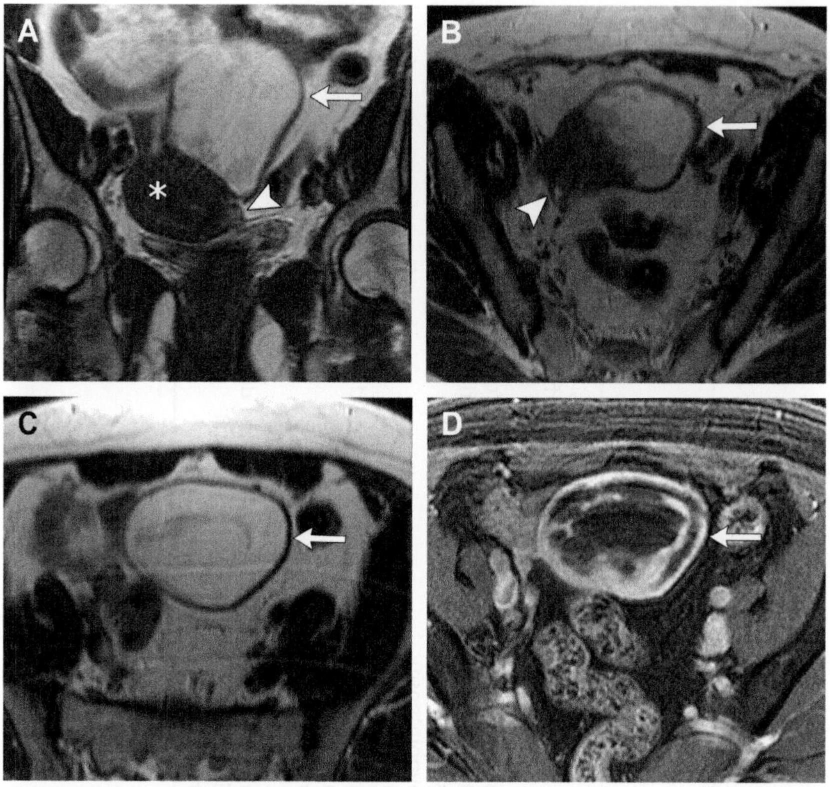

Fig. 10. Fibroid. Coronal (*A*) and axial (*B, C*) T2-weighted images, and postgadolinium fat-saturated T1-weighted image (*D*) of 52-year-old woman with a complex cystic pelvic mass thought to be an ovarian neoplasm at ultrasound. MR images show an 8.5-cm right adnexal mass (*arrow*) superior to the uterus (*asterisk*). The lesion is well circumscribed, has both solid and cystic components, and exhibits robust enhancement within its solid portions. Both ovaries (*arrowhead*) are identified separate from the mass. Pathology confirmed broad ligament degenerated fibroid.

the surrounding pelvic structures, and can envelope the ovary. When such characteristic features are present, the diagnosis of peritoneal inclusion cyst may be confidently made. Paratubal cysts (**Fig. 15**) also appear as fluid collections adjacent to the ovary but are typically unilocular. They represent inclusion cysts originating from the fallopian tube fimbria. Hydrosalpinx (**Fig. 16**) most often occurs in the setting of pelvic adhesions arising from prior infection, bowel inflammation

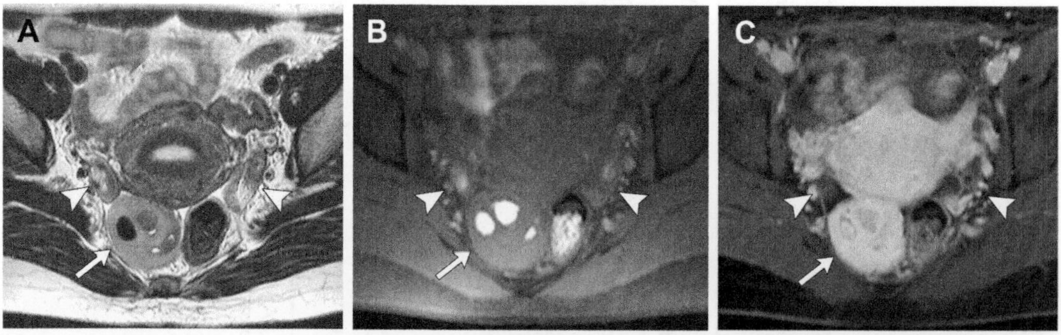

Fig. 11. Adenomyoma. Axial T2-weighted (*A*) and fat-saturated T1-weighted images without (*B*) and with (*C*) gadolinium in a 35-year-old woman with mixed solid and cystic right adnexal mass thought to be an ovarian neoplasm at ultrasound. MR images show a 5-cm right pelvic mass (*arrow*) separate from the ovaries (*arrowheads*). Portions of the mass exhibit high signal on fat-saturated T1-weighted images compatible with blood degradation products, and the solid portions avidly enhance. Diagnosis was confirmed on pathology.

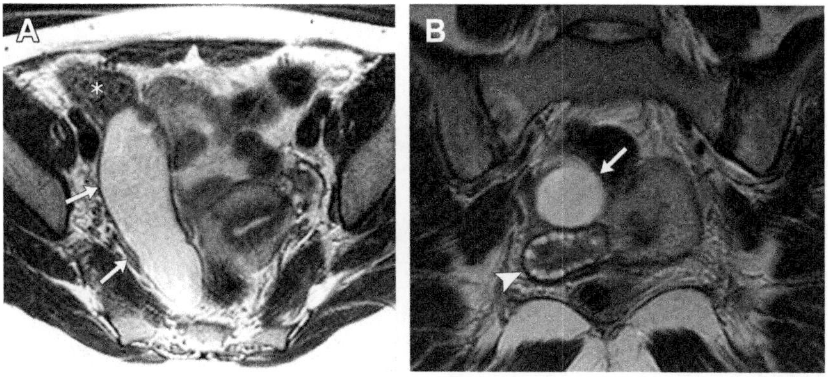

Fig. 12. Appendiceal mucocele. Axial (*A*) and coronal (*B*) T2-weighted images of a complex cystic right pelvic mass in a 32-year-old woman with complex cystic right pelvic mass discovered at ultrasound. MR images show a 5-cm ovoid cystic lesion (*arrows*) with mural nodules arising from the base of the cecum (*asterisk*). The right ovary (*arrowhead*) is separate from this lesion. Pathology showed low-grade mucinous neoplasm of the appendix.

(eg, appendicitis, inflammatory bowel disease), endometriosis, or pelvic surgery.[57,58] At MR, hydrosalpinx is seen as a tubular cystic structure taking an "s" or "c" shape, located medial to the ovary within the broad ligament. Identification of longitudinal folds (plicae) increases the specificity for the diagnosis.[58]

DIAGNOSTIC CRITERIA: MALIGNANT AND BORDERLINE OVARIAN LESIONS

Pathophysiology of Malignant Ovarian Masses

Epithelial ovarian neoplasms constitute most malignant ovarian cancers for women over the age of 30.[47] Of these neoplasms, serous carcinoma is the most common subtype, constituting approximately 70%.[59] Recently, there has been a conceptual shift in the grading and classification of these tumors; they are now described to be either low grade (type I) or high grade (type II). The 2 grades are not 2 ends of a disease spectrum; rather, they are distinct disease states with different clinicopathologic behavior and origins. Low-grade serous ovarian cancers are favored to arise in a stepwise fashion from borderline tumors in the ovary, whereas high-grade serous tumors are now favored to arise from precursor lesions in the fallopian tubes, which subsequently seed the ovaries and peritoneum.[60–62]

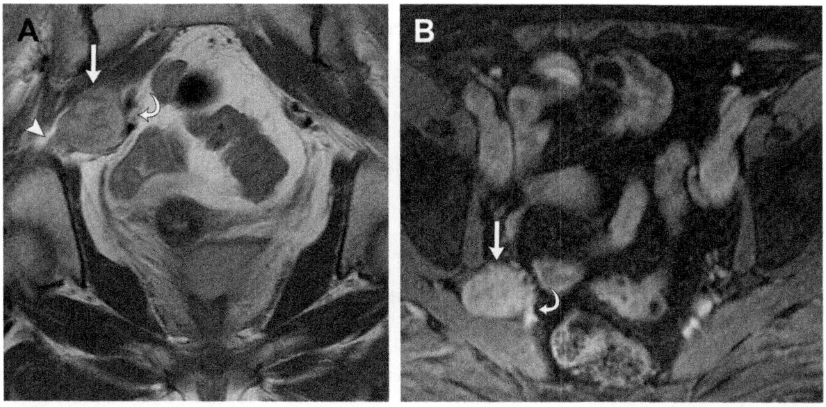

Fig. 13. Nerve sheath tumor. Coronal T2- (*A*) and axial postgadolinium fat-saturated T1- (*B*) weighted images of a 69-year-old woman reveal a normal right ovary (not depicted) and a solid hypervascular 3-cm mass (*straight arrow*) near the right pelvic sidewall. The mass displaces branches of the right internal iliac vessels (*curved arrow*) medially (indicating that it is extraperitoneal in location) and is closely associated with the S2 nerve root (*arrowhead*). The lesion was noted to be stable on follow-up imaging for 5 years.

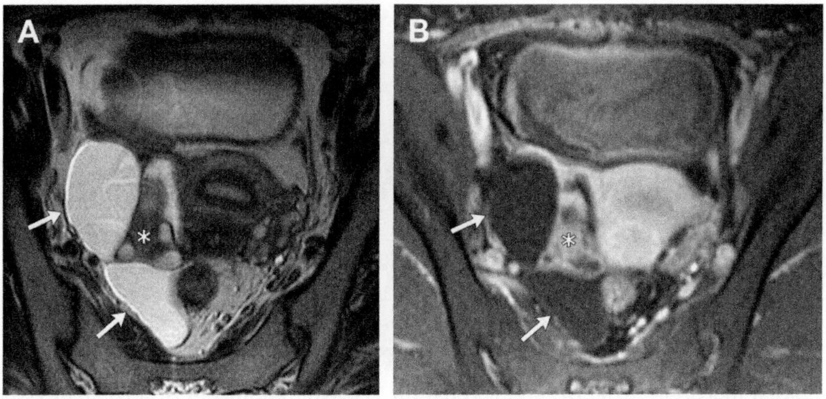

Fig. 14. Peritoneal inclusion cyst. Axial T2- (*A*) and postgadolinium fat-saturated T1- (*B*) weighted images of a 42-year-old woman with chronic pelvic pain show a multiloculated cystic lesion (*arrows*) conforming to the surrounding pelvic structures that is separate from the right ovary (*asterisk*). Diagnosis was confirmed on pathology.

High-grade serous carcinoma, most common in postmenopausal women, has a propensity for early and rapid spread. Less than 2% of high-grade serous carcinomas are stage I at the time of diagnosis.[63,64] This rapid spread is problematic for screening with imaging because many cancers will develop and disseminate in the interim between screening examinations. In 1 of the larger US screening trials, 15% (9/60) arose in the 12-month interval after a normal screening examination. Of these cancers, all had extra ovarian spread at the time of surgical staging.[6] In an earlier trial, all high-grade ovarian carcinomas exhibited growth at the 4- to 6-month follow-up sonographic evaluation.[65]

Similar to high-grade serous carcinomas, malignant germ cell tumors, most common in women under 30 years of age, have a proclivity for rapid growth but tend to be more chemosensitive and of a lower stage at surgery than high-grade serous ovarian carcinomas.[66] Such rapid growth and early dissemination of the common ovarian cancers underscore the importance of expedited imaging characterization (multiparametric MR imaging) and triage rather than longitudinal follow-up (repeat ultrasound) for sonographically indeterminate adnexal masses, as only the former approach will allow for timely intervention for malignancy.

Imaging Findings of Malignant Ovarian Masses

Malignant ovarian tumors have a peak incidence between ages 40 and 80 years. Both low-grade

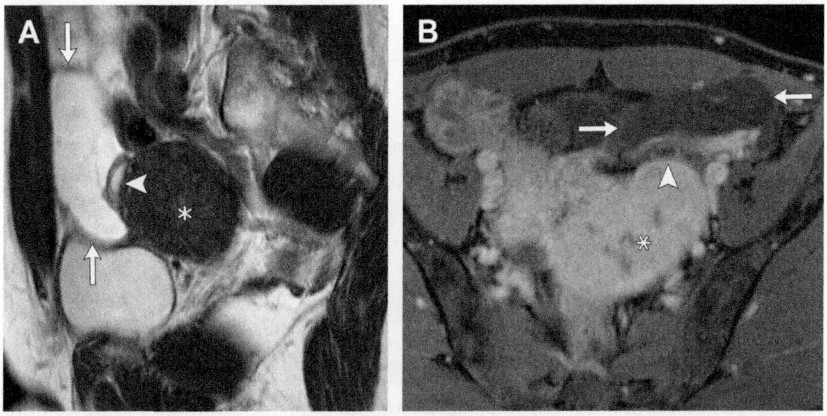

Fig. 15. Paratubal cyst. Sagittal T2- (*A*) and axial postgadolinium fat-saturated T1- (*B*) weighted images of a 48-year-old woman with left adnexal cyst show a 6-cm nonenhancing T2-weighted hyperintense fluid-filled cyst (*arrows*) that is separate from the left ovary (*arrowhead*). Also seen is a uterine fibroid (*asterisk*). Diagnosis was confirmed on pathology.

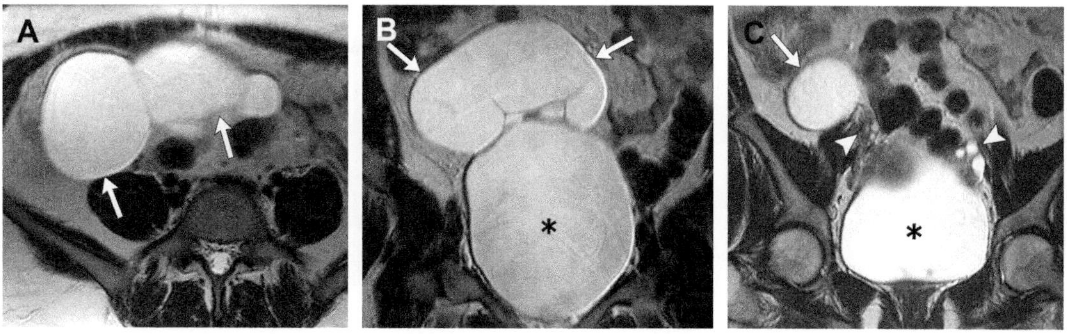

Fig. 16. Hydrosalpinx. Axial (*A*) and coronal (*B*, *C*) T2-weighted images of a 50-year-old woman with a complex cystic pelvic mass thought to be an ovarian neoplasm at ultrasound show a T2-weighted hyperintense fluid-filled tubular right adnexal lesion (*arrows*) above the bladder (*asterisk*) and separate from both ovaries (*arrowheads*). Diagnosis was confirmed on pathology.

(type I) and high-grade (type II) tumors present as large complex mixed solid and cystic adnexal masses. As the majority present with gross extra-ovarian spread (eg, large-volume ascites, peritoneal and omental nodules), they are usually diagnosed at presentation with CT or US. Rarely, a high-grade ovarian carcinoma will present as a predominantly solid mass with a presumptive diagnosis of an atypical or symptomatic fibroid (**Fig. 17**). The nonepithelial ovarian malignancies, which include sex cord stromal tumors (eg, granulosa cell tumor, Sertoli-Leydig tumor) and germ

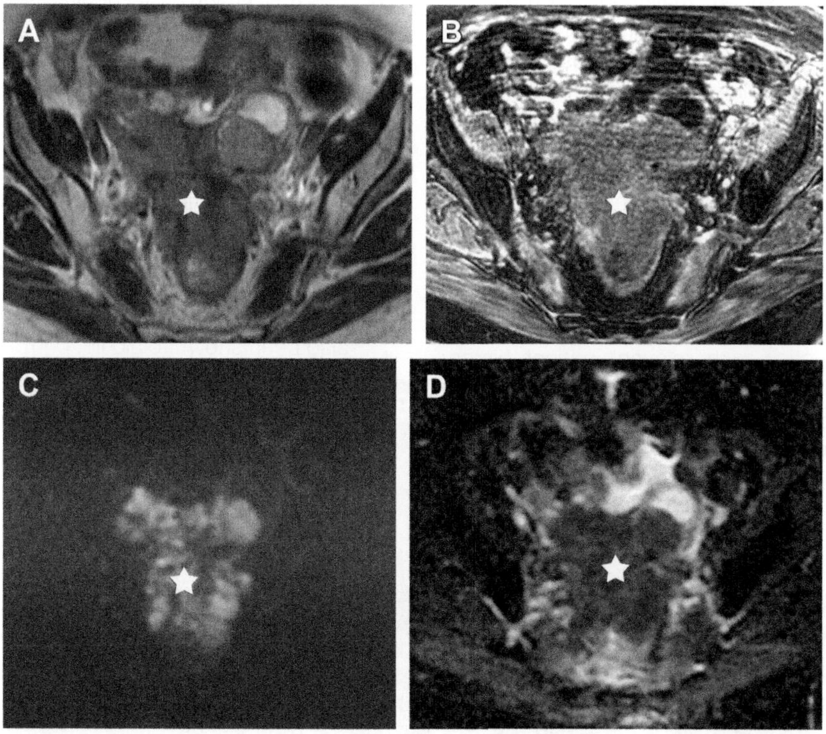

Fig. 17. High-grade serous ovarian carcinoma. Axial T2-weighted (*A*), postgadolinium fat-saturated T1-weighted (*B*), diffusion-weighted (*C*), and ADC map (*D*) images of a 51-year-old woman with abnormal vaginal bleeding attributed to fibroids show a 6-cm predominantly solid irregularly shaped mass (*star*) with isointense T2-weighted signal (*A*) and heterogeneous enhancement postgadolinium (*B*). Hyperintensity on DWI (*C*) and hypointensity on ADC (*D*) indicate restricted diffusion. Pathology showed high-grade serous carcinoma.

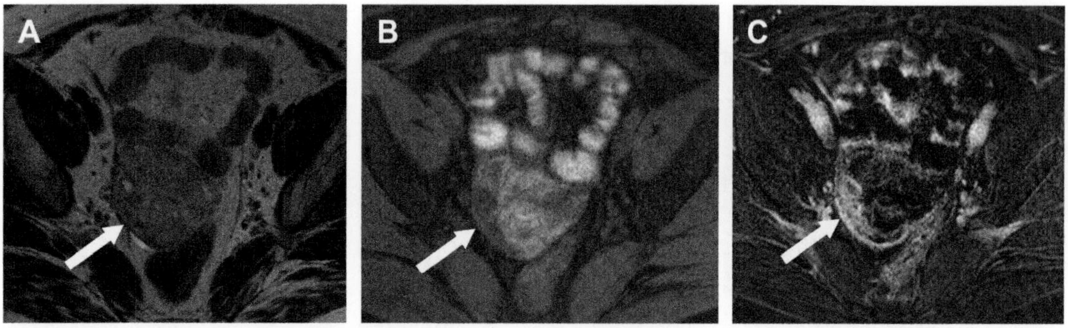

Fig. 18. Granulosa cell tumor. Axial T2-weighted (*A*), pregadolinium fat-saturated T1-weighted (*B*) and postgadolinium subtracted (*C*) images of a 42-year-old woman with a predominantly solid right adnexal mass on ultrasound show a 6-cm right ovarian mass (*arrow*) that is isointense on T2-weighted imaging (*A*) and exhibits internal hyperintensity on fat-saturated T1-weighted imaging (*B*), indicating blood degradation products. Subtraction images (*C*) show solid enhancing tissue. Left ovary (not shown) is normal. Pathology confirmed granulosa cell tumor with hemorrhage.

cell tumors (eg, dysgerminoma), more commonly present as incidental adnexal masses with no evidence for extraovarian metastases. Granulosa cell tumors (**Fig. 18**) typically present between ages 20 and 50 years and are characterized by their propensity for hemorrhage[67]; acute hemoperitoneum has been described as a presenting feature.[68,69] In contrast, malignant germ cell tumors present in adolescent and young women (less than 30 years old). At MR, most malignant tumors will have solid components that are reliably hyperintense or isointense on T2-weighted imaging, enhance, and exhibit diffusion restriction.[27] In the absence of definitive characterization, cancer is the diagnosis of exclusion in MR evaluation of the incidental adnexal mass with solid elements, and any lesion without specific features of benignity should be considered potentially a cancer.

Borderline ovarian tumors are clinically heterogeneous, but demonstrate low malignant potential. When compared with ovarian carcinoma, borderline tumors occur in younger women, present at an earlier stage, and portend a more favorable prognosis with a 10-year survival rate of approximately 95%.[70] Although borderline tumors can present with histologically noninvasive peritoneal implants and mimic carcinoma, the majority are incidental indeterminate ovarian masses (**Fig. 19**). On MR imaging, borderline tumors typically present as complex cysts with irregular septations, mural nodules, or papillary projections. The solid portions of the lesion reliably enhance.[71–73] All adnexal lesions without specific features of benignity after MR imaging evaluation should be considered indeterminate and referred to an oncologist for clinical evaluation and counseling regarding management options.[74]

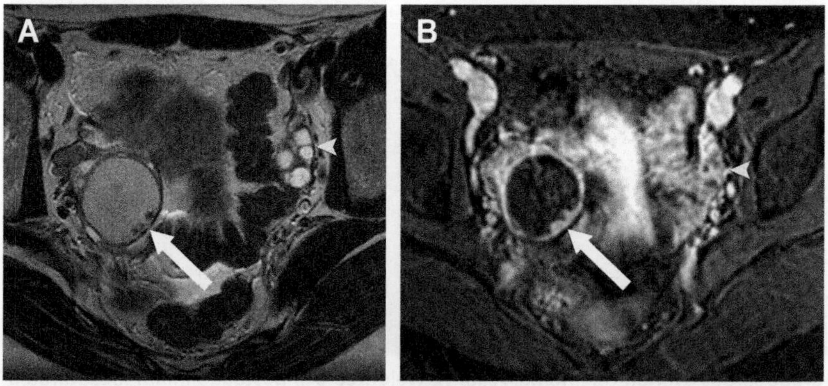

Fig. 19. Ovarian borderline tumor. Axial T2- (*A*) and postgadolinium fat-saturated T1- (*B*) weighted images of a 22-year-old woman with a complex right ovarian cyst on ultrasound show a 3.5-cm cyst in the right ovary with solid mural nodules (*arrow*) that are isointense on T2-weighted (*A*) images and enhance with gadolinium (*B*). Left ovary (*arrowhead*) appears normal. Pathology showed serous papillary borderline tumor.

PEARLS, PITFALLS, AND VARIANTS

Infrequently, cancer may mimic a benign adnexal mass. In such cases, an error in diagnosis can usually be avoided by a meticulous and systematic review of the MR images. Cancer arises in endometriosis, and endometriomas undergo malignant degeneration to cancer from borderline tumors.[60,71,73] Clear cell and endometrioid carcinomas are the most common histologies.[60,75] The usual appearance of cancer arising in an endometrioma is an enhancing mural nodule (**Fig. 20**).[17] Given this, all endometriomas should be assessed on subtraction imaging for evidence of internal enhancement.

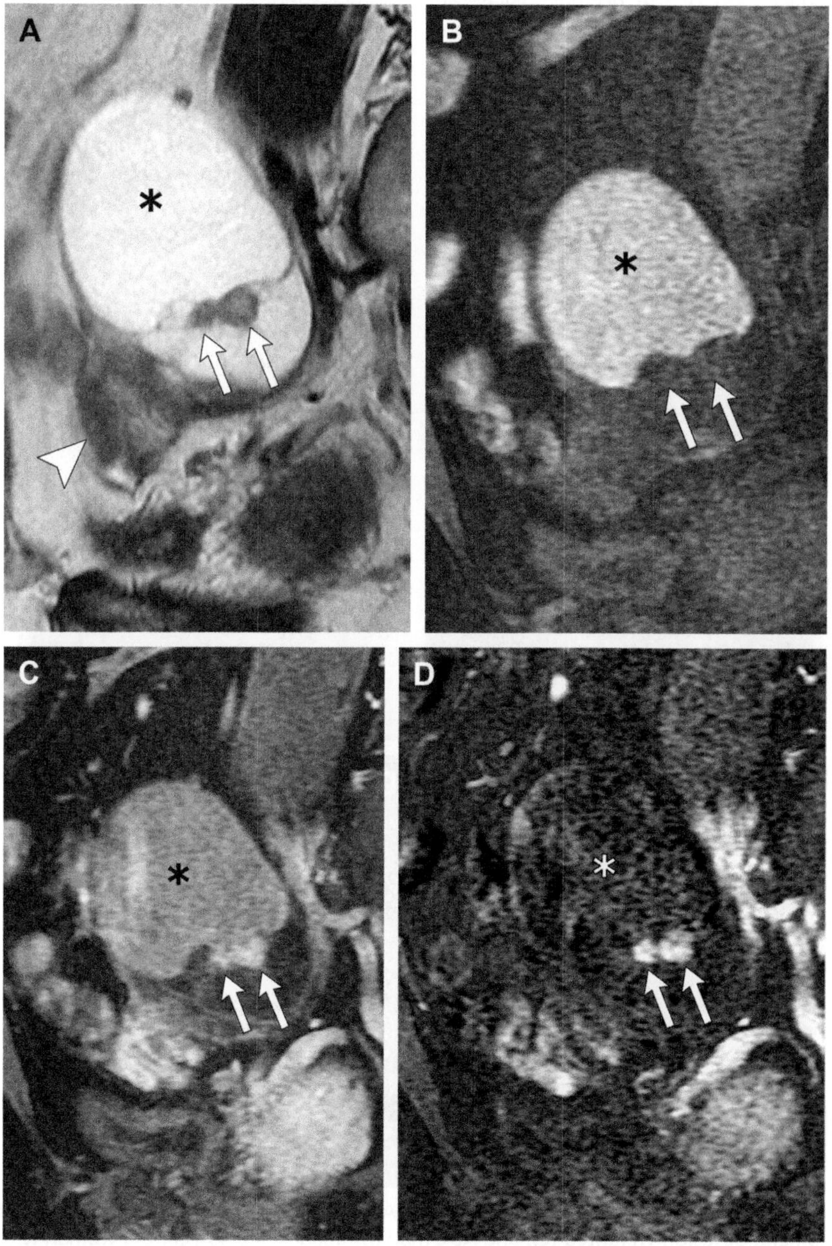

Fig. 20. Malignant transformation of an endometrioma. Sagittal T2-weighted (*A*) and fat-saturated T1-weighted images with fat saturation before (*B*) and after (*C*) intravenous gadolinium of a 48-year-old woman with a history of endometriosis show an 8-cm complex cyst arising from the ovary (*arrowhead*) with homogeneously T1-weighted hyperintense fluid (*asterisk*) compatible with an endometrioma. Subtraction imaging (*D*) best demonstrates enhancement within the solid components (*arrows*). Pathology showed clear cell carcinoma.

Although high-grade ovarian cancer typically presents as a complex cystic mass with high-volume ascites, atypical presentations include predominantly solid lesions with little or no accompanying peritoneal fluid (**Fig. 21**). For many radiologists, there is a temptation to classify all large solid lesions in the female pelvis as fibroids. However, attention must be paid to the MR imaging criteria used to diagnose a lesion as benign (see **Table 1**). Identification of the normal ipsilateral ovary and evaluation of the lesion's features on all pulse sequences, including DWI and postcontrast T1-weighted imaging (see **Table 2**), are important steps in the MR imaging evaluation of an adnexal mass. Careful adherence to image acquisition and interpretation protocols will enable the radiologist to avoid the pitfall of mistaking a malignancy for a benign lesion.

Conversely, many benign lesions may have atypical MR imaging features that may be mistaken for cancer, leading to unnecessarily aggressive surgery. Cystadenofibromas (**Fig. 22**), comprised of epithelial and stromal cells, are benign tumors that are commonly confused for malignancy at MR imaging. They are solid and cystic lesions; the solid portions appear hypointense on T2-weighted imaging, exhibit low-level homogeneous enhancement, and do not restricted diffusion. These characteristic imaging features of cystadenofibroma coupled with a lack of any evidence of extraovarian metastasis will sometimes suggest the diagnosis. However, when presenting the clinical context of Meigs syndrome (benign ovarian tumor, ascites, and pleural effusion),[76] cystadenofibromas cannot be differentiated from ovarian carcinoma. Mature

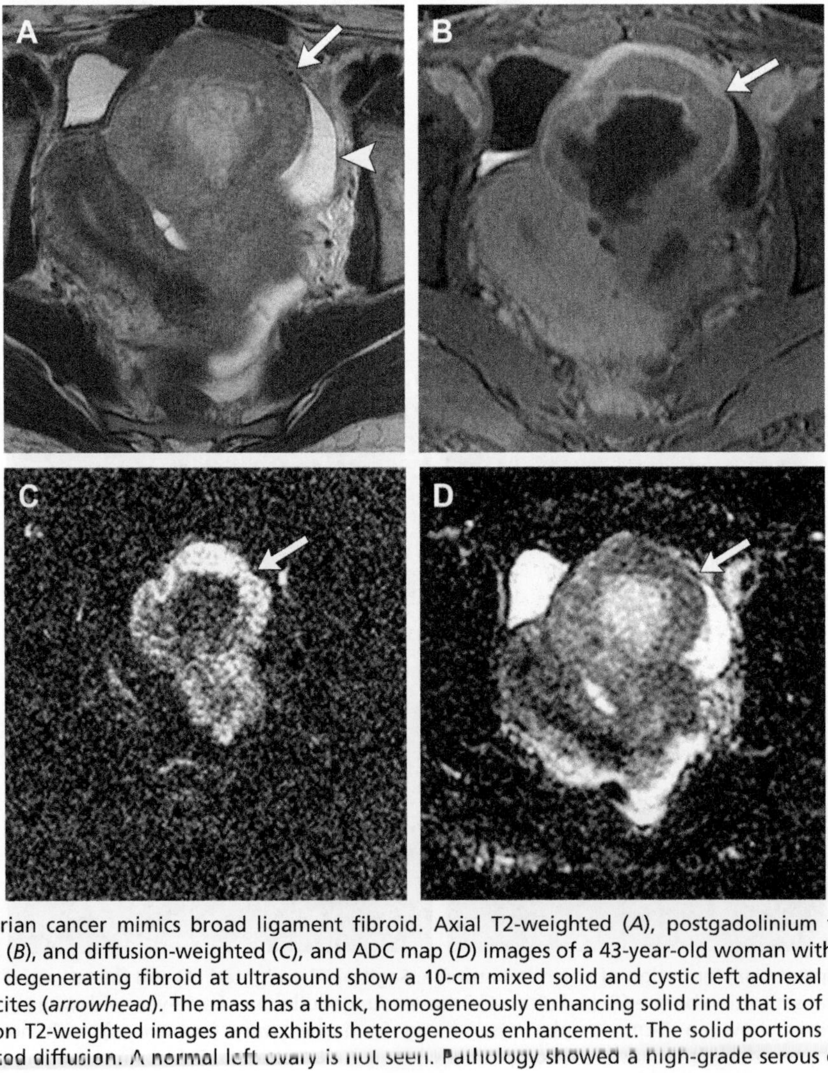

Fig. 21. Ovarian cancer mimics broad ligament fibroid. Axial T2-weighted (*A*), postgadolinium fat-saturated T1-weighted (*B*), and diffusion-weighted (*C*), and ADC map (*D*) images of a 43-year-old woman with a presumed diagnosis of degenerating fibroid at ultrasound show a 10-cm mixed solid and cystic left adnexal mass (*arrow*) and trace ascites (*arrowhead*). The mass has a thick, homogeneously enhancing solid rind that is of intermediate gray signal on T2-weighted images and exhibits heterogeneous enhancement. The solid portions of the lesion show restricted diffusion. A normal left ovary is not seen. Pathology showed a high-grade serous carcinoma of the left ovary.

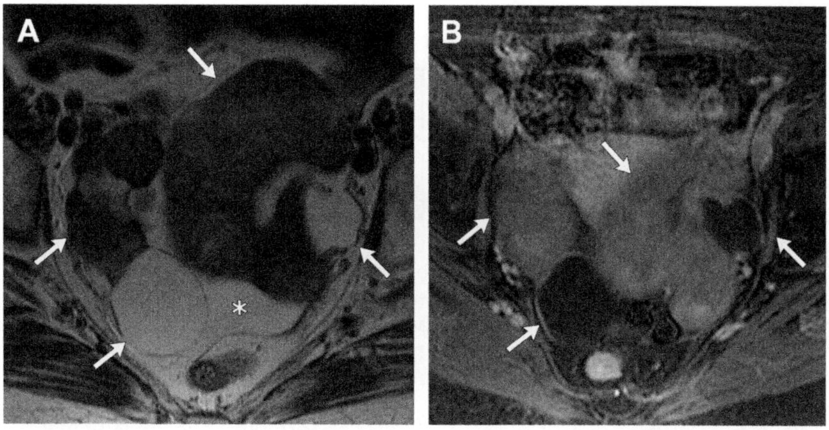

Fig. 22. Cystadenofibromas presenting as Meigs syndrome mimic ovarian cancer. Axial T2- (*A*) and postgadolinium fat-saturated T1- (*B*) weighted images of a 77-year-old woman with a presumed diagnosis of ovarian cancer at ultrasound show 8-cm right and 10-cm left mixed solid and cystic adnexal lesions (*arrows*). The solid portions of the masses are are homogenously hypointense on T2-weighted imaging and exhibit low level enhancement. Normal ovaries are not seen, and ascites (*asterisk*) is noted. Pathology showed bilateral cystadenofibromas.

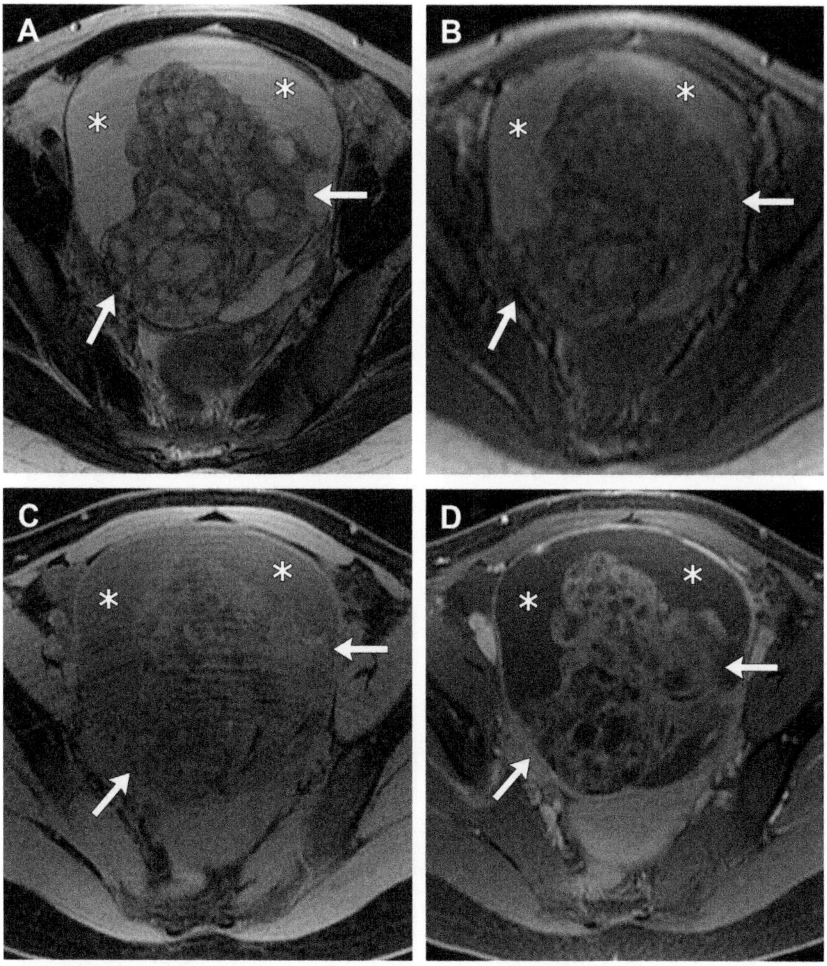

Fig. 23. Benign dermoid cyst mimics malignant transformation. Axial T2- (*A*), T1- (*B*), precontrast fat-saturated T1- (*C*), and postcontrast fat-saturated T1- (*D*) weighted images of a 29-year-old woman with a complex cystic adnexal mass discovered at ultrasound show a 14-cm mixed solid and cystic mass with irregular enhancing components (*arrows*). Loss of hyperintense T1-weighted signal on the fat-saturated sequence (*asterisk*) is consistent with fat. A normal right ovary is not seen. Pathology showed right ovarian dermoid.

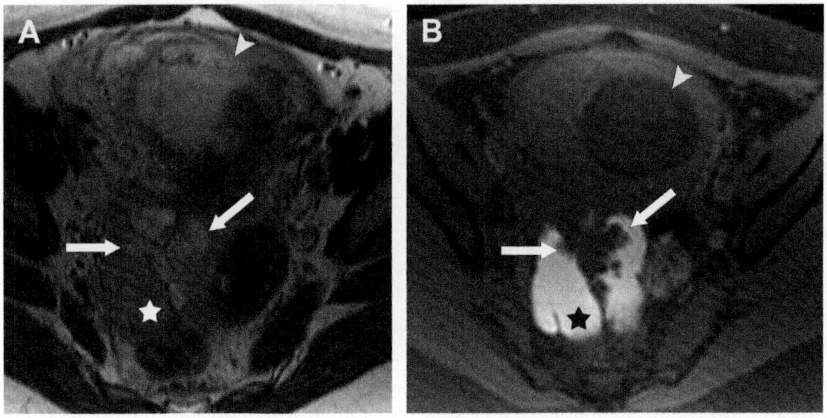

Fig. 24. Decidualized endometrioma mimics ovarian cancer. Axial T2- (*A*) and fat-saturated T1- (*B*) weighted images of a 34-year-old woman at 16 weeks' gestation and complex adnexal mass identified at ultrasound show a 6-cm right adnexal mass with components that are homogeneously hyperintense on T1-weighted imaging and hypointense on T2-weighted imaging (*star*). Solid-appearing mural nodules within the lesion (*arrows*) reflect decidualized tissue. An intrauterine gestation is seen (*arrowhead*). Left ovary (not shown) is normal. Pathology showed endometrioma with pregnancy-related changes.

cystic teratomas (**Fig. 23**) often present as large complex cysts and can resemble high-grade carcinoma. However, tissue diagnosis of macroscopic fat on MR imaging is sufficient to ensure benignity provided no other ancillary features of malignancy (eg, peritoneal nodules, lymphadenopathy) are present. In the setting of pregnancy, decidualized endometrial tissue may result in the presence of suspicious mural nodules in endometriomas (**Fig. 24**). These foci are benign and resolve postpartum. Infectious and inflammatory conditions such as subacute tubo-ovarian abscess (**Fig. 25**) may present as an incidental adnexal mass and mimic cancer. Patients usually provide a history of bowel inflammation (eg, appendicitis, inflammatory bowel disease) or pelvic surgery.

When an incidental adnexal mass mimics a cancer, careful MR imaging review coupled with targeted investigation of the clinical history and laboratory values are necessary for a radiologist to arrive at a non–cancer diagnosis. Nevertheless, if the lesion proves indeterminate after MR evaluation, the patient should be referred to a gynecologic oncologist for clinical evaluation, including physical examination and serum tumor markers, and counseling regarding management options.[74]

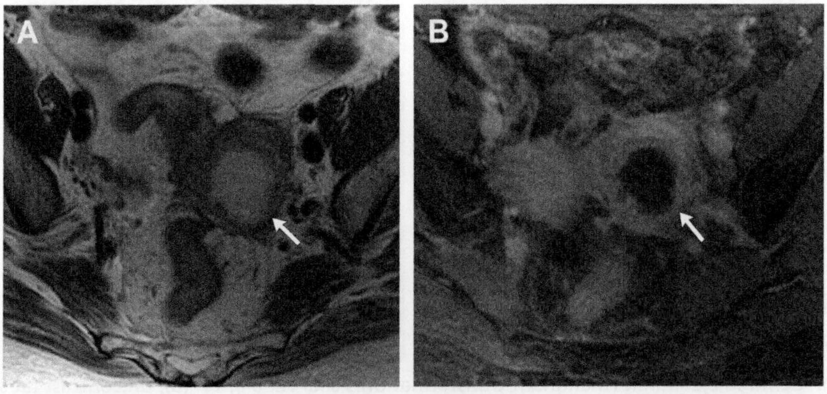

Fig. 25. Tubo-ovarian abscess mimics ovarian cancer. Axial T2- (*A*) and postgadolinium fat-saturated T1- (*B*) weighted images of a 64-year-old woman with a history of perforated appendicitis 6 months prior shows a 5 cm mixed solid and cystic left adnexal mass with a thick irregular enhancing rind (*arrow*). A normal left ovary is not seen. Pathology showed chronic tubo-ovarian abscess with fibrosis.

SUMMARY/WHAT REFERRING CLINICIANS NEED TO KNOW

- MR imaging increases the specificity of the imaging workup of indeterminate adnexal lesions, resulting in decreased rates of false positive cancer diagnoses.
- Tissue characterization with MR imaging often allows for definitive characterization of ovarian lesions as benign. Such lesions include benign physiologic cysts and cystadenomas, endometriomas, mature cystic teratomas, and fibromas.
- Volumetric MR imaging of the entire female pelvis allows for localization of extraovarian lesions relative to normal ovaries. Once a lesion is confirmed to be extraovarian, it is highly likely to be benign.
- MR imaging is safe in pregnancy, but imaging at 3 T and gadolinium-based intravenous contrast material should be avoided.
- Some adnexal lesions considered indeterminate at MR imaging will prove benign. Nevertheless, these should be referred to a gynecologic oncologist for clinical evaluation and patient counseling.

REFERENCES

1. Pickhardt PJ, Hanson ME. Incidental adnexal masses detected at low-dose unenhanced CT in asymptomatic women age 50 and older: implications for clinical management and ovarian cancer screening. Radiology 2010;257(1):144–50.
2. Slanetz PJ, Hahn PF, Hall DA, et al. The frequency and significance of adnexal lesions incidentally revealed by CT. AJR Am J Roentgenol 1997;168(3):647–50.
3. Sharma A, Apostolidou S, Burnell M, et al. Risk of epithelial ovarian cancer in asymptomatic women with ultrasound-detected ovarian masses: a prospective cohort study within the UK collaborative trial of ovarian cancer screening (UKCTOCS). Ultrasound Obstet Gynecol 2012;40(3):338–44.
4. Baser E, Erkilinc S, Esin S, et al. Adnexal masses encountered during cesarean delivery. Int J Gynaecol Obstet 2013;123(2):124–6.
5. Hermans AJ, Kluivers KB, Janssen LM, et al. Adnexal masses in children, adolescents and women of reproductive age in the Netherlands: a nationwide population-based cohort study. Gynecol Oncol 2016;143(1):93–7.
6. van Nagell JR Jr, DePriest PD, Ueland FR, et al. Ovarian cancer screening with annual transvaginal sonography: findings of 25,000 women screened. Cancer 2007;109(9):1887–96.
7. National Institutes of Health Consensus Development Conference Statement. Ovarian cancer: screening, treatment, and follow-up. Gynecol Oncol 1994;55(3 Pt 2):S4–14.
8. Evans EC, Matteson KA, Orejuela FJ, et al. Salpingo-oophorectomy at the time of benign hysterectomy: a systematic review. Obstet Gynecol 2016;128(3):476–85.
9. Solnik MJ, Alexander C. Ovarian incidentaloma. Best practice & research. Clin Endocrinol Metab 2012;26(1):105–16.
10. Dorum A, Blom GP, Ekerhovd E, et al. Prevalence and histologic diagnosis of adnexal cysts in postmenopausal women: an autopsy study. Am J Obstet Gynecol 2005;192(1):48–54.
11. Fishman DA, Cohen L, Blank SV, et al. The role of ultrasound evaluation in the detection of early-stage epithelial ovarian cancer. Am J Obstet Gynecol 2005;192(4):1214–21 [discussion: 1221–2].
12. Iyer VR, Lee SI. MRI, CT, and PET/CT for ovarian cancer detection and adnexal lesion characterization. AJR Am J Roentgenol 2010;194(2):311–21.
13. Kinkel K, Lu Y, Mehdizade A, et al. Indeterminate ovarian mass at US: incremental value of second imaging test for characterization–meta-analysis and Bayesian analysis. Radiology 2005;236(1):85–94.
14. Mohaghegh P, Rockall AG. Imaging strategy for early ovarian cancer: characterization of adnexal masses with conventional and advanced imaging techniques. Radiographics 2012;32(6):1751–73.
15. Sala E, Rockall A, Rangarajan D, et al. The role of dynamic contrast-enhanced and diffusion weighted magnetic resonance imaging in the female pelvis. Eur J Radiol 2010;76(3):367–85.
16. Ha HK, Lim YT, Kim HS, et al. Diagnosis of pelvic endometriosis: fat-suppressed T1-weighted vs conventional MR images. AJR Am J Roentgenol 1994;163(1):127–31.
17. Takeuchi M, Matsuzaki K, Uehara H, et al. Malignant transformation of pelvic endometriosis: MR imaging findings and pathologic correlation. Radiographics 2006;26(2):407–17.
18. Bent CL, Sahdev A, Rockall AG, et al. MRI appearances of borderline ovarian tumours. Clin Radiol 2009;64(4):430–8.
19. Bernardin L, Dilks P, Liyanage S, et al. Effectiveness of semi-quantitative multiphase dynamic contrast-enhanced MRI as a predictor of malignancy in complex adnexal masses: radiological and pathological correlation. Eur Radiol 2012;22(4):880–90.
20. Thomassin-Naggara I, Cuenod CA, Darai E, et al. Dynamic contrast-enhanced MR imaging of ovarian neoplasms: current status and future perspectives. Magn Reson Imaging Clin N Am 2008;16(4):661–72, ix.
21. Mansour SM, Saraya S, El-Faissal Y. Semi-quantitative contrast-enhanced MR analysis of indeterminate ovarian tumours: when to say malignancy? Br J Radiol 2015;88(1053):20150099.

22. Li X, Hu JL, Zhu LM, et al. The clinical value of dynamic contrast-enhanced MRI in differential diagnosis of malignant and benign ovarian lesions. Tumour Biol 2015;36(7):5515–22.
23. Gluskin JS, Chegai F, Monti S, et al. Hepatocellular carcinoma and diffusion-weighted MRI: detection and evaluation of treatment response. J Cancer 2016;7(11):1565–70.
24. Koh DM, Collins DJ. Diffusion-weighted MRI in the body: applications and challenges in oncology. AJR Am J Roentgenol 2007;188(6):1622–35.
25. Thomassin-Naggara I, Darai E, Cuenod CA, et al. Contribution of diffusion-weighted MR imaging for predicting benignity of complex adnexal masses. Eur Radiol 2009;19(6):1544–52.
26. Li W, Chu C, Cui Y, et al. Diffusion-weighted MRI: a useful technique to discriminate benign versus malignant ovarian surface epithelial tumors with solid and cystic components. Abdom Imaging 2012; 37(5):897–903.
27. Davarpanah AH, Kambadakone A, Holalkere NS, et al. Diffusion MRI of uterine and ovarian masses: identifying the benign lesions. Abdom Radiol 2016; 41(12):2466–75.
28. Fujii S, Kakite S, Nishihara K, et al. Diagnostic accuracy of diffusion-weighted imaging in differentiating benign from malignant ovarian lesions. J Magn Reson Imaging 2008;28(5):1149–56.
29. Shellock FG, Crues JV. MR procedures: biologic effects, safety, and patient care. Radiology 2004; 232(3):635–52.
30. Expert Panel on MRS, Kanal E, Barkovich AJ, et al. ACR guidance document on MR safe practices: 2013. J Magn Reson Imaging 2013;37(3):501–30.
31. Thomassin-Naggara I, Aubert E, Rockall A, et al. Adnexal masses: development and preliminary validation of an MR imaging scoring system. Radiology 2013;267(2):432–43.
32. Modesitt SC, Pavlik EJ, Ueland FR, et al. Risk of malignancy in unilocular ovarian cystic tumors less than 10 centimeters in diameter. Obstet Gynecol 2003; 102(3):594–9.
33. Tamai K, Koyama T, Saga T, et al. MR features of physiologic and benign conditions of the ovary. Eur Radiol 2006;16(12):2700–11.
34. Castillo G, Alcazar JL, Jurado M. Natural history of sonographically detected simple unilocular adnexal cysts in asymptomatic postmenopausal women. Gynecol Oncol 2004;92(3):965–9.
35. Bailey CL, Ueland FR, Land GL, et al. The malignant potential of small cystic ovarian tumors in women over 50 years of age. Gynecol Oncol 1998;69(1):3–7.
36. Gerber B, Muller H, Kulz T, et al. Simple ovarian cysts in premenopausal patients. Int J Gynaecol Obstet 1997;57(1):49–55.
37. Giudice LC, Kao LC. Endometriosis. Lancet 2004; 364(9447):1789–99.
38. Bulun SE. Endometriosis. N Engl J Med 2009;360(3): 268–79.
39. Togashi K, Nishimura K, Kimura I, et al. Endometrial cysts: diagnosis with MR imaging. Radiology 1991; 180(1):73–8.
40. Outwater E, Schiebler ML, Owen RS, et al. Characterization of hemorrhagic adnexal lesions with MR imaging: blinded reader study. Radiology 1993; 186(2):489–94.
41. Dias JL, Veloso Gomes F, Lucas R, et al. The shading sign: is it exclusive of endometriomas? Abdom Imaging 2015;40(7):2566–72.
42. Siegelman ES, Oliver ER. MR imaging of endometriosis: ten imaging pearls. Radiographics 2012;32(6): 1675–91.
43. Busard MP, Mijatovic V, van Kuijk C, et al. Magnetic resonance imaging in the evaluation of (deep infiltrating) endometriosis: the value of diffusion-weighted imaging. J Magn Reson Imaging 2010; 32(4):1003–9.
44. Outwater EK, Siegelman ES, Hunt JL. Ovarian teratomas: tumor types and imaging characteristics. Radiographics 2001;21(2):475–90.
45. Comerci JT Jr, Licciardi F, Bergh PA, et al. Mature cystic teratoma: a clinicopathologic evaluation of 517 cases and review of the literature. Obstet Gynecol 1994;84(1):22–8.
46. Park SB, Cho KS, Kim JK. CT findings of mature cystic teratoma with malignant transformation: comparison with mature cystic teratoma. Clin Imaging 2011;35(4):294–300.
47. Koonings PP, Campbell K, Mishell DR Jr, et al. Relative frequency of primary ovarian neoplasms: a 10-year review. Obstet Gynecol 1989;74(6):921–6.
48. Troiano RN, Lazzarini KM, Scoutt LM, et al. Fibroma and fibrothecoma of the ovary: MR imaging findings. Radiology 1997;204(3):795–8.
49. Jung SE, Lee JM, Rha SE, et al. CT and MR imaging of ovarian tumors with emphasis on differential diagnosis. Radiographics 2002;22(6):1305–25.
50. Shinagare AB, Meylaerts LJ, Laury AR, et al. MRI features of ovarian fibroma and fibrothecoma with histopathologic correlation. AJR Am J Roentgenol 2012;198(3):W296–303.
51. Reinhold C, Tafazoli F, Mehio A, et al. Uterine adenomyosis: endovaginal US and MR imaging features with histopathologic correlation. Radiographics 1999;19 Spec No:S147–60.
52. Tamai K, Togashi K, Ito T, et al. MR imaging findings of adenomyosis: correlation with histopathologic features and diagnostic pitfalls. Radiographics 2005;25(1):21–40.
53. Hall T, Lee SI, Boruta DM, et al. Medical device safety and surgical dissemination of unrecognized uterine malignancy: morcellation in minimally invasive gynecologic surgery. oncologist 2015;20(11): 1274–82.

54. Pickhardt PJ, Levy AD, Rohrmann CA Jr, et al. Primary neoplasms of the appendix: radiologic spectrum of disease with pathologic correlation. Radiographics 2003;23(3):645–62.
55. Reed JC, Hallet KK, Feigin DS. Neural tumors of the thorax: subject review from the AFIP. Radiology 1978;126(1):9–17.
56. Jain KA. Imaging of peritoneal inclusion cysts. AJR Am J Roentgenol 2000;174(6):1559–63.
57. Benjaminov O, Atri M. Sonography of the abnormal fallopian tube. AJR Am J Roentgenol 2004;183(3):737–42.
58. Kim MY, Rha SE, Oh SN, et al. MR imaging findings of hydrosalpinx: a comprehensive review. Radiographics 2009;29(2):495–507.
59. McCluggage WG. Morphological subtypes of ovarian carcinoma: a review with emphasis on new developments and pathogenesis. Pathology 2011;43(5):420–32.
60. Koshiyama M, Matsumura N, Konishi I. Recent concepts of ovarian carcinogenesis: type I and type II. Biomed Res Int 2014;2014:934261.
61. Nezhat FR, Apostol R, Nezhat C, et al. New insights in the pathophysiology of ovarian cancer and implications for screening and prevention. Am J Obstet Gynecol 2015;213(3):262–7.
62. Nik NN, Vang R, Shih le M, et al. Origin and pathogenesis of pelvic (ovarian, tubal, and primary peritoneal) serous carcinoma. Annu Rev Pathol 2014;9:27–45.
63. Seidman JD, Horkayne-Szakaly I, Haiba M, et al. The histologic type and stage distribution of ovarian carcinomas of surface epithelial origin. Int J Gynecol Pathol 2004;23(1):41–4.
64. Salvador S, Gilks B, Kobel M, et al. The fallopian tube: primary site of most pelvic high-grade serous carcinomas. Int J Gynecol Cancer 2009;19(1):58–64.
65. van Nagell JR Jr, DePriest PD, Reedy MB, et al. The efficacy of transvaginal sonographic screening in asymptomatic women at risk for ovarian cancer. Gynecol Oncol 2000;77(3):350–6.
66. Low JJ, Ilancheran A, Ng JS. Malignant ovarian germ-cell tumours. Best practice & research. Clin Obstet Gynaecol 2012;26(3):347–55.
67. Kim SH, Kim SH. Granulosa cell tumor of the ovary: common findings and unusual appearances on CT and MR. J Comput Assist Tomogr 2002;26(5):756–61.
68. Jung SE, Rha SE, Lee JM, et al. CT and MRI findings of sex cord-stromal tumor of the ovary. AJR Am J Roentgenol 2005;185(1):207–15.
69. Lee WL, Yuan CC, Lai CR, et al. Hemoperitoneum is an initial presentation of recurrent granulosa cell tumors of the ovary. Jpn J Clin Oncol 1999;29(10):509–12.
70. Sherman ME, Mink PJ, Curtis R, et al. Survival among women with borderline ovarian tumors and ovarian carcinoma: a population-based analysis. Cancer 2004;100(5):1045–52.
71. Tanaka YO, Okada S, Yagi T, et al. MRI of endometriotic cysts in association with ovarian carcinoma. AJR Am J Roentgenol 2010;194(2):355–61.
72. Thomassin-Naggara I, Darai E, Cuenod CA, et al. Dynamic contrast-enhanced magnetic resonance imaging: a useful tool for characterizing ovarian epithelial tumors. J Magn Reson Imaging 2008;28(1):111–20.
73. McDermott S, Oei TN, Iyer VR, et al. MR imaging of malignancies arising in endometriomas and extraovarian endometriosis. Radiographics 2012;32(3):845–63.
74. American College of Obstetricians and Gynecologists Committee on Gynecologic Practice. Committee Opinion No. 477: the role of the obstetrician-gynecologist in the early detection of epithelial ovarian cancer. Obstet Gynecol 2011;117(3):742–6.
75. Leiserowitz GS, Gumbs JL, Oi R, et al. Endometriosis-related malignancies. Int J Gynecol Cancer 2003;13(4):466–71.
76. Classic pages in obstetrics and gynecology. Joe Vincent Meigs and John W. Cass. Fibroma of the ovary with ascites and hydrothorax. With a report of seven cases. Am J Obstet Gynecol 1971;111(7):993.

MR Imaging–Pathologic Correlation in Ovarian Cancer

Erica B. Stein, MD[a,b,*], Ashish P. Wasnik, MD[a], Andrew P. Sciallis, MD[c], Aya Kamaya, MD[d], Katherine E. Maturen, MD, MS[a,e]

KEYWORDS

- Ovarian neoplasm • Ovarian cyst • Epithelial ovarian neoplasms
- Serous tubal intraepithelial carcinoma (STIC) • Ovarian germ cell tumor • Sex cord–stromal tumors
- Magnetic resonance imaging

KEY POINTS

- Multiparametric MR imaging can assist in differentiating subtypes of ovarian cancer.
- Very low T2-weighted signal suggests low-grade or benign disorder.
- Macroscopic fat in a lesion suggests mature teratoma as the diagnosis.
- High-grade serous carcinoma of the ovary arises from a precursor in the fallopian tube mucosa, referred to as serous tubal intraepithelial carcinoma.

INTRODUCTION

The normal ovary contains epithelial, germ cell, and mesenchymal elements. Each of these cell types can undergo neoplasia, resulting in a wide variety of possible tumors arising from a single organ. More than 30 subtypes of ovarian neoplasm have been described. However, most are in one of 3 major categories: epithelial, germ cell, or stromal neoplasms. Some cell types give rise to benign and malignant neoplasms. This article primarily focuses on malignant neoplasms, with some discussion devoted to low-grade and benign ovarian masses.

Ovarian cancer may have nonspecific, subtle, or absent symptoms, and many lesions are detected incidentally. Thus, it is important to recognize concerning imaging features in all types of imaging studies. Ultrasonography has a primary role in adnexal mass detection, whereas MR imaging enables characterization of sonographically indeterminate masses.[1–3] Computed tomography (CT) and PET/CT do not have a primary role in lesion characterization, but are important for staging and follow-up of known ovarian cancer.

With advances in spatial and contrast resolution, and development of functional imaging techniques including perfusion and diffusion,[4] MR imaging has increasing capacity to distinguish benign from malignant adnexal lesions. This article focuses on MR imaging findings concerning for neoplasm, the gross and microscopic features differentiating the subtypes of ovarian malignancy, and correlation between these.

Disclosures: The authors have nothing to disclose.

[a] Department of Radiology, University of Michigan, 1500 East Medical Center Drive, Ann Arbor, MI 48109, USA; [b] Department of Radiology, University of Pittsburgh Medical Center, 200 Lothrop Street, Pittsburgh, PA 15213, USA; [c] Department of Pathology, University of Michigan, 1500 East Medical Center Drive, Ann Arbor, MI 48109, USA; [d] Department of Radiology, Stanford University, 300 Pasteur Drive, Stanford, CA 94305, USA; [e] Department of Obstetrics & Gynecology, University of Michigan, 1500 East Medical Center Drive, Ann Arbor, MI 48109, USA

* Corresponding author. Department of Radiology, University of Pittsburgh Medical Center, Pittsburgh, PA.
E-mail address: steineb@upmc.edu

Magn Reson Imaging Clin N Am 25 (2017) 545–562
http://dx.doi.org/10.1016/j.mric.2017.03.004

MAGNETIC RESONANCE PROTOCOL FOR ADNEXAL MASS CHARACTERIZATION

Imaging parameters at different institutions vary according to equipment and local preference, but the authors consider the following pulse sequences to be important in the evaluation of a suspected ovarian mass. Before imaging, glucagon or another antiperistaltic agent is beneficial in reducing artifact from bowel and uterine peristalsis.

- T1-weighted (T1W) images in the axial plane are obtained without and with fat saturation, to identify foci of macroscopic fat and differentiate them from hemorrhage. T1W chemical shift imaging using dual in-phase and opposed-phase gradient echo (GRE) sequences in the axial plane are useful for confirming the presence of intralesional lipid and macroscopic fat.
- T2-weighted (T2W) images in the axial, sagittal, and coronal planes are obtained without fat saturation. Multiplanar T2W imaging (T2WI) is essential for optimizing tissue characterization and differentiating solid from cystic components. Alternatively, high-resolution single-plane T2WI can be performed as a three-dimensional acquisition, lengthening scan time but enabling isotropic multiplanar reformats. As discussed later, there is a small subset of adnexal masses that are intrinsically low signal on T2WI, which helps narrow the differential diagnosis.
- Multiphase or dynamic contrast-enhanced T1W images using gadolinium-based intravenous contrast agents are critical to evaluate vascularity of any soft tissue elements, including papillary projections, masses and nodules, or thick septations. Postcontrast imaging includes fat-saturated multiphase image acquisitions before contrast, during the arterial and venous phases, and in 1 or more delayed phases. Precontrast and postcontrast imaging should be performed with identical coverage and scan parameters to enable image subtraction, which is of particular importance in hemorrhagic lesions in which intrinsic hyperintensity on T1W imaging (T1WI) can mimic enhancement (**Fig. 1**). In some centers, a true dynamic acquisition through the area of interest is performed, using multiple short acquisitions (15 seconds) repeated over a period of 3 to 4 minutes and enabling visual and quantitative analysis of enhancement kinetics.[1,4,5]
- Diffusion-weighted imaging (DWI) performed at both low and high b values ($>b_{000}$) has some utility for characterization of adnexal masses, and is especially useful in the detection of drop metastases and peritoneal implants. Both omental cake and peritoneal deposits often retain high signal intensity at high b values, increasing the conspicuity of metastases.[5–8] Lymph nodes can also be more easily detected with the assistance of high-b-value DWI. Regarding the primary mass, there is substantial overlap in apparent diffusion coefficient (ADC) values between malignant and highly cellular benign lesions, with false-positives limiting the utility of quantitative comparison. However, there are some specific areas of utility. Fibrous masses with very low ADC values usually also show low signal on DWI, suggesting benignity. Further, masses with benign features on both ADC maps and DWI are most often benign, and demonstration of low DWI signal within a mass may augment diagnostic confidence when features on other sequences favor a benign process.[9]

EPITHELIAL OVARIAN TUMORS

Ovarian cancer is the fifth leading cause of cancer death in women,[10] and most ovarian neoplasms are epithelial in origin. Serous and mucinous histologies are the predominant epithelial subtypes, with serous carcinomas being the most common (60%) and associated with the highest mortality.[11,12]

Epithelial ovarian tumors can also be grouped into 2 broad categories based on genetic lineage: type I and type II. Type I tumors include low-grade serous carcinoma (LGSC), and low-grade endometrioid, clear cell, and mucinous carcinomas, all of which are slow growing and develop from well-established precursor lesions. In general, type I tumors present as large masses confined to the ovary, have an indolent course, and have a good prognosis.[13] In contrast, type II tumors tend to present at advanced stage with a poorer prognosis. Type II tumors include high-grade serous carcinoma (HGSC), high-grade endometrioid carcinoma, carcinosarcoma, and undifferentiated carcinomas. At a molecular level, type I tumors are fairly genetically stable, whereas type II tumors are highly unstable, with p53 mutations present in greater than 95% of cases.[13,14]

Serous Cystadenoma, Borderline Tumor, and Adenocarcinoma

Serous cystadenoma and cystadenofibroma are strictly benign lesions. They are usually smooth walled and unilocular with minimal papillary excrescences (**Fig. 2**). Serous borderline tumor,

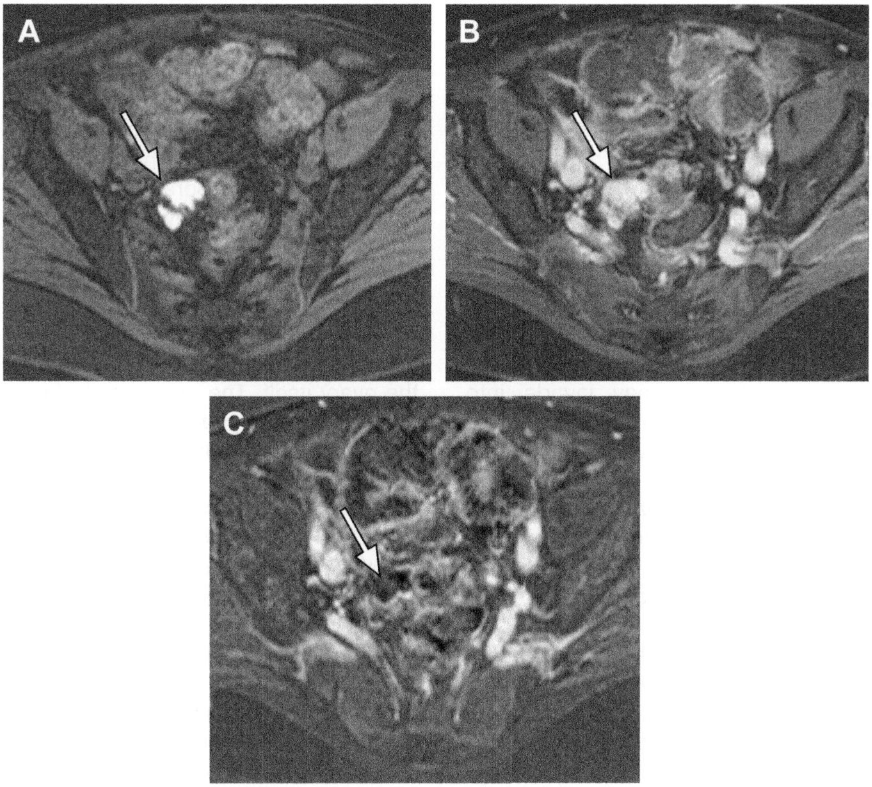

Fig. 1. A 74-year-old woman with long-standing endometrioma. MR imaging was ordered to evaluate for any evidence of neoplastic transformation. (*A*) Precontrast T1WI plus fat saturation (FS) shows a lobulated, very-high-signal right adnexal lesion (*arrow*) containing hemorrhagic products. (*B*) This area remains high signal (*arrow*) on postcontrast T1WI + FS and enhancement is difficult to evaluate. (*C*) Subtraction imaging shows a matched low-signal area (*arrow*), indicating lack of enhancement.

LGSC, and HGSC have increasing degrees of cytologic atypia, and, particularly in the case of HGSC, mitotic activity. The serous cells constituting each subtype closely resemble fallopian tube epithelium, and can contain numerous ciliated cells in cases of cystadenoma/cystadenofibroma, serous borderline tumor, and LGSC. Most frankly malignant serous tumors involve both ovaries pathologically, although 1 or both may be normal in size by imaging. These cancers are typically mixed cystic and solid, and the amount and complexity of the solid tissue correlates with risk of malignancy. Classic papillary architecture and psammomatous calcifications can be appreciated by imaging and under the microscope. These 3 subtypes are discussed later.

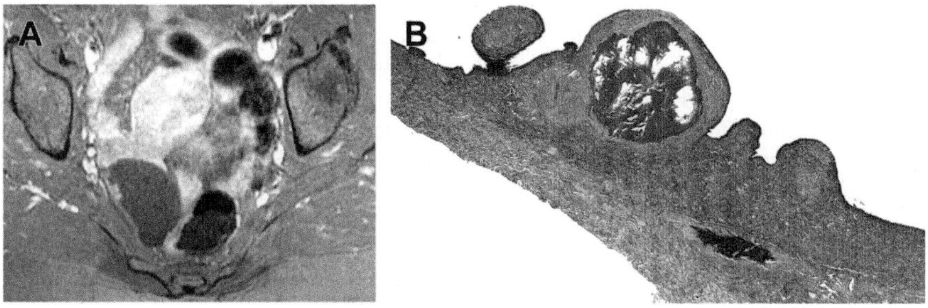

Fig. 2. A 54-year-old woman with benign serous cystadenoma. (*A*) Axial fat-saturated T1WI with contrast shows small enhancing mural nodules at the lateral aspect of an otherwise cystic right ovarian mass. (*B*) At pathologic examination, multiple small, noncomplex papillations were noted, some containing psammomatous calcifications such as this one. (hematoxylin-eosin, original magnification ×20).

Serous borderline tumors are thought to develop from neoplastic transformation of serous cystadenomas, usually through acquisition of either BRAF or KRAS mutations.[15] In general, these tumors are characterized by slow growth with overall excellent prognosis. These tumors usually form cysts containing intracystic excrescences that resemble broad-based papillary buds. These buds are often branched and are composed of fibrotic stroma lined by serous epithelium, subsets of which are ciliated. They can also form fine papillary soft tissue elements within cysts not supported by stromal buds. The serous epithelial cells may invade into ovarian stroma; however, the invasive areas are small and focal by definition (<5 mm in greatest dimension).[16] Although it was originally introduced as a provisional category between cystadenoma and carcinoma, "borderline" is now a formal pathologic designation rather than an indication of uncertainty.[17] Borderline serous carcinoma can manifest with peritoneal implants (**Fig. 3**) and metastatic lymphadenopathy in 35% and 27% of patients respectively.[18,19] Regardless, the 10-year survival of patients with serous borderline tumor remains high at 96% to 100%.[17]

The pathogenesis of LGSC is also unclear but cases may develop from serous borderline tumors. These tumors share similar pathologic and molecular features (eg, KRAS mutations) with serous borderline tumors, and tend to have a better prognosis than HGSC given their indolent growth, possibly secondary to lack of p53 mutations.[18] LGSC are well differentiated, frequently contain calcifications, and maintain a cystic and papillary architecture with little necrosis, evident both on MR imaging and gross pathologic examination. At imaging, these tumors are often large, complex, cystic masses with well-marginated septa and solid components, potentially distinguishable from HGSCs when contralateral masses, ascites, omental caking, and lymphadenopathy are absent.

Terminology regarding LGSC has historically been confusing because cases can closely resemble borderline tumors, and thus pathologic discrimination can be difficult. In general, LGSC is reserved for cases in which the primary tumor shows definitive stromal invasion (≥5 mm).[20] However, noninvasive forms of LGSC, characterized by areas of confluent epithelial growth (≥5 mm) but without stromal invasion, are also recognized by gynecologic pathologists. Pathologic terminology in these cases is especially confusing because the terms noninvasive LGSC and serous borderline tumor, micropapillary/cribriform variant, are regarded as equivalent. In addition, transformation of LGSC to HGSC is a very rare phenomenon.[21]

HGSC are type II tumors frequently associated with early p53 mutations. Although most BRCA-related hereditary ovarian cancers are HGSCs,[18] BRCA mutation carriers have a better prognosis than women with sporadic ovarian HGSCs.[17] In general, these are very aggressive tumors that often present at advanced stage with overall poor prognosis. It is now well established that HGSC of the ovary arises from a precursor in the fallopian tube mucosa, or at least tubal-type epithelium, rather than from low-grade lesions of the ovary itself. The precursor lesion in the fallopian tube is referred to as serous tubal intraepithelial carcinoma (STIC). Further supporting the connection, STIC is absent in nonserous ovarian carcinomas, such as mucinous and endometrioid types.[22,23] At imaging, HGSCs often appear as complex cystic masses with solid components (**Fig. 4**), but some are completely solid.[24] There is rapid intracoelomic spread, with peritoneal and multiorgan surface involvement sometimes even in the context of normal-sized or minimally enlarged ovaries. The origin of HGSC in the fallopian tube could help explain the high incidence of peritoneal disease at time of diagnosis.

Mucinous Cystadenoma, Borderline Tumor, and Adenocarcinoma

In contrast with the bimodal lineage of serous tumors, ovarian mucinous neoplasms probably progress sequentially from cystadenoma, to borderline, to carcinoma. This process has been theorized given the presence of adenoma, borderline, and carcinomatous components in cases of mucinous carcinoma, as well as identical KRAS mutations in each component.[25] Overall, mucinous neoplasms are the second most common ovarian epithelial neoplasm. On histology, most mucinous neoplasms are benign or borderline (80%), with carcinoma representing a small fraction.[17] In contrast with serous tumors, which are commonly bilateral, most ovarian mucinous tumors are unilateral. These tumors may attain a very large size while remaining benign.

Mucinous cystadenoma is predominantly cystic at imaging, unilocular, multilocular, or with multiple thin, smooth septations (**Fig. 5**). On histology, the epithelial cells lining the cysts comprise a population of well-differentiated mucinous cells arranged in a simple, nonstratified pattern. There is some variation in the appearance in the epithelial cells, with some resembling colorectal mucosa (including goblet cells), small intestine (sometimes featuring Paneth cells), or upper gastrointestinal

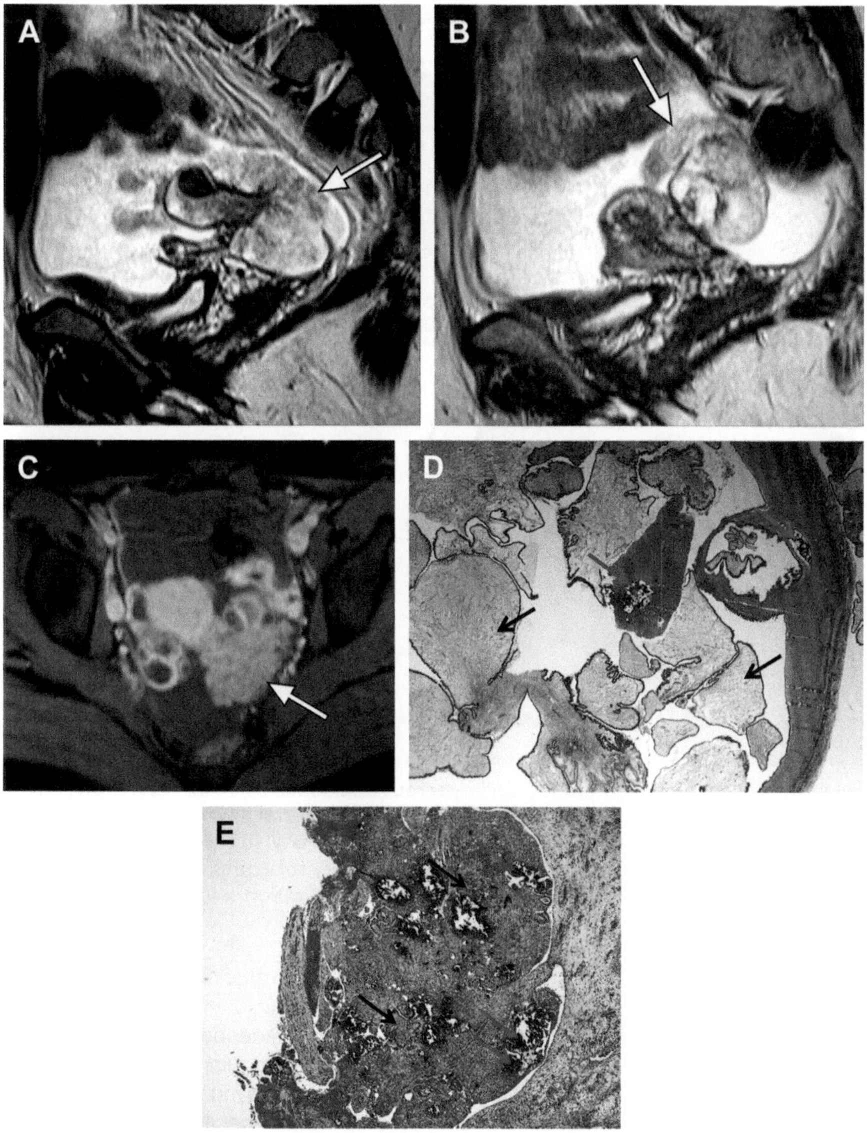

Fig. 3. A 24-year-old woman with serous borderline tumor and noninvasive peritoneal implants. (*A, B*) Sagittal T2WI shows ascites, exophytic but orderly papillary soft tissue arising from the left ovary (*arrow, A*), and a small amount of abnormal soft tissue adherent to the right ovary (*arrow, B*). (*C*) Postcontrast imaging confirms enhancement (*arrow*). (*D*) There are multiple fibrotic intracystic papillations (*black arrows*) within a cyst. These excrescences are lined by cells resembling fallopian tube epithelium. Calcifications are common (*red arrows*). (hematoxylin-eosin, original magnification ×20). (*E*) Extraovarian implants took the form of noninvasive nodules that appeared to be stuck on to the peritoneal surfaces, with internal nodular excrescences (*black arrows*) identical to the primary tumor. Calcifications are also present (*red arrows*). (hematoxylin-eosin, original magnification ×40).

pyloric mucosa. It had been thought that ovarian mucinous cystadenomas could also contain endocervical-type (müllerian) mucinous epithelium, but it is likely that these are mucinous cells of an upper gastrointestinal phenotype mimicking endocervical epithelium. Seromucinous ovarian neoplasms are likely to be fundamentally different from mucinous cystadenomas, because the former often arise in a background of endometriosis, which is an uncommon phenomenon in ovarian mucinous tumors.[26] Mucinous borderline tumors are usually large, with smooth capsules and no grossly evident papillations/excrescences. As such, they are likely to be indistinguishable from mucinous cystadenoma by imaging, because both tumors may be multicystic and large. Microscopically, mucinous borderline tumors are also composed of gastrointestinal-type epithelium,

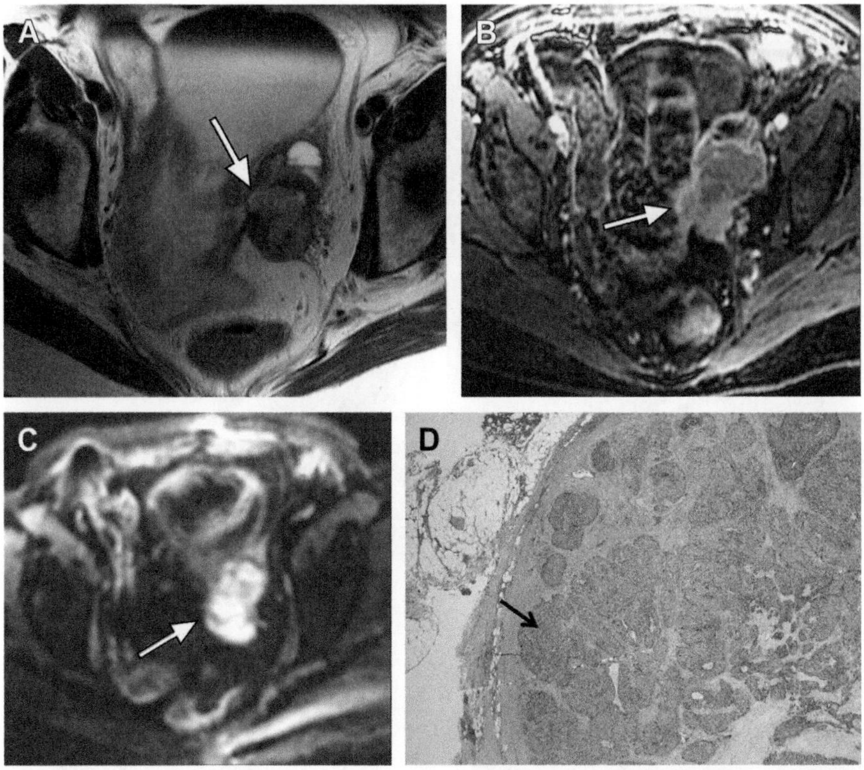

Fig. 4. A 74-year-old woman with high-grade papillary serous carcinoma. (*A*) Axial T2WI shows an irregular mass with substantial solid components (*arrow*) in the left pelvis. (*B*) Postcontrast T1WI shows enhancement of most of the mass as well as direct involvement of adjacent sigmoid (*arrow*). (*C*) DWI (b = 800) shows high signal within the mass. (*D*) Although high-grade serous carcinoma can form papillary structures, it can also form dense nodules with rare papillae (*black arrow*). (hematoxylin-eosin, original magnification ×40).

usually with a colorectal or intestinal appearance. The pathologic diagnosis of mucinous borderline tumor is rendered when proliferative areas comprise greater than 10% of the epithelial volume[27]; compared with mucinous cystadenoma, borderline tumors have a greater amount of the epithelial component, which manifests as closely packed cells with architectural complexity (microscopic tufting). Similarly, mucinous borderline tumors also tend to show a greater degree of cytologic atypia compared with cystadenomas. Mucinous borderline tumors can show striking nuclear atypia to the point at which there is intraepithelial carcinoma (mucinous borderline tumor with intraepithelial carcinoma), and microinvasion may also be present (by definition, the invasive foci must be small, measuring <5 mm in greatest linear extent). The long-term disease-related survival nears 100%, even in patients with intraepithelial carcinoma, because older descriptions of so-called invasive mucinous borderline tumors are now thought to most likely represent metastases from the gastrointestinal tract. There are insufficient data regarding the behavior of mucinous borderline tumors with microinvasion.

Mucinous adenocarcinoma is also cystic, but shows thick, nodular septa. Historically, the prevalence of invasive mucinous tumors was significantly overestimated, because mucinous gastrointestinal metastases to the ovary are now known to be much more common than primary mucinous ovarian carcinoma.[17,28] Classically, metastases are usually bilateral, whereas primary invasive mucinous cancer is usually unilateral. However, metastases can present clinically as a unilateral ovarian mass with bilateral involvement only encountered microscopically. In contrast with benign mucinous tumors, cystadenocarcinoma shows frank ovarian stromal invasion microscopically. Metastatic tumors to the ovary are usually smaller than primary ovarian tumors but, similarly to laterality, the range of size in metastatic cases is broad and overlaps with primary ovarian tumors.[29] Gross or radiographic ovarian surface involvement and presence of extraovarian disease (including clinical pseudomyxoma peritonei [PMP]) at presentation should also prompt

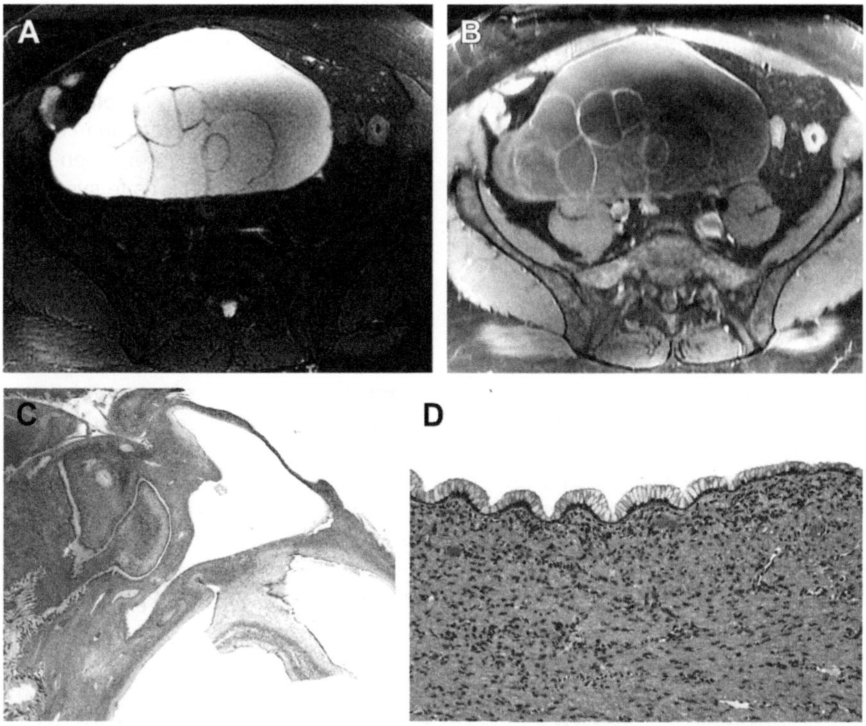

Fig. 5. A 55-year-old woman with mucinous cystadenoma. (*A*) T2WI + FS shows a dominant cystic mass in central pelvis with multiple thin, smooth septations. (*B*) Postcontrast T1WI + FS shows enhancement of these fine septations, but no nodular elements. (*C*) Low-power image shows a multilocular cystic tumor with thin septations. (hematoxylin-eosin, original magnification ×20). (*D*) Higher-power image shows a thin, bland, mucinous epithelium with no nuclear atypia. (hematoxylin-eosin, original magnification ×100).

investigation for a nongynecologic primary. Primary ovarian mucinous adenocarcinomas are characterized by destructive stromal invasion (>5 mm) and/or expansile epithelial growth, the latter defined by confluent glands with little intervening stroma. Mucinous adenocarcinoma may also show mural nodules grossly and radiographically characterized by solid growths arising adjacent to or within cysts. Microscopically, these mural nodules often manifest as an infiltrative proliferation of poorly-differentiated carcinoma cells (anaplastic carcinoma) or cells resembling a sarcoma (sarcomalike mural nodule). All 3 patterns may exist in the same tumor, and all carry a risk for recurrence.[30] The pattern of spread differs from serous cancer, because there is less transcoelomic growth along the peritoneal surfaces.[17] Instead, invasive mucinous cancers tend to invade into the abdominal wall and metastasize to solid organs (liver and spleen). PMP is a clinical term for a specific type of intraperitoneal disease that is usually secondary to a nongynecologic mucinous tumor (eg, metastatic appendiceal mucinous neoplasm).[31,32] Cases of PMP may manifest as abundant extracellular mucin with a minority of bland gastrointestinal-type epithelial cells, and symptoms are usually related to tumor bulk.

Endometrioid Ovarian Carcinoma

Endometrioid ovarian cancer is associated with long-standing endometriosis, and endometriomas and endometriotic cysts are probably its benign precursors. After serous carcinoma, endometrioid is the second most common type of ovarian carcinoma, although mucinous tumors (usually benign) are more common overall. The risk of malignancy is proportional to size of endometriotic deposit and patient age. In some series, endometriosis in the same ovary or elsewhere in the pelvis is observed in up to 42% of cases.[33] Endometrioid ovarian adenocarcinoma is associated with microsatellite instability, usually via loss of MLJ1 or MLH2 expression, and can be seen in patients with Lynch syndrome.[34,35]

Endometrioid neoplasms of the ovary also follow a benign, borderline, and malignant subclassification scheme. Specifically, these include endometrioid adenofibroma, atypical proliferative (borderline) endometrioid tumor, and endometrioid adenocarcinoma. Because of its clear association with endometriosis, there are various other lesions that, although not representative of outright carcinoma, are atypical enough to earn designations as atypical endometriosis. This term has been used in endometriotic cysts lined by cytologically atypical cells, as well as cases of endometriosis with features identical to those seen in atypical endometrial hyperplasia. Endometrioid adenocarcinoma is usually a smooth-walled, multiseptate cystic mass containing blood products, variable amounts of fibrotic stroma, and friable soft tissue elements on gross examination that manifest on MR imaging as enhancing intracystic soft tissue components (**Fig. 6**). Thus, it is important to carefully assess for the presence of enhancement within all endometriomas. Microscopically, these tumors closely resemble their counterparts in the endometrium. Most of these tumors are low grade, resembling FIGO (International Federation of Gynecology and Obstetrics) grade 1 endometrial endometrioid adenocarcinoma; however, grading of endometrioid ovarian carcinoma is controversial. Although these tumors are histologically malignant, most present as early-stage unilateral tumors confined to the ovary without extraovarian disease.

Approximately 40% of women with endometrioid ovarian carcinoma have synchronous endometrial hyperplasia and approximately 15% to 20% present with concurrent endometrial carcinoma.[17,36] Differentiating ovarian metastasis from an endometrial primary versus synchronous primaries can be difficult. Often, pathologic features such as the depth of invasion in the endometrial primary, grade of the endometrial tumor, size of the ovarian lesion (larger ovarian tumors at presentation are thought to be more indicative of a synchronous primary rather than metastasis), presence of endometriosis in the ovarian tumor, presence of pelvic or lymph node disease (pelvic disease is more indicative of metastasis of an endometrial primary), and presence of lymphovascular space invasion in the uterus can help

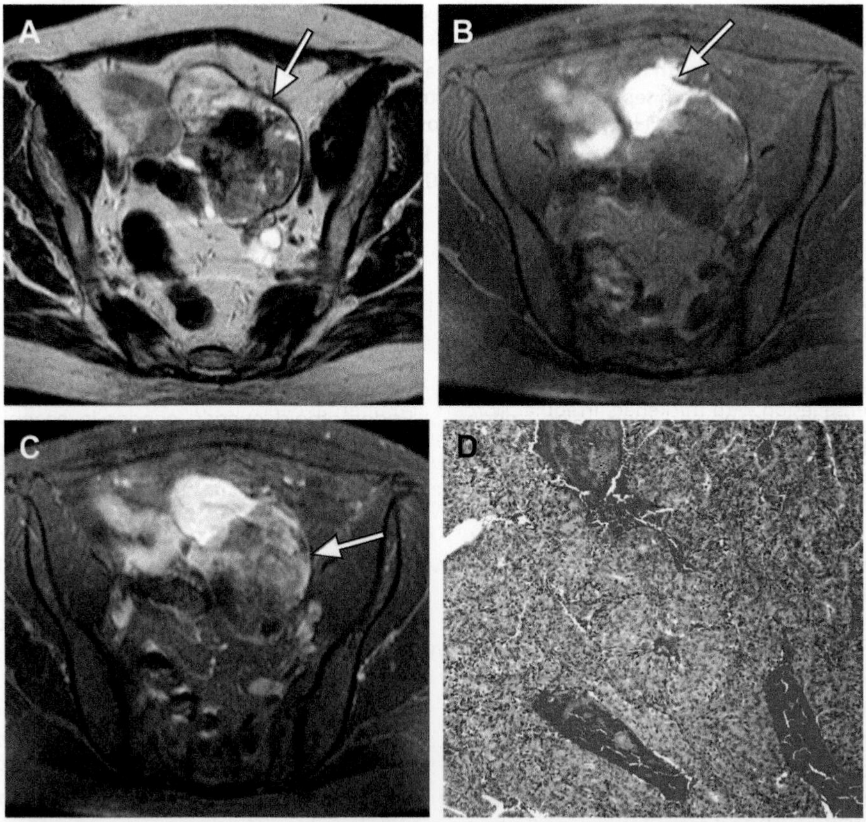

Fig. 6. A 57-year-old with endometrioid ovarian cancer arising in endometriosis. (*A*) T2WI shows a well-circumscribed cystic mass with hemosiderin rim (*arrow*) and large internal solid component. (*B*) The anterior cystic component of the mass is very high signal (*arrow*) on precontrast T1WI because of blood products. (*C*) The posterior solid component enhances heterogeneously (*arrow*) on postcontrast T1WI. (*D*) Microscopic image reveals cords of tissue forming endometrial-type glands, interspersed with large vascular spaces. (hematoxylin-eosin, original magnification ×100).

reconcile this issue. However, some cases may still pose a diagnostic dilemma, even with molecular genetics, because endometrioid tumors of the ovary and endometrium share many similar molecular abnormalities. For radiologists, it is important to evaluate the endometrial stripe in all patients with ovarian cancer given the associations with hyperplasia and carcinoma (**Fig. 7**).

Clear Cell Ovarian Carcinoma

Like endometrioid ovarian cancer, clear cell carcinoma of the ovary is also associated with endometriosis. It almost always manifests as a carcinoma, and borderline tumors (clear cell borderline tumor) are very rare. Clear cell carcinoma of the ovary usually presents with disease confined to the ovary. The imaging appearance is usually cystic, often with coexisting endometriosis; however, some manifest grossly and radiographically as solid masses. On histology, these tumors are characterized by glycogen-containing clear cells and so-called hobnail cells with various architectural patterns, including tubulocystic, solid, and papillary, either arising within a cyst or as an adenofibromatous mass.[24]

Brenner (Transitional Cell) Tumor

Overall, transitional cell tumors constitute up to 10% of ovarian epithelial tumors, almost all of which are benign.[17] The name arises from the histologic resemblance to urothelium; however, despite the appearance, the epithelium likely represents a metaplastic transformation of müllerian epithelium. Most are small, solid, fibrous, and incidentally detected at imaging. The gross appearance is a well-circumscribed solid mass with correlative MR features of low signal on T2WI and DWI (**Fig. 8**). The rare high-grade variant is both solid and cystic, and behaves much like a high-grade serous tumor. Malignant Brenner tumors are rare, and although patients with disease confined to the ovary have an excellent prognosis, studies of cases with extraovarian disease are lacking.[37]

Mixed Epithelial Tumor

Many carcinomas show areas of varying morphology but are named according to the dominant pattern; for example, a serous carcinoma with clear cell features. However, when 2 or more epithelial cell types each make up 10% of the total tumor volume, it is designated a mixed epithelial tumor. Epithelial cancers with mixed histology are treated according to the most aggressive cell type unless it constitutes only a very small percentage of the whole. This degree of microscopic nuance is beyond the capacity of MR imaging to capture, and these tumors present as mixed cystic and solid lesions like other epithelial carcinomas.

Carcinosarcoma (Malignant Mixed Mesodermal/Müllerian Tumor)

Ovarian carcinosarcoma is rare, accounting for 1% to 2% of ovarian epithelial malignancies. It is pathologically identical to uterine carcinosarcoma, and is characterized by an often haphazard mixture of epithelial and sarcomatoid components. The epithelial component tends to manifest as HGSC but other histologic types can be seen. The sarcomatoid component is classified as homologous when it has a nonspecific sarcomalike spindle cell appearance lacking morphologic

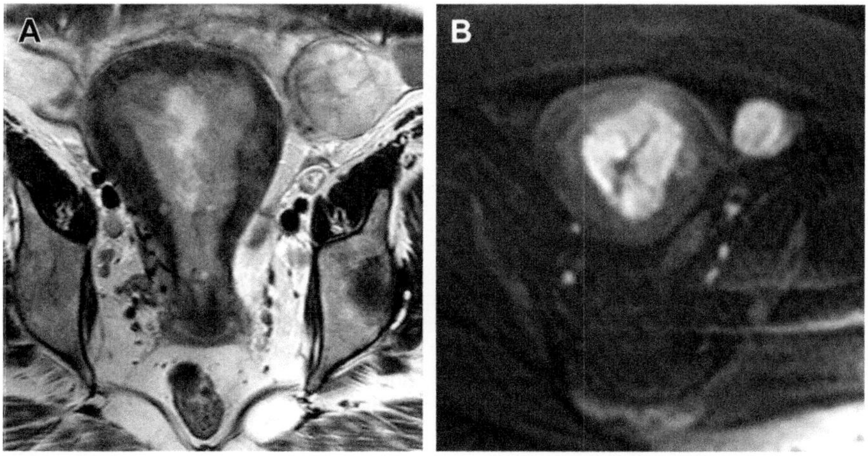

Fig. 7. A 48-year-old woman with synchronous endometrioid ovarian carcinoma and endometrioid endometrial carcinoma. The endometrial mass (and right obturator node) and left ovarian mass show identical imaging features: (*A*) intermediate signal intensity between normal endometrium and myometrium on T2WI, and (*B*) high signal on DWI.

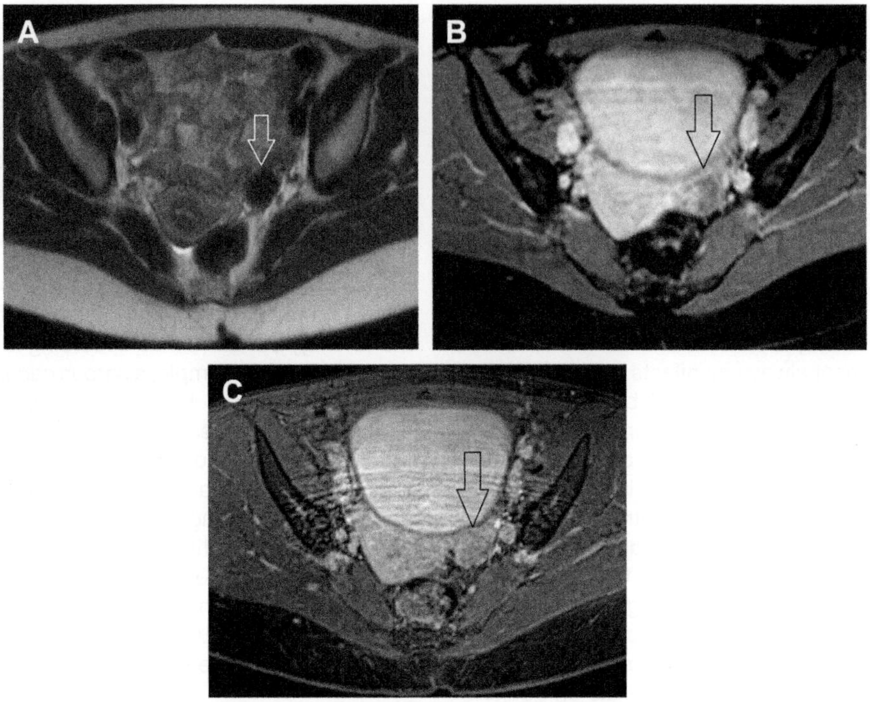

Fig. 8. A 48-year-old woman with incidentally detected Brenner tumor. (*A*) Axial T2WI shows a rounded mass in the left adnexa (*arrow*) that shows homogeneous low signal. (*B*) Axial T1WI postcontrast shows enhancement of the left adnexal mass (*arrow*). (*C*) Axial T1WI delayed postcontrast shows progressive accumulation of contrast in the left adnexal mass (*arrow*).

features of a particular line of differentiation, or heterologous when there is skeletal muscle (rhabdomyosarcomatous), cartilaginous (chondrosarcomatous), bone (osteosarcomatous), or other lines of differentiation.[38] Ovarian carcinosarcomas often present as large masses (15–20 cm) with extraovarian disease. The relative amount of carcinomatous and sarcomatoid components can vary considerably, and some cases show focal sarcomatoid areas, whereas others have only a few epithelial structures. This variability can render pathologic classification difficult, because carcinosarcoma is considered fundamentally a high-grade carcinoma rather than sarcoma, and thus would have therapeutic ramifications.[39] Imaging may show complex masses with mixed internal signal characteristics (**Fig. 9**), but there are few specific or distinctive features.

GERM CELL OVARIAN TUMORS

Malignant ovarian germ cell tumors (GCTs) tend to arise in younger women than do ovarian epithelial carcinomas. Some grow very rapidly and many elaborate serum tumor markers such as alpha-fetoprotein (αFP) and human chorionic gonadotropin (hCG) that are helpful for both diagnosis and monitoring. In contrast with the cyst with mural nodule morphology typical of the epithelial category, GCTs often show solid components with elements of hemorrhage and necrosis. However, with the exception of fat in teratomas, there are few specific MR imaging features enabling distinction between the tumor cell types within the GCT category.

Dysgerminoma

Dysgerminoma is the most common malignant ovarian GCT. It is considered the ovarian equivalent of testicular seminoma and can sometimes be associated with gonadal dysgenesis. There is usually no increase in αFP level and hCG level is rarely increased. Dysgerminomas occur bilaterally in 10% to 15% of cases and may metastasize to retroperitoneal lymph nodes.[40] At gross inspection, the tumor is often well encapsulated, solid, and large; mean diameter is 15 cm. When sectioned, the tissue is lobulated, soft, fleshy, and white to tan in color.[41,42] There may be foci of necrosis, calcifications, or hemorrhage, with or without cystic changes. At histology, the tumor cells are separated by fibrous or fibrovascular septa often containing mature lymphocytes.

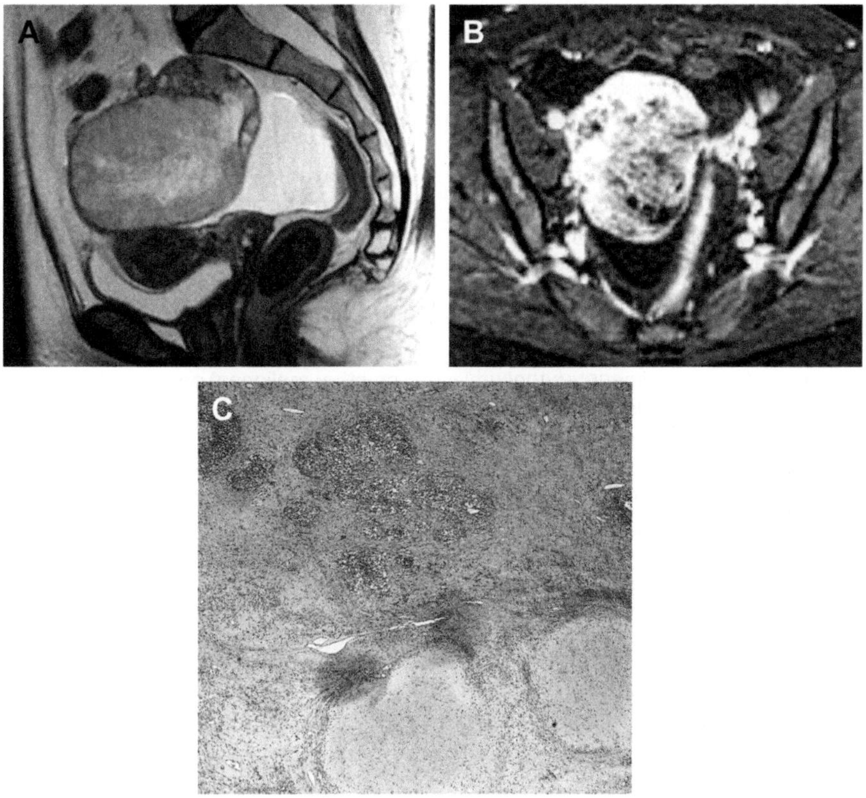

Fig. 9. A 58-year-old woman with carcinosarcoma (also called malignant mixed mesodermal tumor). (*A*) Sagittal T2WI shows minimally complex ascites and a large intermediate-signal mass extending inferiorly from the intact right ovary. (*B*) Postcontrast T1WI confirms heterogeneous enhancement of this mass. (*C*) Microscopic image reveals a biphasic mass with epithelial elements (purple glandular structures) in the upper half of the image and mesenchymal elements, including cartilage, in the lower half of the image. (hematoxylin-eosin, original magnification ×40).

Accordingly, the characteristic imaging appearance is a multilobulated solid mass with prominent fibrovascular septa. At MR, the septa appear as hypointense lines at T2WI and may show postcontrast enhancement. The solid component often shows low signal on T1WI relative to muscle and is isointense or slightly hyperintense on T2WI.[41,43,44] The necrosis, calcifications, hemorrhage, and cystic changes that can be seen at gross inspection are also commonly seen at MR.

Yolk Sac Tumor (Endodermal Sinus Tumor)

The second most common ovarian germ cell tumor, yolk sac tumor is notable for its very rapid growth and early spread to the abdominopelvic cavity. Yolk sac tumor is often associated with increased αFP. At gross inspection, the tumors often have mixed solid and cystic components. The solid component is soft gray to yellow, with areas of hemorrhage and necrosis. The cystic components are typically diffusely scattered throughout the tumor, giving it a honeycombed/meshlike appearance.[41] Like its testicular counterpart, ovarian yolk sac tumor can show a variety of microscopic appearances, the most common of which is proliferation of cells with clear cytoplasm arranged in a loose, microcystic network with numerous blood vessels. It is a notorious mimic of other ovarian tumors, particularly clear cell carcinoma. The tumors are usually pure but can coexist with other germ cell components (including teratoma). Increased incidence of capsular tears has been observed with yolk sac tumors both at surgery and pathology, possibly owing to the very rapid growth rate.

At MR, tumors are typically large and unilateral, containing enhancing solid components and cystic components. Foci of internal hemorrhage and necrosis may be present. The imaging features are not particularly specific, but radiologists should consider a yolk sac tumor in a younger woman with a unilateral predominantly solid ovarian mass and increased serum αFP level.

Immature Teratoma

Immature teratoma is the third most common malignant ovarian GCT, but only constitutes 1% of all teratomas. The peak incidence is in the teen years, with median age of presentation 17 years. Malignant degeneration of a mature cystic teratoma is very rare (<1%) and peaks at age 60 to 70 years.[41] Serum markers are usually negative, but increased αFP level has been reported.[42] Like mature cystic teratomas, immature teratomas contain 2 to 3 embryonic layers, but with primitive elements intermixed. The primitive elements usually manifest as variable amounts of immature neuroepithelium. Grading of these tumors depends on the amount of the immature component, with grade 1 tumors containing only rare foci and grade 3 tumors showing large amounts occupying greater than 3 low-power (40×) fields.[45] These tumors tend to be unilateral and large. At MR, they often appear as a heterogeneous mass with predominantly solid or mixed solid and cystic lesions (**Fig. 10**). Foci of macroscopic fat and calcifications are common.

Embryonal Tumor

This rare tumor generally presents in children and adolescents. The tumor is generally unilateral, large, and predominantly solid.[41] Both αFP and hCG levels can be increased. At gross pathology and MR imaging, the average size is 17 cm, with extensive areas of hemorrhage and necrosis and cystic spaces containing mucoid material (**Fig. 11**). The tumors tend to have a smooth outer surface. At histology, the tumor comprises a proliferation of high-grade, poorly differentiated cells with epithelial differentiation. The tumor is rarely pure and often appears mixed with other malignant germ cell types.[42]

Choriocarcinoma

Non gestational choriocarcinoma is rare and has a worse prognosis than malignant gestational trophoblastic disease (GTD). Like benign GTD, choriocarcinoma is associated with increased hCG level. At microscopy, a mixture of multinucleated syncytiotrophoblastic and mononuclear

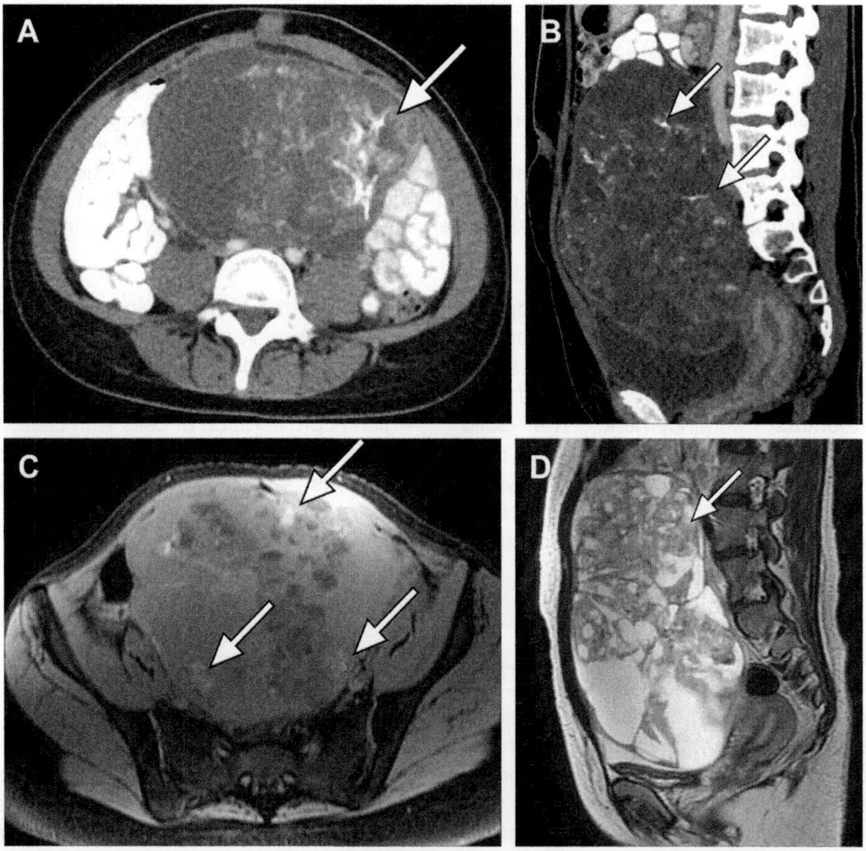

Fig. 10. A 24-year-old woman with immature teratoma, who presented with abdominal swelling and bilateral hydronephrosis. (*A*) Axial contrast-enhanced CT (CECT) shows a large partially cystic mass with calcifications (*arrow*). (*B*) Sagittal CECT confirms the large size and calcifications (*arrows*). (*C*) Axial precontrast T1WI shows minimal hemorrhage (*arrows*). (*D*) Sagittal T2WI shows a large mass with cystic and solid (*arrow*) elements.

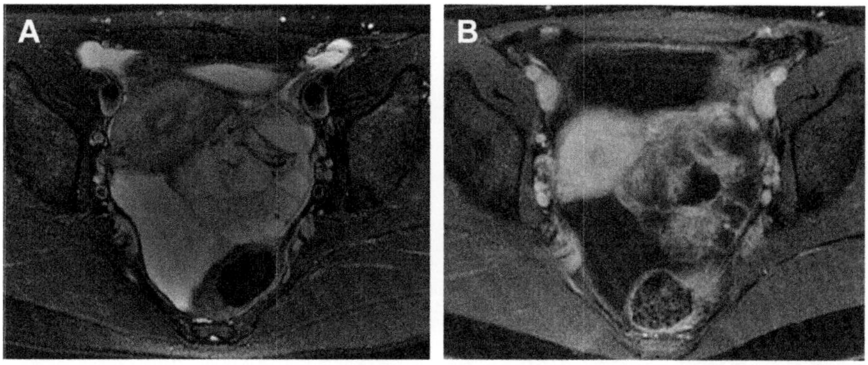

Fig. 11. A 25-year-old woman with embryonal tumor of left ovary. (*A*) Axial T2WI shows pelvic ascites and a multiloculated mass with some low-signal linear areas suggesting hemosiderin from prior hemorrhage. (*B*) Axial T1WI postcontrast shows enhancement of thick, irregular septa.

cytotrophoblastic cells surrounding hemorrhage is the most common appearance.[41] The presence of the mononuclear cytotrophoblastic component is vital to diagnosis, because scattered syncytiotrophoblastic cells can be seen in other nonchoriocarcinomatous GCTs, such as dysgerminoma. At cross-sectional imaging, nongestational choriocarcinoma is often a highly vascular

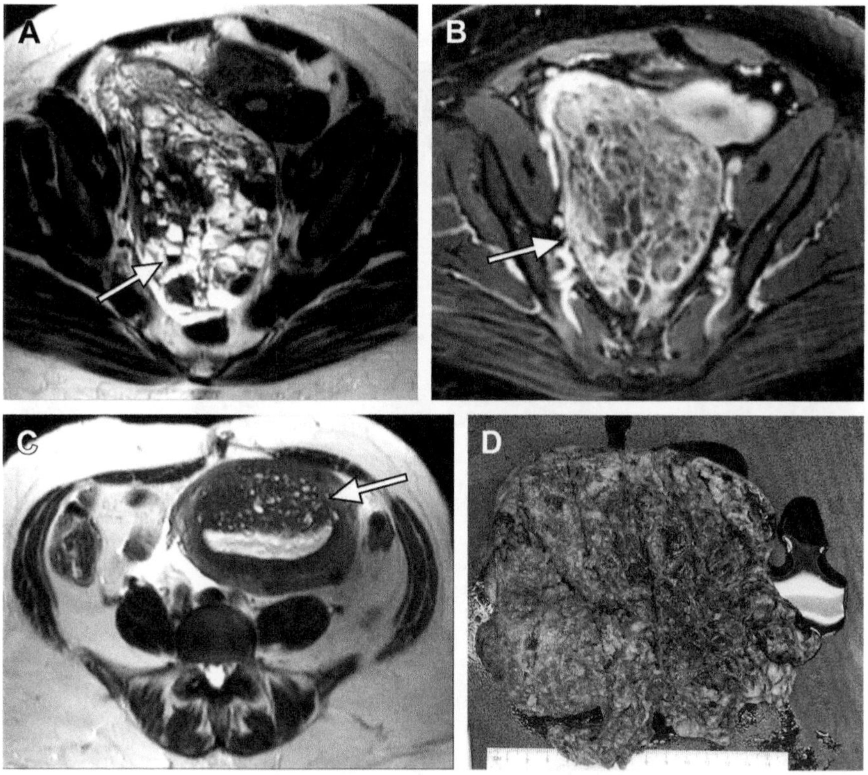

Fig. 12. A 50-year-old woman with adult granulosa tumor, adenomyosis, and endometrial hyperplasia. (*A*) Axial T2WI through the ovarian mass shows innumerable cystic spaces, some with layering blood products (*arrow*). (*B*) Postcontrast T1WI shows spongiform enhancement. (*C*) Axial T2WI through the enlarged uterus shows marked asymmetric thickening of anterior myometrium with multiple tiny subendometrial cysts, compatible with adenomyosis. This finding and the accompanying endometrial hyperplasia noted at pathology are likely attributable to the high levels of estrogen secreted by the granulosa cell tumor and the frequent presentation of vaginal bleeding. (*D*) Gross specimen (bivalved ovary) has multiple blood-filled cysts, in correlation with the MR appearance.

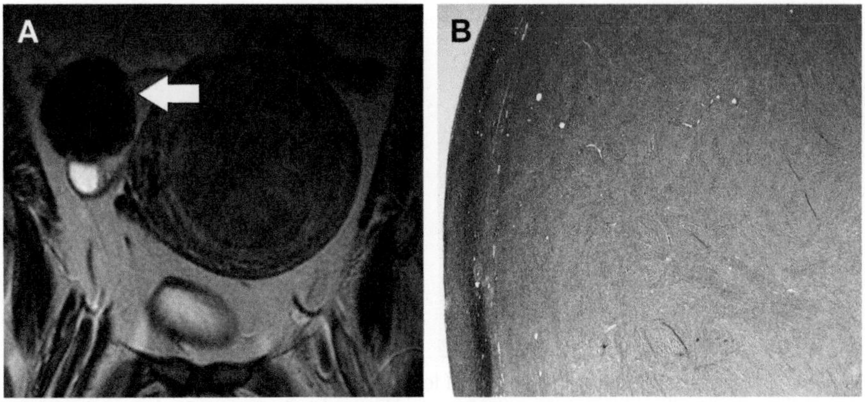

Fig. 13. A 55-year-old woman with both a right ovarian fibroma and a fibroid uterus. (*A*) Coronal T2WI shows a very-low-signal, well-circumscribed right ovarian mass (*arrow*) and an enlarged uterus with intermediate to low signal intensity. (*B*) Microscopic image shows a solid, circumscribed mass with a storiform architecture. (hematoxylin-eosin, original magnification ×20).

solid mass. At MR, signal voids at T2WI may be seen, representing vascular structures. Central cystic cavities and/or hemorrhage may also be present.

Mixed Germ Cell Tumor

Mixed GCTs are much less common in the ovary than in the testis. Dysgerminoma and yolk sac

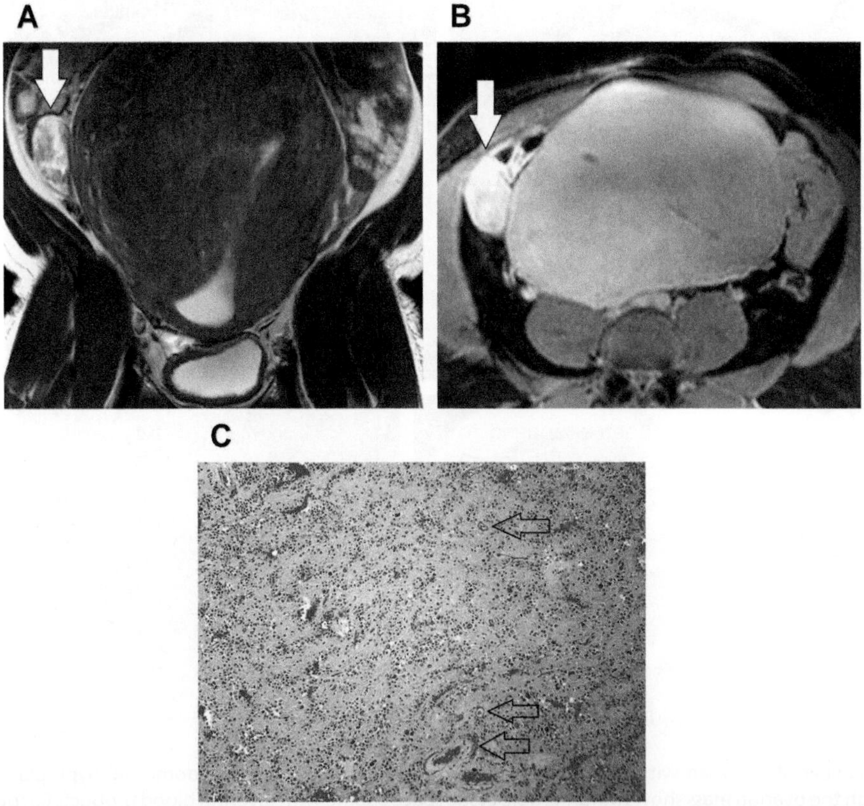

Fig. 14. A 55-year-old woman with Leydig tumor and clinical virilization. (*A*) Coronal T2WI shows massive myometrial hypertrophy and a small, mixed-signal right ovarian mass (*arrow*). The ovarian mass is a Leydig tumor and secretes testosterone, which is peripherally converted to estrogen and results in the uterine enlargement. (*B*) The mass (*arrow*) enhances avidly on postcontrast T1WI. (*C*) Microscopic section shows a solid, vascular tumor with characteristic vividly eosinophilic concentric perivascular fibrin deposition (*arrows*). (hematoxylin-eosin, original magnification ×40).

tumor are the most common elements. As with mixed epithelial cancers, the more aggressive cell type dictates therapy and prognosis. There are no specific imaging criteria for mixed GCTs, because the tissue composition can vary. When immature teratoma elements are present, intralesional fat and/or calcifications may be present.

SEX CORD–STROMAL OVARIAN TUMORS

Sex cord–stromal tumors (SCSTs) arise from the soft tissue matrix that surrounds and supports the germ cells. Many SCSTs produce steroids and present with estrogenic or androgenic clinical syndromes, although they are often benign or of low malignant potential. Although SCSTs account for only 7% of malignant ovarian neoplasms, they constitute 90% of all hormonally functioning ovarian neoplasms.[46]

Granulosa Cell Tumor

There are 2 discrete clinical subtypes: adult (95%) and juvenile (5%) granulosa tumor, with the latter occurring almost exclusively in children and adolescents (girls and teens). Estrogenic effects are common and include precocious puberty in girls, and vaginal bleeding caused by endometrial hyperplasia in women. Microscopically, juvenile granulosa cell tumors show a nodular and diffuse proliferation of cells without cytoplasmic grooves. Often there are folliclelike spaces filled with light pink fluid. The cells are mitotically active and can resemble high-grade epithelial tumors. Adult granulosa cell tumors are composed of ovoid cells with variable amounts of cytoplasm and prominent longitudinal nuclear grooves resembling coffee beans, sometimes forming glandlike structures called Call-Exner bodies. Like some ovarian epithelial tumors, adult granulosa cell tumors can show variable architectural patterns, including solid, nested, cystic, macrofollicular, and microfollicular types. Granulosa cell tumor often presents at an early stage of the disease with excellent long-term prognosis. However, it does have a unique feature of recurrence after prolonged intervals of years to decades. Both types are often unilateral and large. At gross pathologic examination and MR, the tumors have a characteristic spongelike appearance with solid areas and multicystic blood-filled spaces (**Fig. 12**).

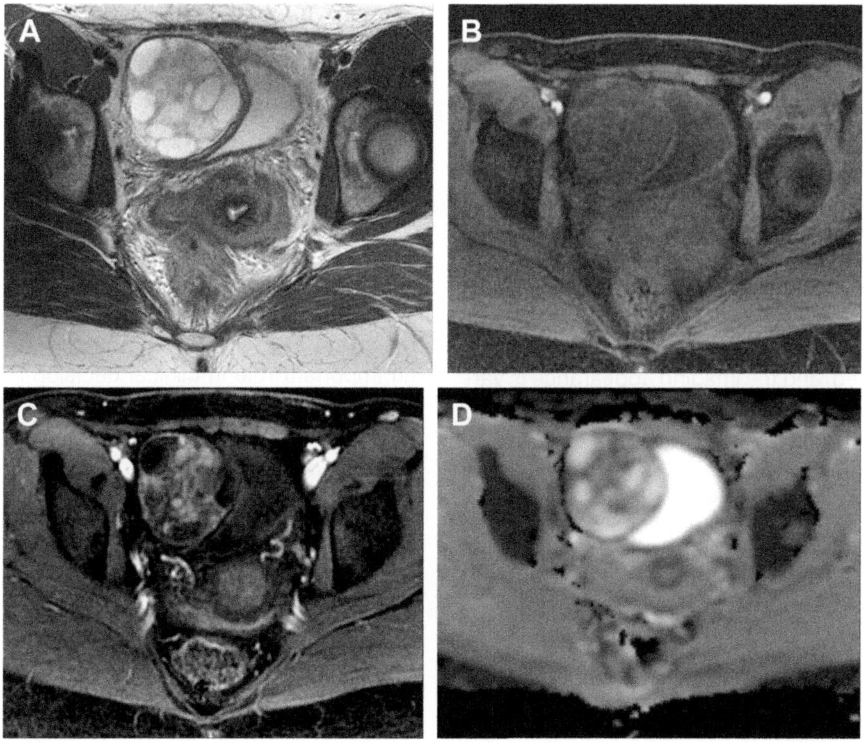

Fig. 15. A 30-year-old woman with Sertoli-Leydig tumor, who presented with abdominal pain and ongoing vaginal spotting. (*A*) Axial T2WI shows a heterogeneous right ovarian mass with mixed signal intensity. (*B*) Precontrast T1WI shows a predominantly hypointense mass. (*C*) Postcontrast T1WI shows enhancing solid components. (*D*) ADC map shows focal areas of low signal confirming impeded diffusion.

Thecoma-Fibroma Tumors

Thecoma-fibroma tumors are a spectrum that includes thecomas, fibrothecomas, and fibromas. Ovarian thecoma and fibroma are pure stromal tumors. Thecomas consist of lipid-laden stromal cells analogous to those seen with ovarian follicles. These cells are endocrinologically functional and can produce estrogen, explaining the frequent presentation of vaginal bleeding. Fibroma is the most common sex cord tumor and can occur in both premenopausal and postmenopausal women. Fibromas and tumors with fibroma elements arise from spindle collagen-producing cells and are rarely associated with hormone production.[42] Fibromas have a solid appearance at imaging with prolonged enhancement that depends on the amount of fibrous content. Classically, these solid tumors are typically low signal on T1WI and very low signal on T2WI (**Fig. 13**) because of their collagen content. Dense calcifications can be seen as well. Large tumors can be associated with Meigs syndrome, which is characterized by ascites and right-sided pleural effusion. It is common for tumors to have areas resembling both thecoma and fibroma, and many are classified as fibrothecoma. Malignant ovarian pure stromal tumors manifest as fibrosarcoma, are very rare, and portend a poor prognosis.

Sertoli and Sertoli-Leydig Tumors

Sertoli cell tumors average 9 cm in size and are typically solid. They present with estrogen excess. Leydig cell tumors are rare, varying widely in size, and most commonly present with virilization caused by androgen excess. When small they may be detectable only as a hyperenhancing focus in an otherwise normal ovary. Even at very large sizes, they have low malignant potential and favorable long-term outcomes. Often the two cell types are intermixed, and the imaging appearance is variable.[47] Most commonly, the tumor is a well-defined, enhancing solid mass with intratumoral cysts (**Figs. 14** and **15**). T1W and T2W signal intensity depends on the amount of fibrous content, and the low T2WI signal characteristic of fibromas is not characteristically seen.

DISCUSSION/SUMMARY

The variety of ovarian cancer subtypes gives rise to a range of gross and MR appearances. However, some fundamental concepts extend across multiple histologies and can provide guidance to radiologists. First, the presence of lipid within a lesion usually indicates a mature teratoma and a benign histology. If there are dominant or invasive enhancing components, an immature teratoma is possible, but is most common in younger women and girls. Malignant degeneration of mature teratoma is very rare and is generally squamous cell carcinoma arising in a postmenopausal woman. Second, very low signal on T2WI is a favorable prognostic sign because it is associated with benign fibromas, exophytic fibroids, and occasionally Brenner tumors. In the absence of fat or reassuringly low signal on T2WI, most other predominantly solid masses usually need surgical removal for diagnosis, particularly in the setting of any internal hemorrhage or necrosis. Third, unilocular cystic masses with 1 or a few purely endophytic mural nodules are usually benign cystadenomas and cystadenofibromas. These masses grow slowly if at all, and can safely be observed in poor operative candidates. Fourth, serous borderline tumors, LGSC, and HGSCs arise in a separate and more aggressive lineage. They are poorly differentiated from one another by imaging but clinical suspicion for aggressive malignancy should increase in the presence of soft tissue papillations that are multiple, large, or exophytic; bilateral masses; confluent tumor cloaking adjacent structures such as fallopian tubes; and ascites. Fifth, the presence of substantial blood products within a lesion often means endometriosis, but any enhancing components within an endometriotic cyst should be viewed with suspicion because they may indicate secondary neoplasia.

In general, the gross pathologic appearance of a mass most closely correlates with the imaging appearance, but the superior contrast sensitivity of MR enables depiction of both gross and microscopic tissue constituents. Contemporary MR imaging has the capacity to characterize and risk stratify ovarian masses, and radiologists aware of the range of ovarian cancer histologies can play an important role in clinical decision making and patient management.

REFERENCES

1. Thomassin-Naggara I, Aubert E, Rockall A, et al. Adnexal masses: development and preliminary validation of an MR imaging scoring system. Radiology 2013;267(2):432–43.
2. Adusumilli S, Hussain HK, Caoili EM, et al. MRI of sonographically indeterminate adnexal masses. AJR Am J Roentgenol 2006;187(3):732–40.
3. Spencer JA, Ghattamaneni S. MR imaging of the sonographically indeterminate adnexal mass. Radiology 2010;256(3):677–94.
4. Thomassin-Naggara I, Balvay D, Rockall A, et al. Added value of assessing adnexal masses with

advanced MRI techniques. Biomed Res Int 2015; 2015:785206.
5. Thomassin-Naggara I, Toussaint I, Perrot N, et al. Characterization of complex adnexal masses: value of adding perfusion- and diffusion-weighted MR imaging to conventional MR imaging. Radiology 2011; 258(3):793–803.
6. Sala E, Rockall AG, Freeman SJ, et al. The added role of MR imaging in treatment stratification of patients with gynecologic malignancies: what the radiologist needs to know. Radiology 2013;266(3):717–40.
7. Thomassin-Naggara I, Darai E, Cuenod CA, et al. Contribution of diffusion-weighted MR imaging for predicting benignity of complex adnexal masses. Eur Radiol 2009;19(6):1544–52.
8. Fujii S, Matsusue E, Kanasaki Y, et al. Detection of peritoneal dissemination in gynecological malignancy: evaluation by diffusion-weighted MR imaging. Eur Radiol 2008;18(1):18–23.
9. Rockall AG. Diffusion weighted MRI in ovarian cancer. Curr Opin Oncol 2014;26(5):529–35.
10. American Cancer Society. Cancer facts and figures 2016. Atlanta (GA): American Cancer Society; 2016.
11. World Health Organization classification of tumors. Pathology and genetics of tumors of the breast and female genital organ. Lyon (France): IARC Press; 2003.
12. Lalwani N, Shanbhogue AK, Vikram R, et al. Current update on borderline ovarian neoplasms. AJR Am J Roentgenol 2010;194(2):330–6.
13. Kurman RJ, Shih Ie M. Molecular pathogenesis and extraovarian origin of epithelial ovarian cancer–shifting the paradigm. Hum Pathol 2011;42(7):918–31.
14. Ahmed AA, Etemadmoghadam D, Temple J, et al. Driver mutations in TP53 are ubiquitous in high grade serous carcinoma of the ovary. J Pathol 2010;221(1):49–56.
15. Malpica A, Wong KK. The molecular pathology of ovarian serous borderline tumors. Ann Oncol 2016; 27(Suppl 1):i16–9.
16. Salvador S, Gilks B, Kobel M, et al. The fallopian tube: primary site of most pelvic high-grade serous carcinomas. Int J Gynecol Cancer 2009;19(1): 58–64.
17. Barakat RR, Berchuck A, Markman M, et al. Principles and practice of gynecologic oncology. 6th edition. Philadelphia: Lippincott Williams & Wilkins; 2013.
18. Heaps JM, Nieberg RK, Berek JS. Malignant neoplasms arising in endometriosis. Obstet Gynecol 1990;75(6):1023–8.
19. Fadare O. Recent developments on the significance and pathogenesis of lymph node involvement in ovarian serous tumors of low malignant potential (borderline tumors). Int J Gynecol Cancer 2009; 19(1):103–8.
20. Seidman JD, Bell DA, Crum CP, et al. Serous tumours. In: Kurman RJ, Carcangiu ML, Herrington CS, et al, editors. World Health Organization classification of tumours. pathology and genetics of tumours of female reproductive organs. Lyon (France): IARC Press; 2014. p. 17–24.
21. Bell DA. Low-grade serous tumors of ovary. Int J Gynecol Pathol 2014;33(4):348–56.
22. Dietl J. Revisiting the pathogenesis of ovarian cancer: the central role of the fallopian tube. Arch Gynecol Obstet 2014;289(2):241–6.
23. Przybycin CG, Kurman RJ, Ronnett BM, et al. Are all pelvic (nonuterine) serous carcinomas of tubal origin? Am J Surg Pathol 2010;34(10):1407–16.
24. Lalwani N, Prasad SR, Vikram R, et al. Histologic, molecular, and cytogenetic features of ovarian cancers: implications for diagnosis and treatment. Radiographics 2011;31(3):625–46.
25. Garrett AP, Lee KR, Colitti CR, et al. k-ras mutation may be an early event in mucinous ovarian tumorigenesis. Int J Gynecol Pathol 2001;20(3):244–51.
26. Shappell HW, Riopel MA, Smith Sehdev AE, et al. Diagnostic criteria and behavior of ovarian seromucinous (endocervical-type mucinous and mixed cell-type) tumors: atypical proliferative (borderline) tumors, intraepithelial, microinvasive, and invasive carcinomas. Am J Surg Pathol 2002;26(12): 1529–41.
27. Longacre TA, Bell DA, Malpica A, et al. Mucinous tumours. In: Kurman RJ, Carcangiu ML, Herrington CS, et al, editors. World Health Organization classification of tumours. pathology and genetics of tumours of female reproductive organs. Lyon (France): IARC Press; 2014. p. 25–8.
28. Zaino RJ, Brady MF, Lele SM, et al. Advanced stage mucinous adenocarcinoma of the ovary is both rare and highly lethal: a Gynecologic Oncology Group study. Cancer 2011;117(3):554–62.
29. Yemelyanova AV, Vang R, Judson K, et al. Distinction of primary and metastatic mucinous tumors involving the ovary: analysis of size and laterality data by primary site with reevaluation of an algorithm for tumor classification. Am J Surg Pathol 2008;32(1):128–38.
30. Tabrizi AD, Kalloger SE, Kobel M, et al. Primary ovarian mucinous carcinoma of intestinal type: significance of pattern of invasion and immunohistochemical expression profile in a series of 31 cases. Int J Gynecol Pathol 2010;29(2):99–107.
31. Young RH. Pseudomyxoma peritonei and selected other aspects of the spread of appendiceal neoplasms. Semin Diagn Pathol 2004;21(2):134–50.
32. Carr NJ. Current concepts in pseudomyxoma peritonei. Ann Pathol 2014;34(1):9–13.
33. Mostoufizadeh M, Scully RE. Malignant tumors arising in endometriosis. Clin Obstet Gynecol 1980;23(3):951–63.
34. Liu J, Albarracin CT, Chang KH, et al. Microsatellite instability and expression of hMLH1 and hMSH2

proteins in ovarian endometrioid cancer. Mod Pathol 2004;17(1):75–80.
35. Chui MH, Gilks CB, Cooper K, et al. Identifying Lynch syndrome in patients with ovarian carcinoma: the significance of tumor subtype. Adv Anat Pathol 2013;20(6):378–86.
36. Gilks CB, Prat J. Ovarian carcinoma pathology and genetics: recent advances. Hum Pathol 2009; 40(9):1213–23.
37. Gilks CB, Prat J, Carinelli SG. Brenner tumours. In: Kurman RJ, Carcangiu ML, Herrington CS, et al, editors. World Health Organization classification of tumours. pathology and genetics of tumours of female reproductive organs. Lyon (France): IARC Press; 2014. p. 35–7.
38. Ellenson LH, Cho KR, Soslow R. Mesenchymal tumours and mixed epithelial and mesenchymal tumours. In: Kurman RJ, Carcangiu ML, Herrington CS, et al, editors. World Health Organization classification of tumours. pathology and genetics of tumours of female reproductive organs. Lyon (France): IARC Press; 2014. p. 41–3.
39. Jin Z, Ogata S, Tamura G, et al. Carcinosarcomas (malignant mullerian mixed tumors) of the uterus and ovary: a genetic study with special reference to histogenesis. Int J Gynecol Pathol 2003;22(4):368–73.
40. Meisel JL, Woo KM, Sudarsan N, et al. Development of a risk stratification system to guide treatment for female germ cell tumors. Gynecol Oncol 2015; 138(3):566–72.
41. Shaaban AM, Rezvani M, Elsayes KM, et al. Ovarian malignant germ cell tumors: cellular classification and clinical and imaging features. Radiographics 2014;34(3):777–801.
42. Heo SH, Kim JW, Shin SS, et al. Review of ovarian tumors in children and adolescents: radiologic-pathologic correlation. Radiographics 2014;34(7): 2039–55.
43. Kim SH, Kang SB. Ovarian dysgerminoma: color Doppler ultrasonographic findings and comparison with CT and MR imaging findings. J Ultrasound Med 1995;14(11):843–8.
44. Tanaka YO, Kurosaki Y, Nishida M, et al. Ovarian dysgerminoma: MR and CT appearance. J Comput Assist Tomogr 1994;18(3):443–8.
45. Prat J, Nogales FF, Cao D. Germ cell tumors. In: Kurman RJ, Carcangiu ML, Herrington CS, et al, editors. World Health Organization classification of tumours. pathology and genetics of tumours of female reproductive organs. Lyon (France): IARC Press; 2014. p. 41–3.
46. Barakat RR, Berchuck A, Markman M, et al. Principles and practice of gynecologic oncology. 6th edition. Philadelphia: Wolters Kluwer; 2013.
47. Horta M, Cunha TM. Sex cord-stromal tumors of the ovary: a comprehensive review and update for radiologists. Diagn Interv Radiol 2015;21(4):277–86.

MR Imaging of Müllerian Fusion Anomalies

Jeffrey D. Olpin, MD, Aida Moeni, MD, Roderick J. Willmore, MD, Marta E. Heilbrun, MD*

KEYWORDS

• Female genital tract anomalies • Urogenital anomalies • Congenital uterine anomalies
• Müllerian duct anomalies • MR imaging methods • Pregnancy outcomes • Reproductive outcomes

KEY POINTS

- Müllerian duct developmental anomalies are clinically relevant in patients with a history of infertility and pregnancy-related complications.
- Müllerian duct developmental anomalies are readily characterized on MR imaging.
- Understanding the various classification systems for müllerian duct developmental anomalies is critical in providing accurate descriptions of the spectrum of anomalies and directing management.

INTRODUCTION

This article reviews the classification of müllerian duct anomalies (MDAs), the clinical impact of these diagnoses as related to fertility and pregnancy loss, and the MR imaging appearance of the spectrum of these congenital anomalies.[1–4] MDAs are a group of congenital uterine disorders resulting from abnormalities in the embryologic development of the müllerian ducts. The prevalence of MDAs in the general population ranges between 4% and 7%.[5–7] In a population of women with recurrent pregnancy loss, however, the incidence increases to as much as 18%.[4,6,8] Most women with MDAs have little difficulty in conceiving. MDAs are associated with a higher rate of reproductive complications, however, including spontaneous abortion, intrauterine growth restriction, abnormal fetal lie, and preterm labor and birth.[2,9] MDAs are commonly associated with other congenital anomalies of the urinary tract.[10]

EMBRYOLOGY

During early embryonic development, the male and female genitals are indistinguishable, with 2 sets of paired ducts that are present by 6 weeks: the mesonephric (wolffian) and paramesonephric (müllerian) ducts. In the absence of müllerian inhibiting factor from male primitive gonads, the mesonephric ducts regress and the paramesonephric ducts begin to develop along the lateral aspect of the primitive kidneys. The müllerian ducts begin to develop in a bidirectional fashion, are open to the coelomic or peritoneal cavity superiorly, and are closed inferiorly.

During the 8th to 12th weeks of embryologic development, the müllerian ducts extend caudally into the primitive pelvic region where they eventually meet the urogenital sinus at the müllerian tubercle. The inferior aspect of the müllerian ducts develop into the uterus, cervix, and upper two-thirds of the vagina. The superior aspect of the müllerian ducts develops into the fallopian tubes.

By weeks 12 to 16, the septum that separates the inferior müllerian ducts begins to regress, resulting in fusion of the ducts to form a primitive uterus. Failure in septal regression results in a spectrum of MDAs. Fusion of the inferior müllerian ducts was traditionally thought to occur in a caudal to cranial direction. During formation of the uterovaginal canal, the sinus tubercle thickens and forms the sinovaginal bulbs, which create the lower 20% of the vagina. The uterovaginal canal

The authors have nothing to disclose.
Department of Radiology and Imaging Sciences, University of Utah, 30 North 1900 East, #1A071, Salt Lake City, UT 84132-2140, USA
* Corresponding author.
E-mail address: marta.heilbrun@hsc.utah.edu

Magn Reson Imaging Clin N Am 25 (2017) 563–575
http://dx.doi.org/10.1016/j.mric.2017.03.008
1064-9689/17/

remains separated from the sinovaginal bulbs by the horizontal vaginal plate. The vaginal plate interface with the urogenital sinus at the third month to fifth month forms the hymen.

This description, however, does not account for certain variant MDAs, such as a vertically oriented vaginal septum with an otherwise unremarkable uterus. Newer theories of septal regression that entail simultaneous bidirectional fusion in both cranial and caudal directions help explain the spectrum of anomalies.[11]

IMAGING TECHNIQUES

Over the past few decades, a variety of imaging techniques have been developed for the characterization and classification of MDAs, including hysterosalpingography (HSG), ultrasound (US), and MR imaging.

Hysterosalpingography

Prior to the advent of US and MR imaging, the most widely accepted imaging technique for the assessment of MDAs was HSG. The study is performed by injecting iodinated contrast material into the uterine cavity under fluoroscopic observation. A series of spot images are generally obtained as the contrast material fills the uterine cavity and passes through the fallopian tubes (**Fig. 1**). HSG can provide reasonable evaluation of the endometrial cavity and can reliably establish tubal patency. This technique has several limitations, however. The procedure is more invasive than other imaging modalities, necessitating the insertion of a cannula into the external os or balloon-tip catheter into the endometrial cavity. More importantly, the study is of limited use in the depiction of MDAs because the myometrium and external uterine contour are not visualized. There is frequent overlap in the HSG imaging findings between different anomalies. Additionally, there is the inherent disadvantage of exposing young women to ionizing radiation. Currently, HSG plays little role in the evaluation of MDAs.

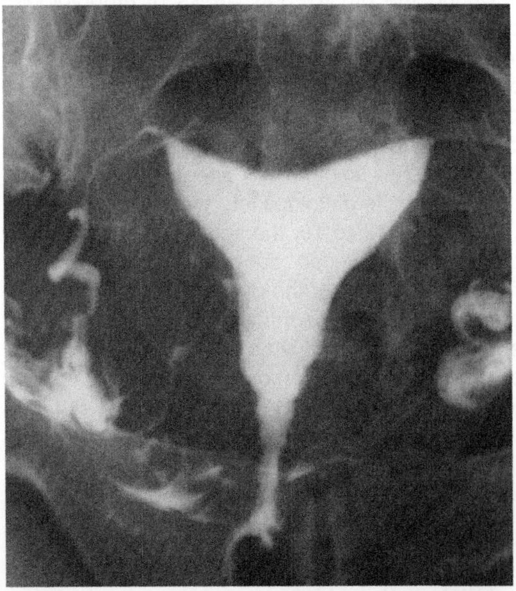

Fig. 1. Normal hysterosalpingogram. A single image from a hysterosalpingogram demonstrates opacification of the endometrial cavity with contrast material. Contrast material is also noted within both fallopian tubes.

Ultrasonography

Technical advances in US have allowed for increasingly accurate evaluation of MDAs, particularly with 3-D techniques. MDAs are best evaluated during the secretory phase of the menstrual cycle when the endometrial thickness and echo complex are optimally visualized. Although conventional sagittal and transverse images of the uterus are essential, orthogonal images of the long axis of the uterus are crucial to assess the overall uterine contour. When performing US to evaluate a suspected MDA, transabdominal US should be attempted, although image acquisition may be limited by the patient's body habitus, bowel peristalsis, bowel gas, or variation in uterine lie. Transvaginal US can provide better spatial resolution, although the field of view is inherently limited.

Endovaginal 3-D US allows for the creation of 3-D images from a uterine volume acquisition. After the acquisition, the data set can be manipulated to provide 3-D images of the uterus from virtually any angle. Coronal images provide essential detail regarding both the endometrial cavity and serosal surface of the uterus (**Fig. 2**). In experienced hands, a sensitivity of 98.3% and a specificity of 99.4% have been reported in the assessment of MDAs.[12] A high degree of concordance between 3D US and MR imaging has been shown.[13,14] A recent study of surgically proved MDA cases reported a higher level of accuracy with 3-D US in comparison to MR imaging.[15] Key advantages of this technique are lower cost and shorter examination time in experienced hands as opposed to MR imaging. Major disadvantages include the relative lack of sonographers and sonologists with adequate training in 3-D image acquisition and postprocessing techniques.

MR Imaging

MR imaging has emerged as the universally accepted gold standard in the imaging evaluation

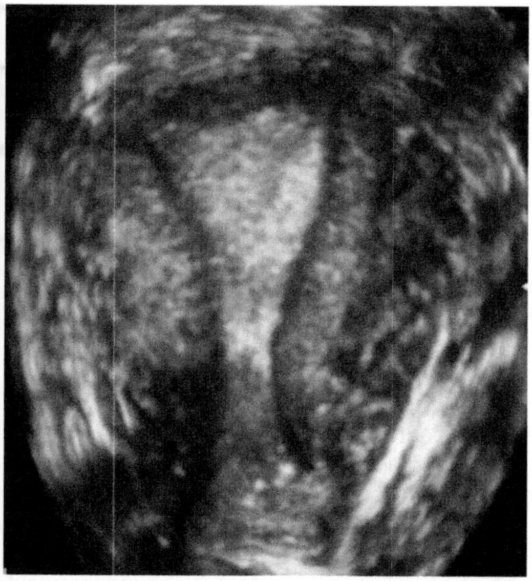

Fig. 2. Normal 3-D US uterus. Coronally reconstructed 3-D US image provides excellent depiction of the endometrium as well as the external uterine fundal contour.

of MDAs. Accuracies up to 100% in the evaluation of MDAs have been reported.[16] MR imaging provides excellent delineation of both internal and external uterine anatomy. T2-weighted images are the mainstay of pelvic imaging. The endometrium is uniformly hyperintense on T2-weighted images. The junctional zone surrounds the endometrium and is readily identified as a hypointense band measuring up to 8 mm to 10 mm in thickness. The uterine myometrium surrounds the junctional zone and is of intermediate signal intensity on T2-weighted images (**Fig. 3**). T2-weighted imaging is best performed without fat suppression due to the inherent contrast between the signal intensity of the uterus and the surrounding fat. T1-weighted images are of limited value in the evaluation of uterine zonal anatomy because the uterus is uniformly hypointense. T1-weighted images can be useful, however, for detecting hyperintense blood products in the setting of hematocolpos or endometriosis.

An inert, viscous contrast agent, such as Surgilube (HR Pharmaceuticals, Inc) or US gel, is commonly administered to distend the vagina prior to scan acquisition for a suspected MDA. Failure to adequately distend the vagina prior to imaging may preclude accurate diagnosis of complex vaginal anomalies, such as vaginal septations or vaginal duplication. Disadvantages of MR imaging are few but include high cost and potentially lengthy examination time relative to other imaging modalities. Patients with claustrophobia, excessively large body habitus, or implantable ferromagnetic medical devices may not be candidates for an MR imaging examination.

CLASSIFICATION SYSTEMS OF MÜLLERIAN DUCT ANOMALIES

Various classification systems have been proposed over the past several decades to describe MDAs:

- The American Fertility Society, now the American Society of Reproductive Medicine, (ASRM) system[1]

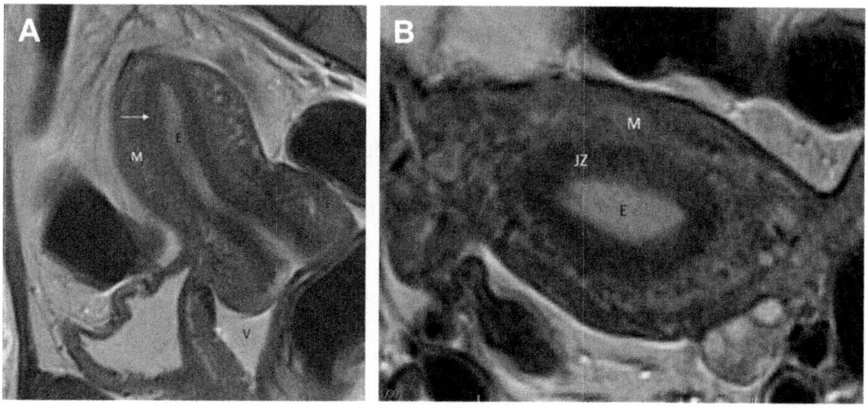

Fig. 3. (*A*) Normal sagittal MR uterine zonal anatomy. Sagittal T2-weighted MR image of the uterus demonstrates normal uterine zonal anatomy. The endometrium (E) is uniformly hyperintense. The junctional zone (*arrow*) is a uniformly hypointense ring surrounding the endometrium. The intermediate signal myometrium (M) is seen surrounding the junctional zone. Surgilube is seen within the distended vagina (V). (*B*) Normal coronal MR uterine zonal anatomy. Coronal T2-weighted MR image of the uteris demonstrates normal uterine zonal anatomy. The endometrium (E) is centrally hyperintense. The junctional zone (JZ) is uniformly hypointense ring surrounding the endometrium. The intermediate signal myometrium (M) is seen surrounding the junctional zone.

- The vagina, cervix, uterus, adnexa, and associated malformations (VCUAM) classification[17]
- The European Society of Human Reproduction and Embryology (ESHRE)/European Society for Gynaecologic Endoscopy (ESGE) classification[18]

The most widely accepted classification system is the ASRM classification, initially proposed by Buttram and Gibbons in 1979.[19] The system was later modified in 1988 by a subcommittee of the American Fertility Society and remains the most universally accepted system to date for classification of MDAs.[1] This simple system is based on the degree of failure of normal development. The anomalies are divided into categories that demonstrate similar clinical manifestations and treatment (**Table 1**).

Although the ASRM classification remains widely accepted, the system has several drawbacks. Some particularly complex MDAs demonstrate multiple features that may encompass several ASRM categories. In a patient with disparate genital tract anomalies, it is imperative to describe each anomaly as a component part rather than attempt to classify according to the most dominant anatomic feature. Additionally, the system does not thoroughly classify vaginal anomalies. Finally, the ASRM system does not provide accurate measurements to confidently classify a uterus as bicornuate, septate, or arcuate.

The VCUAM system[5] is designed to categorize complex malformations that defy classification by the traditional ASRM system. In the VCUAM system, each component of the genital tract is classified separately, much like the tumor-nodes-metastasis (TNM) classification for malignancies.[17] A disadvantage of the VCUAM system is its inherent complexity, in which 56,700 individual combinations of anomalies are possible (**Table 2**).

The ESHRE/ESGE published a new classification in 2013 (**Table 3**).[18] An important characteristic of ESHRE/ESGE system is the independent classification of uterine, cervical, and vaginal abnormalities. Deviations of uterine anomaly rising from the same embryologic origins are the basis

Table 1
Classification of müllerian duct anomalies based on the American Society for Reproductive Medicine system

Classification	Description	Subcategories
I. Hypoplasia/agenesis	Early developmental failure of the müllerian ducts	Vaginal (I-A) Cervical (I-B) Fundal (I-C) Tubal (I-D) Combined (I-E)
II. Unicornuate uterus	Arrested development of one of the 2 müllerian ducts	Rudimentary horn with: Communicating uterine cavity (II-A)[a] Noncommunicating uterine cavity (II-B) No uterine cavity (II-C) No rudimentary horn (II-D)
III. Uterus didelphys	Complete failure of müllerian duct fusion	—
IV. Bicornuate uterus	Incomplete or partial fusion of the müllerian ducts	Complete (IV-A)[b] Partial (IV-B)
V. Septate uterus	Complete or partial failure of resorption of the uterovaginal septum	Complete (V-A) Partial (V-B)
VI. Arcuate uterus	Near complete resorption of the uterovaginal septum	—
VII. DES uterus	Related to the use of DES during the late 1940s to 1971	—

[a] Endometrial cavity that communicates with the normal side.
[b] Complete type has accompanying cervical duplication.
Adapted from ASRM. The American Fertility Society classifications of adnexal adhesions, distal tubal occlusion, tubal occlusion secondary to tubal ligation, tubal pregnancies, mullerian anomalies and intrauterine adhesions. Fertil Steril 1988;49(6):952; with permission.

Table 2
The vagina, cervix, uterus, adnexa, and associated malformations classification: description of the individual malformations relative to the portion of the organ system

Vagina	
0	Normal
1a	Partial hymenal atresia
1b	Complete hymenal atresia
2a	Incomplete septate vagina <50%
2b	Complete septate vagina
3	Stenosis of the introitus
4	Hypoplasia
5a	Unilateral atresia
5b	Complete atresia
S1	Sinus urogenitalis (deep confluence)
S2	Sinus urogenitalis (middle confluence)
S3	Sinus urogenitalis (high confluence)
C	Cloacae
+	Other
#	Unknown
Cervix	
0	Normal
1	Duplex cervix
2a	Unilateral atresia/aplasia
2b	Bilateral atresia/aplasia
+	Other
#	Unknown
Uterus	
0	Normal
1a	Arcuate
1b	Septate <50% of the uterine cavity
1c	Septate >50% of the uterine cavity
2	Bicornate
3	Hypoplastic uterus
4a	Unilaterally rudimentary or aplastic
4b	Bilaterally rudimentary or aplastic
+	Other
#	Unknown
Adnexa	
0	Normal
1a	Unilateral tubal malformation, ovaries normal
1b	Bilateral tubal malformation, ovaries normal
2a	Unilateral hypoplasia/gonadal streak (including tubal malformation if appropriate)
2b	Bilateral hypoplasia/gonadal streak (including tubal malformation if appropriate)
3a	Unilateral aplasia
3b	Bilateral aplasia
+	Other
#	Unknown
Associated Malformation	
0	None
R	Renal system
S	Skeleton
C	Cardiac
N	Neurologic
+	Other
#	Unknown

Adapted from Oppelt P, Renner SP, Brucker S, et al. The VCUAM (Vagina Cervix Uterus Adnex-associated Malformation) classification: a new classification for genital malformations. Fertil Steril 2005;84(5):1494; with permission.

for the design of the main classes, and the different degrees of clinically relevant uterine deformity are the basis for the design of the main subclasses. Cervical and vaginal anomalies are classified into independent supplementary subclasses. Recent studies have demonstrated that the ESHRE/ESGE system provides an effective and comprehensive classification for almost all the currently known MDAs and overcomes the limits of previous classifications.[12,18,20]

MR IMAGING FEATURES OF MÜLLERIAN DUCT ANOMALIES

Although there are multiple classification schemes, are outlined previously, the principle anomalies of the female genital tract are presented according to the ASRM classification system, with differences between systems highlighted in the text.

Uterine Hypoplasia/Agenesis

Uterine hypoplasia/agenesis is a class I MDA according to the ASRM classification.[1] Uterine and vaginal hypoplasia, or agenesis, occurs due to early failure of the paramesonephric ducts to develop prior to fusion. These disorders account for approximately 5% to 10% of all MDAs. The most common manifestation is the Mayer-Rokitansky-Küster-Hauser syndrome. This syndrome entails vaginal agenesis as well as uterine agenesis in 90% of individuals. The ovaries are normal in a majority of cases.

Uterine agenesis or hypoplasia is optimally visualized on sagittal MR images whereas vaginal agenesis is best visualized on axial MR images. No identifiable uterus is seen in the setting of

Table 3
The European Society of Human Reproduction and Embryology/European Society for Gynaecologic Endoscopy classification of female genital tract anomalies

	Uterine Anomaly		Cervical/Vaginal Anomaly
	Main Class	**Main Subclass**	**Coexistent Subclass**
Class 0	Normal uterus		Cervix C0 Normal
Class I	Dysmorphic uterus	a. T-shaped b. Infantilis	C1 Septate C2 Double "normal"
Class II	Septate uterus	a. Partial b. Complete	C3 Unilateral aplasia/dysplasia C4 Aplasia/dysplasia
Class III	Dysfused uterus (including dysfused "septate")	a. Partial b. Complete	 Vagina
Class IV	Unilaterally formed uterus	a. Rudimentary horn with cavity (communicating or not) b. Rudimentary horn without cavity/aplasia (no horn)	V0 Normal vagina V1 Longitudinal nonobstructing vaginal septum V2 Longitudinal obstructing vaginal septum
Class V	Aplastic/dysplastic	a. Rudimentary horn with cavity (bilateral or unilateral) b. Rudimentary horn without cavity (bilateral or unilateral)/aplasia	V3 Transverse vaginal septum/ imperforate hymen V4 Vaginal aplasia
Class VI	Unclassified malformations		

Adapted from Grimbizis GF, Gordts S, Di Spiezio Sardo A, et al. The ESHRE/ESGE consensus on the classification of female genital tract congenital anomalies. Hum Reprod 2013;28(8):2036; with permission.

uterine agenesis (**Fig. 4**) A small uterine remnant with a lack of normal uterine zonal anatomy may be seen on T2-weighted images in the setting of uterine hypoplasia (**Fig. 5**).

Unicornuate Uterus

Unicornuate uterus is a class II MDA according to the ASRM classification. The unicornuate uterus accounts for approximately 20% of all müllerian

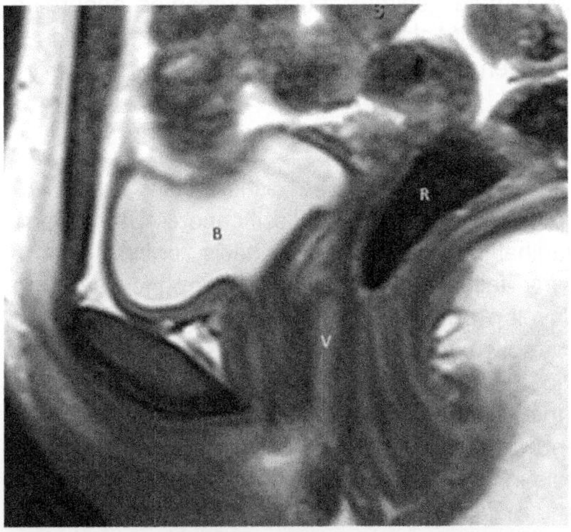

Fig. 4. Uterine agenesis. Sagittal T2-weighted MR image of the pelvis demonstrates a partially distended urinary bladder (B) and stool-filled rectum (R). The vagina (V) is foreshortened. No identifiable uterus is seen.

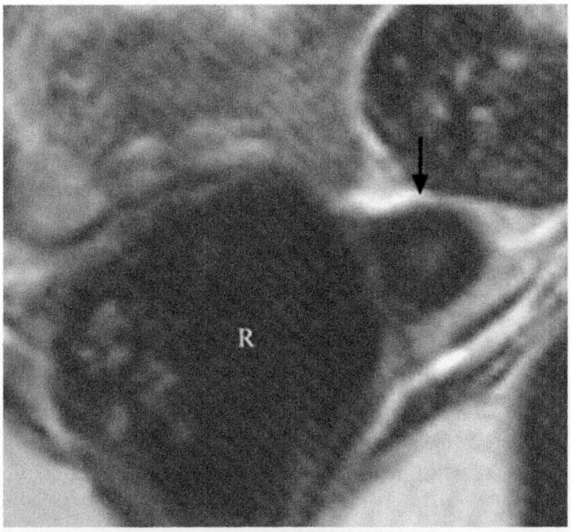

Fig. 5. Uterine hypoplasia. Coronal T2-weighted MR image demonstrates leftward deviation of a rudimentary uterus (*arrow*). A stool-filled rectum (R) is noted in the midline.

duct anomalies. The condition is present when 1 müllerian duct fails to elongate while the other duct develops in a normal fashion. A solitary uterine horn can be observed in up to 35% of patients. More commonly, a small rudimentary horn is seen arising from the primary single horn in 65% of cases. Within this subset of patients with rudimentary horns, the rudimentary horn may contain endometrium in 50% of patients. The endometrium of the rudimentary horn may communicate with the dominant horn in up to 33% of cases. Conversely, there is no communication between rudimentary and primary horns in 66% of cases. No identifiable endometrium is seen in the remaining 50% of patients with rudimentary horns.

There is a higher incidence of unicornuate horns occurring within the right hemipelvis that is not fully understood.[21] Renal anomalies are more commonly seen in association with unicornuate uterus than with other MDAs and have been reported in up to 40% of the cases.[10] The most common anomaly is unilateral renal agenesis, which is consistently ipsilateral to the rudimentary horn. Other anomalies, such as duplicated collecting systems, ectopic kidney, horseshoe kidney, and cystic renal dysplasia have been described.[22]

A unicornuate uterus is diagnosed by the presence of a solitary deviated and often atrophic horn. The solitary horn is typically fusiform or banana-shaped, the endometrium is narrow and described as bullet-shaped, which tapers at the apex. This is usually best visualized in the axial plane on T2-weighted images (**Fig. 6**). MR imaging is the most sensitive imaging modality for determining the presence of a rudimentary horn. Additionally, when endometrium in a rudimentary horn is present, the zonal anatomy is generally well visualized on T2-weighted images. It is essential to include at least cursory images (such as coronal SSFSE) through the upper abdomen when performing a study for a suspected MDA, given the high incidence of associated renal anomalies (**Fig. 7**).

Uterus Didelphys

Uterus didelphys is a class III müllerian anomaly based on the ASRM classification. This disorder accounts for approximately 5% of MDAs. Uterus didelphys occurs as a result of a complete or near-complete lack of müllerian duct fusion. Each duct develops into an independent hemiuterus and cervix, although partial cervical fusion is generally seen. The endometrial cavities do not communicate in this condition. A longitudinal vaginal septum can be seen in up to 75% of cases. The presence of a vaginal septum may result in unilateral vaginal obstruction, which is generally not clinically apparent until menarche. There might be also an associated unilateral transverse hemivaginal septum, which can cause ipsilateral obstruction and hematometrocolpos.

MR imaging reliably demonstrates 2 separate, widely divergent uterine horns with 2 separate cervices (**Fig. 8**). A longitudinally oriented septum is commonly seen within the upper vagina (**Fig. 9**). Normal zonal anatomy is generally well preserved in each uterine horn. In the setting of an obstructed unilateral vaginal septum, hematometrocolpos may be seen with resultant asymmetric dilatation of the obstructed vagina (**Fig. 10**). Uterus didelphys can also be associated

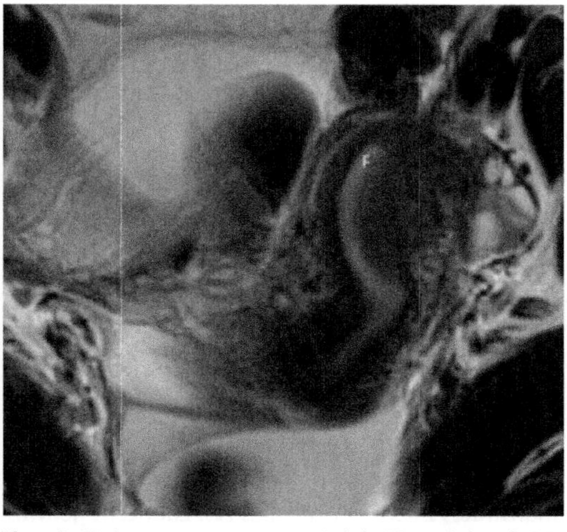

Fig. 6. Unicornuate uterus. Axial T2-weighted MR demonstrates leftward deviation of a solitary uterine horn. Uterine fundus (F).

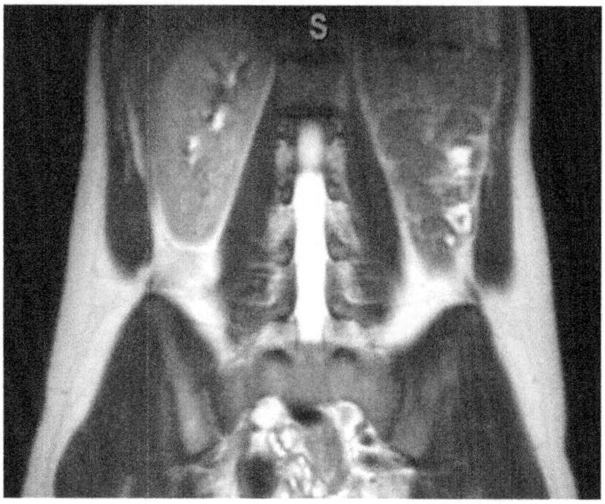

Fig. 7. Unilateral renal agenesis. Coronal T2 HASTE through the upper abdomen demonstrates a normal appearing right kidney. The left kidney is congenitally absent. S, spine.

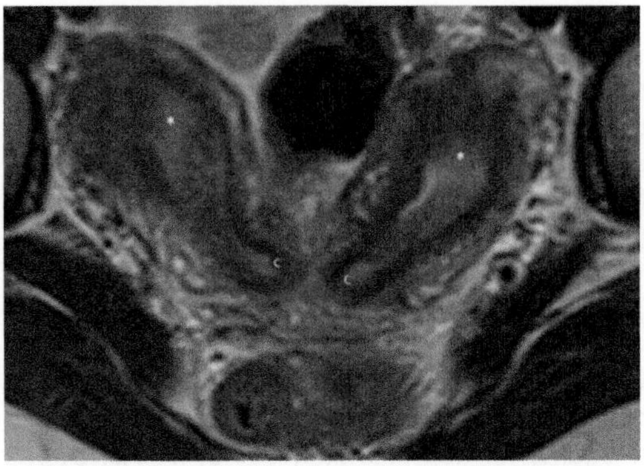

Fig. 8. Uterus didelphys. Axial T2-weighted image demonstrates 2 widely divergent uterine horns (*asterisk*). Two separate cervices are (C) are likewise visualized on this image.

with renal anomalies, usually ipsilateral to the transverse vaginal septum. This combination has been named obstructed hemivagina and ipsilateral renal agenesis.

Bicornuate Uterus

The bicornuate uterus is classified as a class IV MDA. This condition is the result of incomplete fusion of the uterovaginal horns at the level of the uterine fundus. This anomaly is associated with an increased risk of spontaneous abortion, intrauterine growth restriction, and perinatal mortality.[4] This disorder accounts for approximately 10% of all MDAs and is characterized by 2 divergent uterine horns that fuse at the level of the lower uterine segment or uterine isthmus. Longitudinal septa within the upper vagina have been described in approximately 25% of women with bicornuate uteri (**Fig. 11**). The ASRM has proposed that an external fundal indentation greater than 1.0 cm is indicative of a bicornuate uterus.[8]

In the setting of a bicornuate unicollis uterus, the endometrial cavities within each horn fuse at the level of the uterine isthmus to form a solitary endocervical canal (**Fig. 12**). A bicornuate bicollis uterus implies cervical duplication, and is comprised of 2 distinct endometrial cavities that arise from separate endocervical canals, although a certain degree of communication between the 2 horns is usually maintained (**Fig. 13**). At least 6 separate variations of the bicornuate uterus have been described in the literature.[23] On the T2-weighted images through the long axis of the uterine corpus, it is important to look for the widely divergent horns with an external fundal cleft greater than 1.0 cm (**Fig. 14**A) and normal uterine zonal anatomy within both horns (**Fig. 14**B).

Septate Uterus

The septate uterus is classified as a class V MDA. It is the most common of these disorders, comprising up to 55% of MDAs. This condition results from partial or complete failure of resorption of the uterovaginal septum after fusion of the paramesonephric ducts. In addition to being the most common of all MDAs, it is also associated with pregnancy-related complications. The true impact of a septum on fertility and recurrent pregnancy loss remains an area of debate. Recent practice guidelines by the ASRM state that the current evidence is insufficient to conclude that the septum is associated with infertility.[8] A 2014 meta-analysis

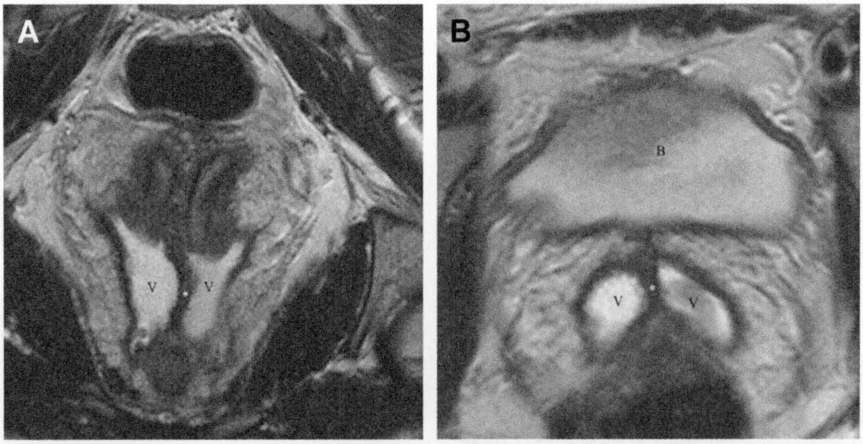

Fig. 9. (*A*) Uterus didelphys. Coronal T2-weighted image demonstrates 2 separate vaginas (V). Lubricant gel was administered intravaginally prior to image acquisition. A prominent, longitudinally oriented septum (*asterisk*) is noted that divides the 2 distinct vaginas. (*B*) Uterus didelphys. Axial T2 weighted image depicts the lumen of 2 separate, distinct vaginas (V). The vaginas are separated by a prominent septum (*asterisk*). Urinary bladder (B).

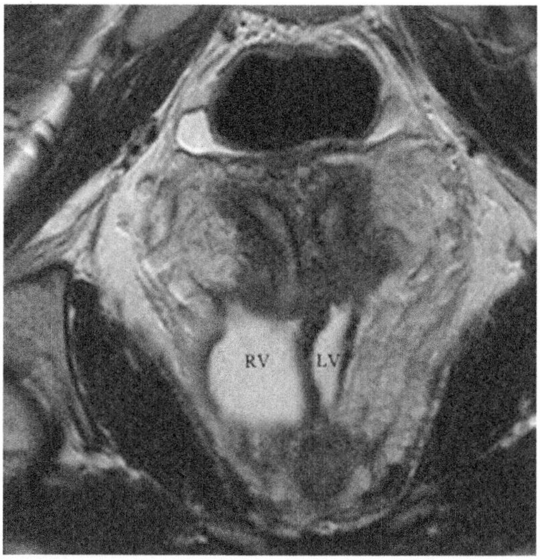

Fig. 10. Uterus didelphys. Coronal T2-weighted image demonstrates asymmetric dilatation of the right vagina (RV) in this patient with an obstructing vaginal septum. A normal caliber left vagina (LV) is noted.

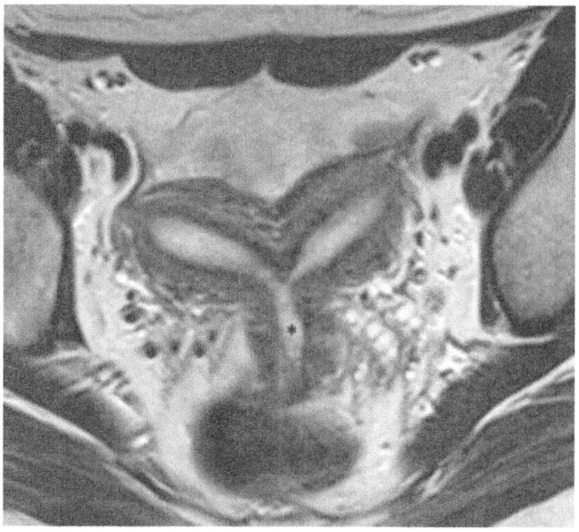

Fig. 12. Bicornuate unicollis. Axial T2-weighted image demonstrates 2 widely divergent uterine horns. Two distinct endometrial cavities are noted that fuse within the lower uterine segment to form a solitary endocervical canal (*asterisk*).

concludes that there does seem to be an impact of a uterine septum on first-trimester and second-trimester pregnancy losses.[4] The length of the septum does not seem to correlate with poor obstetric outcome.[24] Observational studies suggest that hysteroscopic removal of the septum improves clinical pregnancy rates and that the rate of spontaneous abortion decreases following resection of the septum.[4,25,26]

Septate uteri are classified as possessing either a complete or partial septum. A septate uterus is considered complete when the septum extends from the fundus to the external cervical os (**Fig. 15**). The septum can extend even further caudally into the vagina in approximately 25% of cases.[27] In a partial septate uterus, the septum can be of widely variable length. A short septum extends from the fundus and terminates within the body of the uterine (**Fig. 16**). A longer incomplete septum may extend beyond the internal cervical os into the endocervical canal but terminates proximal to the external cervical os. In rare instances, the cervix is duplicated in a septate uterus.

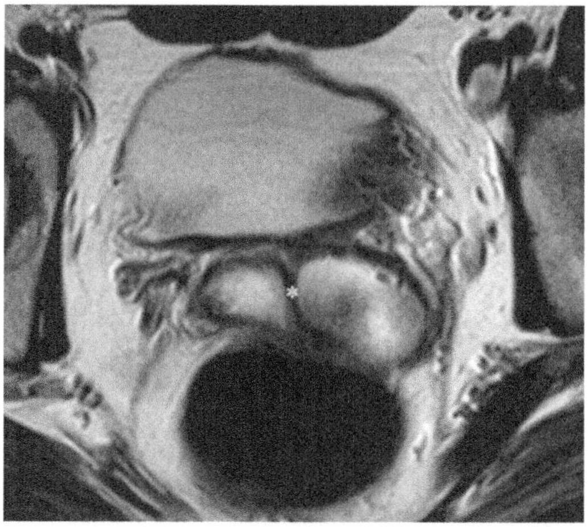

Fig. 11. Bicornuate uterus. Axial T2-weighted image through the level of the proximal vagina in a patient with a known bicornuate uterus. A prominent vaginal septum (*asterisk*) is noted.

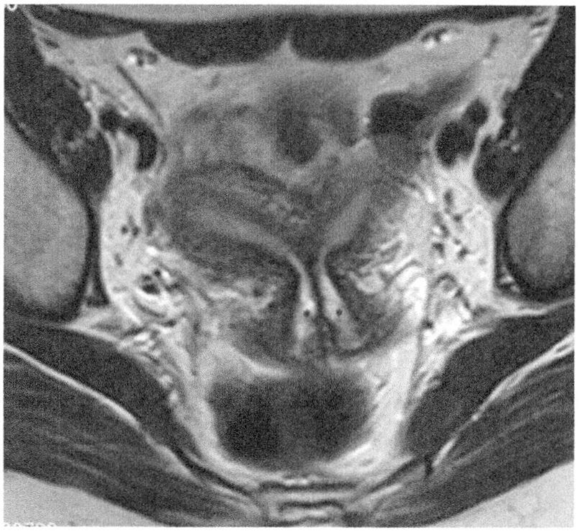

Fig. 13. Bicornuate bicollis uterus. Axial T2-weighted image demonstrates 2 widely divergent uterine horns. Two distinct endometrial cavities and endocervical canals are noted (*asterisk*).

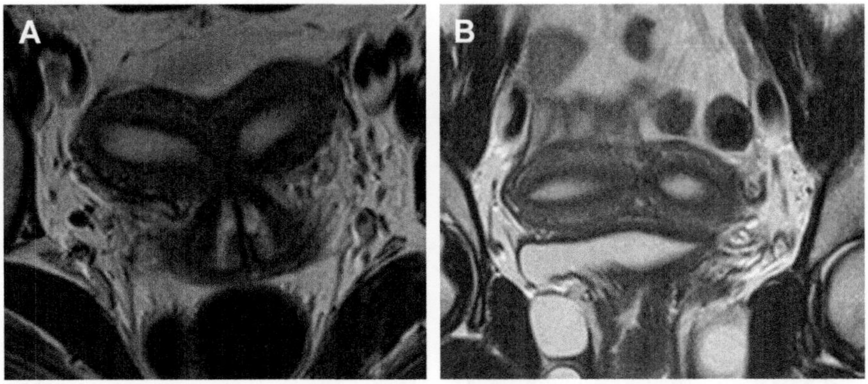

Fig. 14. (*A*) Bicornuate bicollis uterus. Axial T2-weighted image through the long axis of the uterine corpis demonstrates widely divergent horns with a fundal cleft greater than 1.0 cm. (*B*) Bicornuate uterus. Coronal T2-weighted image demonstrates 2 widely divergent uterine horns with normal zonal anatomy within both horns. The uterus is anteflexed, and the uterine corpus lies along the axial or transverse plane.

Visualization of the uterine fundus is crucial to reliably differentiate between a septate and bicornuate uterus. Accurate classification is essential because the treatment options for these 2 disorders are significantly different. A septate uterus is generally amenable to hysteroscopic resection of the septum, whereas the bicornuate uterus generally requires no surgical intervention.

In a septate uterus, the external uterine contour may be convex, flat or mildly concave (less than 1 cm). In 2016 the ASRM proposed a definition for a septate uterus.[8] This is defined by a depth from the interstitial line to the apex of the fundal indentation that is greater than 1.5 cm and an angle of the indentation that is greater than 90°.[8] The ESHRE/ESGE criteria for a septate uterus is an internal indentation extending greater than 50% of the myometial thickness.[18] These recommendations are based on both laparoscopy and hysteroscopy, where there is an emerging consensus of opinion that an external fundal indentation less than 1.0 cm suggests a septate uterus.[28,29]

MR imaging remains the gold standard in the evaluation of this disorder, although 3D-US is increasingly effective.[15] MR reliably depicts the external uterine fundal contour. Additionally, the length and extent of the uterine septum is well-visualized by this technique. Prior to the advent

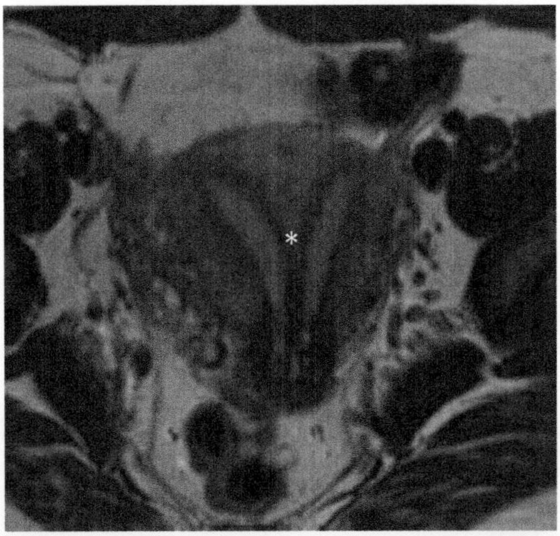

Fig. 15. Complete septate uterus. Axial T2-weighted MR image demonstrates a prominent midline septum (*asterisk*) extending from the uterine fundus to the external cervical os.

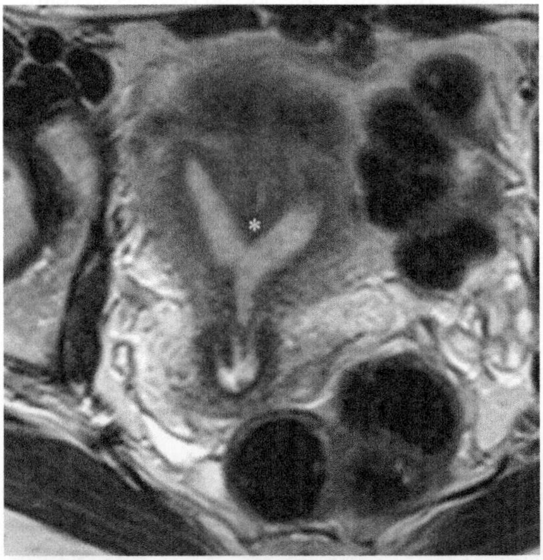

Fig. 16. Partial septate uterus. Axial T2-weighted MR image demonstrates prominence of the fundal myometrium with a deep cleft separating 2 fundal endometrial cavities. A truncated septum is noted (*asterisk*) that terminates within the body of the uterus.

of MR, it was generally assumed that poor obstetric outcomes of this condition were attributable to the fibrous and avascular nature of the septum. MR imaging revealed, however, that the septum demonstrates signal intensity similar to that of the myometrium.

Arcuate Uterus

The arcuate uterus is classified as a class VI MDA in the ASRM system. This disorder is characterized by mild myometrial thickening at the uterine fundus and occurs as a result of incomplete resorption of the uterovaginal septum. This entity remains somewhat controversial; some investigators believe it represents a true anomaly, whereas others consider it a normal anatomic variant. The original Buttram and Gibbons classification[19] described this entity as a subcategory of the bicornuate uterus. The entity became a discrete MDA on the ASRM revision, which describes a distinction between the 2 entities based on the degree of fundal union.[1] Data regarding the clinical relevance of this anomaly are somewhat disparate. Most investigators currently agree that the disorder is associated with minimal adverse reproductive outcome. Because of the limited impact on pregnancy outcomes, and the lack of a consensus definition, the ESHRE/ESGE system does not have a unique classification for arcuate uterus.[18]

MR reliably depicts the characteristic thickening of the fundal myometrium with preservation of the convex external fundal contour (**Fig. 17**). The signal intensity of the fundal myometrium is isointense to background myometrium.

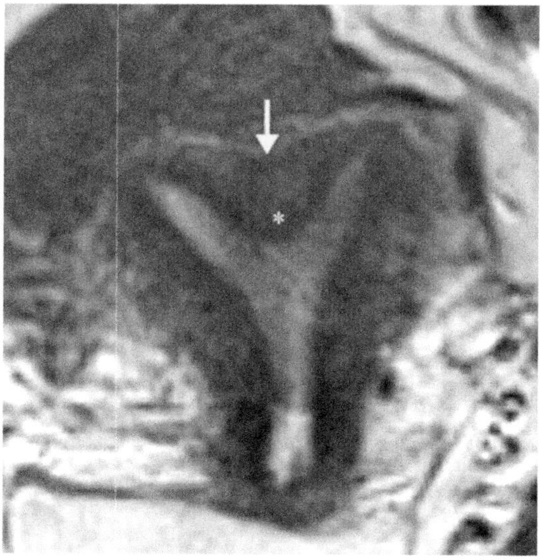

Fig. 17. Arcuate uterus. Oblique axial T2 weighted MR image through the long axis of the uterine corpus demonstrates a broad, saddle shaped indentation of the fundal myometrium (*asterisk*). Slight concavity is likewise noted involving the external uterine fundus (*arrow*).

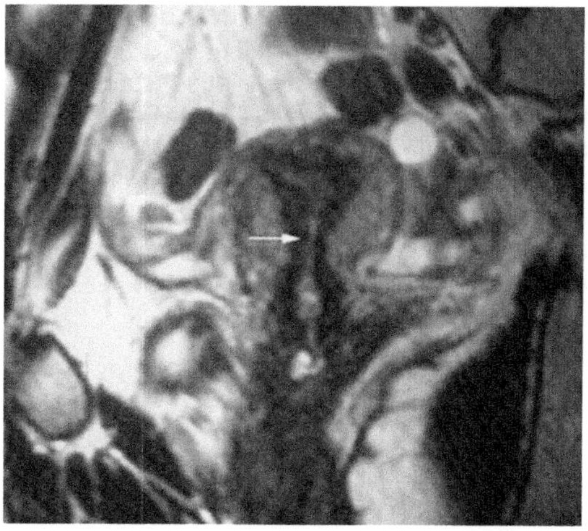

Fig. 18. DES exposed uterus. T2-weighted MR image through the long axis of the uterus demonstrates an unusually small endometrial cavity with a T-shaped configuration. Areas of focal endometrial stenosis are likewise noted (*arrow*).

Diethylstilbestrol-exposed Uterus

Diethylstilbestrol (DES) is a synthetic estrogen that was first introduced in 1948 in an effort to decrease the risk of pregnancy loss. The DES-exposed uterus is classified as a class VII MDA. The drug was prescribed to women who had experienced prior spontaneous abortions or other poor reproductive outcomes. The drug was discontinued in 1971 after an association between in utero DES exposure and clear cell carcinoma of the vagina as well as MDAs was established.[30]

MR imaging accurately portrays the structural abnormalities related to DES exposure. The T-shaped uterine configuration is easily demonstrated on MR imaging, as is uterine hypoplasia. Another frequently seen disorder in the DES-exposed uterus is the presence of constriction bands or areas of focal stenosis of the endometrium. These are characterized by focal thickening of the junctional zone with resultant narrowing and irregularity of the endometrial cavity (**Fig. 18**).

SUMMARY

The imaging of MDAs has evolved significantly over the past few decades. Accurate classification of these diverse anomalies is essential for clinicians to provide the most appropriate treatment options and counseling to women. It is important for radiologists to be aware of the current classification systems to accurately describe the spectrum of MDAs. Although these disorders may be rudimentarily characterized at HSG or conventional pelvic US, newer techniques, such as 3-D US, will continue to provide better insight into this spectrum of disorders. MR imaging remains the imaging gold standard and will likely remain the imaging modality of choice because of its multiplanar capability and excellent spatial resolution.

REFERENCES

1. ASRM. The American Fertility Society classifications of adnexal adhesions, distal tubal occlusion, tubal occlusion secondary to tubal ligation, tubal pregnancies, mullerian anomalies and intrauterine adhesions. Fertil Steril 1988;49(6):944–55.
2. Olpin JD, Heilbrun M. Imaging of Mullerian duct anomalies. Clin Obstet Gynecol 2009;52(1):40–56.
3. Troiano RN, McCarthy SM. Mullerian duct anomalies: imaging and clinical issues. Radiology 2004;233(1):19–34.
4. Venetis CA, Papadopoulos SP, Campo R, et al. Clinical implications of congenital uterine anomalies: a meta-analysis of comparative studies. Reprod Biomed Online 2014;29(6):665–83.
5. Chan YY, Jayaprakasan K, Zamora J, et al. The prevalence of congenital uterine anomalies in unselected and high-risk populations: a systematic review. Hum Reprod Update 2011;17(6):761–71.
6. Grimbizis GF, Camus M, Tarlatzis BC, et al. Clinical implications of uterine malformations and hysteroscopic treatment results. Hum Reprod Update 2001;7(2):161–74.
7. Saravelos SH, Cocksedge KA, Li TC. Prevalence and diagnosis of congenital uterine anomalies in women with reproductive failure: a critical appraisal. Hum Reprod Update 2008;14(5):415–29.
8. Practice Committee of the American Society for Reproductive Medicine, Electronic Address Aao, Practice Committee of the American Society for Reproductive Medicine. Uterine septum: a guideline. Fertil Steril 2016;106(3):530–40.
9. Deutch TD, Abuhamad AZ. The role of 3-dimensional ultrasonography and magnetic resonance imaging in the diagnosis of mullerian duct anomalies: a review of the literature. J Ultrasound Med 2008;27(3):413–23.
10. Epelman M, Dinan D, Gee MS, et al. Mullerian duct and related anomalies in children and adolescents. Magn Reson Imaging Clin N Am 2013;21(4):773–89.
11. Acien P, Acien M, Sanchez-Ferrer M. Complex malformations of the female genital tract. New types and revision of classification. Hum Reprod 2004;19(10):2377–84.
12. Grimbizis GF, Di Spiezio Sardo A, Saravelos SH, et al. The Thessaloniki ESHRE/ESGE consensus on diagnosis of female genital anomalies. Gynecol Surg 2016;13:1–16.
13. Bermejo C, Martinez Ten P, Cantarero R, et al. Three-dimensional ultrasound in the diagnosis of Mullerian duct anomalies and concordance with magnetic resonance imaging. Ultrasound Obstet Gynecol 2010;35(5):593–601.
14. Graupera B, Pascual MA, Hereter L, et al. Accuracy of three-dimensional ultrasound compared with magnetic resonance imaging in diagnosis of Mullerian duct anomalies using ESHRE-ESGE consensus on the classification of congenital anomalies of the female genital tract. Ultrasound Obstet Gynecol 2015;46(5):616–22.
15. Ergenoglu AM, Sahin C, Simsek D, et al. Comparison of three-dimensional ultrasound and magnetic resonance imaging diagnosis in surgically proven Mullerian duct anomaly cases. Eur J Obstet Gynecol Reprod Biol 2016;197:22–6.
16. Carrington BM, Hricak H, Nuruddin RN, et al. Mullerian duct anomalies: MR imaging evaluation. Radiology 1990;176(3):715–20.
17. Oppelt P, Renner SP, Brucker S, et al. The VCUAM (Vagina Cervix Uterus Adnex-associated Malformation) classification: a new classification for genital malformations. Fertil Steril 2005;84(5):1493–7.
18. Grimbizis GF, Gordts S, Di Spiezio Sardo A, et al. The ESHRE/ESGE consensus on the classification of female genital tract congenital anomalies. Hum Reprod 2013;28(8):2032–44.
19. Buttram VC Jr, Gibbons WE. Mullerian anomalies: a proposed classification. (An analysis of 144 cases). Fertil Steril 1979;32(1):40–6.
20. Di Spiezio Sardo A, Giampaolino P, Scognamiglio M, et al. An exceptional case of complete septate uterus with unilateral cervical aplasia (class U2bC3V0/ESHRE/ESGE classification) and isolated Mullerian remnants: combined hysteroscopic and laparoscopic treatment. J Minim Invasive Gynecol 2016;23(1):16–7.
21. Heinonen PK. Unicornuate uterus and rudimentary horn. Fertil Steril 1997;68(2):224–30.
22. Brody JM, Koelliker SL, Frishman GN. Unicornuate uterus: imaging appearance, associated anomalies, and clinical implications. AJR Am J Roentgenol 1998;171(5):1341–7.
23. Toaff ME, Lev-Toaff AS, Toaff R. Communicating uteri: review and classification with introduction of two previously unreported types. Fertil Steril 1984;41(5):661–79.
24. Kupesic S, Kurjak A. Septate uterus: detection and prediction of obstetrical complications by different forms of ultrasonography. J Ultrasound Med 1998;17(10):631–6.
25. Homer HA, Li TC, Cooke ID. The septate uterus: a review of management and reproductive outcome. Fertil Steril 2000;73(1):1–14.

26. Saygili-Yilmaz E, Yildiz S, Erman-Akar M, et al. Reproductive outcome of septate uterus after hysteroscopic metroplasty. Arch Gynecol Obstet 2003;268(4):289–92.
27. Propst AM, Hill JA 3rd. Anatomic factors associated with recurrent pregnancy loss. Semin Reprod Med 2000;18(4):341–50.
28. Fedele L, Ferrazzi E, Dorta M, et al. Ultrasonography in the differential diagnosis of "double" uteri. Fertil Steril 1988;50(2):361–4.
29. Ludwin A, Pitynski K, Ludwin I, et al. Two- and three-dimensional ultrasonography and sonohysterography versus hysteroscopy with laparoscopy in the differential diagnosis of septate, bicornuate, and arcuate uteri. J Minim Invasive Gynecol 2013;20(1):90–9.
30. Herbst AL, Ulfelder H, Poskanzer DC. Adenocarcinoma of the vagina. Association of maternal stilbestrol therapy with tumor appearance in young women. N Engl J Med 1971;284(15):878–81.

Benign Gynecologic Conditions of the Uterus

Zahra Kassam, MD[a], Iva Petkovska, MD[b,c], Carolyn L. Wang, MD[d], Angela M. Trinh, MD[e], Aya Kamaya, MD[f,*]

KEYWORDS

• Leiomyoma • Fibroid • Adenomyosis • Retained products of conception
• Uterine arteriovenous malformation

KEY POINTS

- Adenomyosis is a common, frequently debilitating condition affecting women in their later reproductive years.
- Uterine leiomyomas are the most common tumor of the uterus, affecting up to 80% of women, and can be a cause of abnormal uterine bleeding, pelvic pain and mass effect, and reproductive or sexual dysfunction.
- Differentiating retained products of conception, a common cause of postpartum hemorrhage, from uterine arteriovenous malformation is important in order to allow for optimal treatment.
- Although ultrasound is the first line imaging modality in evaluation of the uterus, MR imaging has become a useful and reliable noninvasive tool in diagnosis and problem solving in all of these entities.

BACKGROUND

Relevant Uterine Anatomy

The anatomy of the normal, premenopausal uterus is traditionally divided into 2 distinct components: the endometrium and the myometrium. MR imaging has the advantage of further stratifying the anatomic layers into 3 well-depicted zones on T2-weighted imaging (T2WI), as follows (**Fig. 1**):

1. *Endometrium*: It has high signal on T2WI due to the presence of secretions and abundant cytoplasm. In reproductive-aged women, normal endometrial thickness varies between 3 and 6 mm in the proliferative phase and 5 and 13 mm in the secretory phase.
2. *Inner myometrium/junctional zone (JZ)*: This superficial myometrial layer consists of myocytes with a high nuclear-to-cytoplasmic ratio and reduced water content, relative to the deeper myometrial myocytes.[1] This unique morphology results in an intrinsic, lower signal on T2WI. The concentric orientation of smooth muscle fibers, in contrast to the longitudinal arrangement in the outer myometrium, also contributes to the lower signal of the JZ. The JZ is the presumed site of origin of uterine contractions and peristalsis.[2]
3. *Outer myometrium*: The outer myometrium consists of myocytes with a lower nuclear-to-cytoplasmic ratio. The relative increase in water content and the longitudinal orientation of smooth muscle fibers results in a higher T2 signal than the JZ.

Physiologic variation of the JZ may occur with age or with changes in hormone levels. In postmenopausal patients, there is progressive

The authors have nothing to disclose.

[a] Radiology and Oncology, Department of Medical Imaging, University of Western Ontario, Western University, St Joseph's Health Care London, 268 Grosvenor Street, London, ON N6A 4V2, Canada; [b] Department of Radiology, Memorial Sloan Kettering Cancer Center, 1275 York Avenue, Box 29, New York, NY, 10065, USA; [c] Department of Medical Imaging, University of Arizona, 1501 North Campbell Avenue, Tucson, AZ 85724, USA; [d] Department of Radiology, University of Washington, 1959 Northeast Pacific Street, Seattle, WA 98195, USA; [e] Sutter Medical Foundation, 1500 Expo Parkway, Sacramento, CA 95815, USA; [f] Department of Radiology, Stanford University Medical Center, 300 Pasteur Drive, H1307, Stanford, CA 94305, USA
* Corresponding author.
E-mail address: kamaya@stanford.edu

Magn Reson Imaging Clin N Am 25 (2017) 577–600
http://dx.doi.org/10.1016/j.mric.2017.03.005

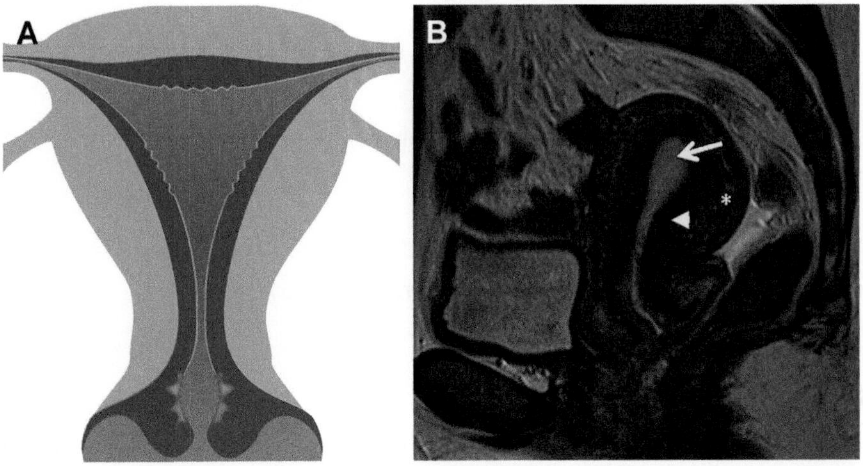

Fig. 1. Zonal anatomy of uterus. (*A*). Endometrial-subendometrial unit of uterus. Endometrial-subendometrial unit is composed of glandular/stromal portion of endometrium (*green*) and stratum subvasculare of myometrium, with predominantly circular muscular fibers (*yellow*). (*B*). Sagittal T2WI demonstrates 3 distinct uterine layers visible on MR imaging: endometrium (*arrow*), JZ (inner myometrium, *arrowhead*), and outer myometrium (*asterisks*). ([*A*] *Courtesy of* Amy N. Thomas, Stanford University; *Modified from* Leyendecker G, Kunz G, Kissler S, et al. Adenomyosis and reproduction. Best Pract Res Clin Obstet Gynecol 2006;20(4):528; with permission.)

dehydration of the outer myometrium, which lowers the T2 signal and, therefore, the distinction between the JZ and outer myometrium.[1] With increasing age, the smooth muscle of the myometrium undergoes progressive atrophy. Therefore, the JZ may not be delineated in up to 30% of postmenopausal patients.[3]

Patient Preparation

Bladder emptying is recommended immediately before the examination in order to reduce artifacts related to bladder filling and patient discomfort.[4] Motion artifacts related to small bowel peristalsis may be minimized using antiperistaltic agents, such as hyoscine butylbromide (20 mg intramuscularly [IM]/intravenously [IV]) or glucagon (0.5–1.0 mg IM/IV). Routine use of antiperistaltic agents in pelvic MR imaging has been shown to significantly improve image quality.[5]

MR Imaging Protocol

Uterine evaluation is optimized using high-resolution, thin-section MR imaging with images acquired at 1.5 T or 3.0 T. Optimal signal-to-noise ratio may be achieved using a phased-array surface coil.

Recommended sequences include

- High-resolution, free-breathing T2 sequences in the axial, oblique, sagittal, and coronal planes is recommended. (High-resolution, 3-dimensional [3D], T2WI with multi-planar reformatting may also be used.) Sagittal T2WI best depicts the zonal anatomy of the uterus. T2WI acquisitions in more than one plane are helpful to avoid misinterpretation of transient uterine contractions.
- Axial T1-weighted sequence with and without fat suppression is recommended.
- Contrast-enhanced axial T1-weighted images (T1WI) of the pelvis with fat saturation is recommended.

ADENOMYOSIS

Discussion of Problem/Clinical Presentation

- Adenomyosis of the uterus is a common gynecologic condition, affecting 1% of women in the fourth and fifth decades of life and 20% to 35% of women undergoing hysterectomy for benign gynecologic disorders.[6] Most affected women are multiparous.
- The condition occurs at the endometrial-myometrial interface and is characterized by the presence of ectopic endometrial glands and stroma within the myometrium, with adjacent smooth muscle hyperplasia.
- Up to one-third of patients are asymptomatic. Symptomatic patients most frequently present with menorrhagia (50%), dysmenorrhea (30%), and metrorrhagia (20%). Occasionally, dyspareunia may be a presenting complaint.[7]
- Adenomyosis is associated with female infertility due to the overlapping pathophysiology and association with endometriosis.[8]

Pathophysiology

Adenomyosis is characterized by the ectopic, intramyometrial location of endometrial glands and stroma. The ectopic glands are surrounded by reactive hypertrophy of the myometrium, often leading to globular enlargement of the myometrium and uterus. Occasionally, extravasated blood products may accumulate within cystic intramyometrial spaces.[7] At surgery, foci of ectopic endometrial tissue may be macroscopically visible on the serosal surface of a hysterectomy specimen (**Fig. 2**).[7] At the microscopic level, adenomyosis is arrayed randomly within the myometrium, usually at least 2 mm deep to the basal endometrial layer (**Fig. 3**).[7]

The pathogenesis of adenomyosis is unclear, but several mechanisms have been proposed[7,9]:

1. *Uterine autotraumatization*: This widely accepted theory suggests that chronic uterine peristaltic activity and hyperperistalsis induce microtraumatizations at the endometrial-myometrial interface. The endometrial/myometrial interface is structurally a point of weakness and is, therefore, susceptible to microtrauma, usually due to hyperperistalsis (iatrogenic microtrauma is also a potential inciting factor). This autotraumatization by peristaltic activity, in turn, activates a cycle of tissue injury and repair, resulting in local production of estrogen.[9] The relative increase in local estrogen production by the uterus, which increases uterine peristalsis, competes with a function normally controlled by the ovaries. These interactions lead to a state of perpetual hyperperistalsis and a cyclical disease process. This theory is supported by evidence indicating that estradiol levels are elevated in the menstrual blood of women with adenomyosis.[10]
2. *Impairment of repair mechanisms normally involving the basal endometrial layer*: Endometrial stroma invaginates into the myometrium at structural points of weakness along the basal endometrial layer. This invagination may be due to focal disruption; however, absence of enzymatic activity required specifically to maintain the contiguity of the basal layer is also a possible cause.
3. *Lymphatic contamination*: Invagination of the basal endometrial layer into the myometrium may occur via the local lymphatic channels, resulting in ectopic endometrial tissue.
4. *Metaplastic transformation*: As Müllerian tissue is pluripotent, this theory proposes that myometrial tissue within the JZ differentiates into the glandular and stromal tissue characteristic of the endometrium.

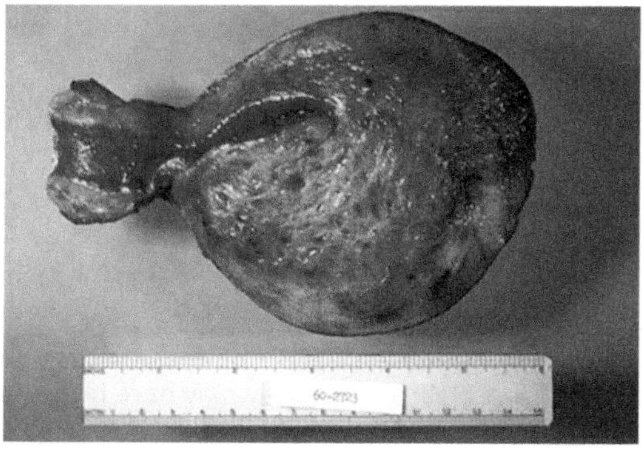

Fig. 2. Diffuse adenomyosis of anterior wall of uterus. Note coarsely trabeculated, diffusely hypertrophied myometrium, stippled with foci of ectopic endometrium (original magnification × 4). (*From* Bergeron C, Amant F, Ferenczy A. Pathology and physiopathology of adenomyosis. Best Pract Res Clin Obstet Gynaecol 2006;20:511–21; with permission.)

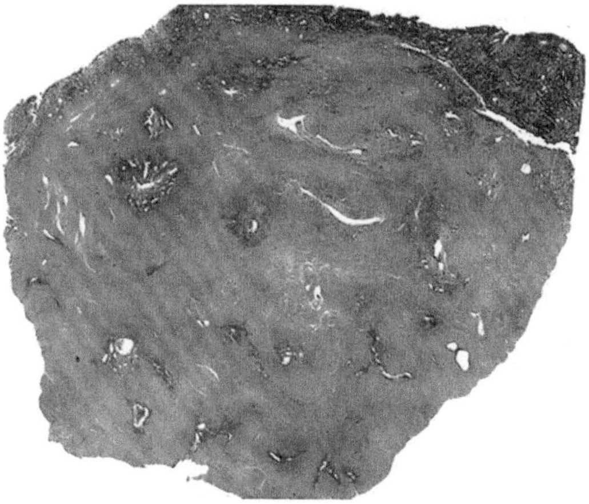

Fig. 3. Whole section of endomyometrium. Adenomyotic foci scattered throughout myometrium (original magnification × 25). (*From* Bergeron C, Amant F, Ferenczy A. Pathology and physiopathology of adenomyosis. Best Pract Res Clin Obstet Gynaecol 2006;20:511–21; with permission.)

Histologic examination of the myometrium in patients with and without adenomyosis suggests that a chronic state of hyperperistalsis may alter the myometrial ultrastructure, causing distortion of the myocytes, nuclear enlargement, and reduced prominence of collagen fibrils due to expansion of the extracellular space. Intracellular calcium is also increased in myocytes harboring adenomyosis, which has been shown to affect contractility. This dysfunctional contractility may manifest clinically as dysmenorrhea.[11]

MR Imaging Features and Diagnostic Criteria

Studies evaluating the diagnostic performance of MR imaging in adenomyosis describe a sensitivity of 70% to 86%, specificity of 86% to 93%, and mean accuracy of 87.5%.[12] In contrast, accuracy of clinical diagnosis alone ranges from 2.6% to 26.0%, due to the nonspecific clinical presentation.[13]

Features of adenomyosis on MR imaging may be stratified into direct and indirect signs.[1] *Direct signs* have specific correlation with the presence of endometrial glands within the myometrium, whereas *indirect signs* are the result of reactive changes in the myometrium (**Table 1**).

Direct Signs

1. *Submucosal microcysts*: They are focal pools of fluid embedded within the myometrium, varying in size from 2 to 7 mm. These microcysts typically demonstrate water signal on T1WI and T2WI. While considered a specific sign of adenomyosis, they are detected in only 50% of cases.[13] Occasionally, toward the end of the luteal phase, hemorrhagic content may accumulate within the cysts, manifesting as T1 shortening[1] (**Fig. 4**).
2. *Adenomyoma*: Masslike consolidation of adenomyotic glands within the myometrium, appearing distinct from the JZ. The distinction from leiomyoma may be challenging; adenomyomas are usually low signal on T2WI but may contain punctate foci of high T2 signal. They do not typically have feeding vessels in the vicinity, in contrast to leiomyomas. Recognition of this entity is important for patient management, as myomectomy or polypectomy may be curative for leiomyomas but ineffective for adenomyomas (**Fig. 5**).

Indirect Signs

1. *Thickening of the JZ* results from smooth muscle hypertrophy, secondary to the presence of ectopic endometrial glands within the myometrium. When the entire JZ is thickened, diffuse adenomyosis is likely (**Fig. 6**); if only a portion of the JZ is thickened, focal adenomyosis is considered. The most widely accepted diagnostic criterion in establishing the diagnosis of adenomyosis is a JZ thickness of greater than 12 mm.[12] This criterion reveals a diagnostic accuracy of 85%, specificity of 96%, and sensitivity of 63%.[12] The relatively low sensitivity may relate to reduced T2 signal contrast between the JZ and dehydrated outer myometrium in some patients. Focal JZ thickening greater than 12 mm may also indicate adenomyosis but should be distinguished from transient uterine contraction.[14]
2. The JZ *differential* was described by Dueholm and colleagues[15] in 2001 as the difference between maximal and minimal thicknesses in the anterior and posterior uterine JZ. The investigators described a differential of greater than 5 mm as a more reliable measure than a JZ thickness of greater than 12 mm.

Pearls, Pitfalls, and Variants

Problem-solving pearls

The following problem-solving techniques may be used in challenging cases:

1. *Diffusion-weighted imaging* is useful for distinguishing between endometrial carcinoma and focal adenomyosis.[16] Adenomyoma demonstrates high signal on both T2WI and apparent diffusion coefficient in contrast to cellular leiomyomas and carcinoma.[16]
2. *Cine MR imaging* may aid in differentiating between transient myometrial contraction and focal adenomyosis.[17,18]
3. *Susceptibility-weighted imaging* is useful for detection of hemosiderin deposits in adenomyosis (**Fig. 7**), particularly when leiomyoma is in the differential diagnosis.[19]

Table 1
Adenomyosis: MR imaging features of direct and indirect signs

Direct Signs	Indirect Signs	MR Imaging Features
Microcysts	—	Intramyometrial cysts measuring 2–7 mm (average 3 mm); usually simple fluid signal on T1WI and T2WI, occasionally may have high signal on T1WI
Adenomyoma	—	Focal consolidation of ectopic endometrial glands, often distinct from JZ; often contain foci of high signal on T2WI
—	JZ thickening	Smooth muscle hypertrophy reactive to presence of ectopic endometrial tissue; >12 mm thickness
—	JZ differential	>5 mm differential between maximal and minimal uterine JZ thicknesses

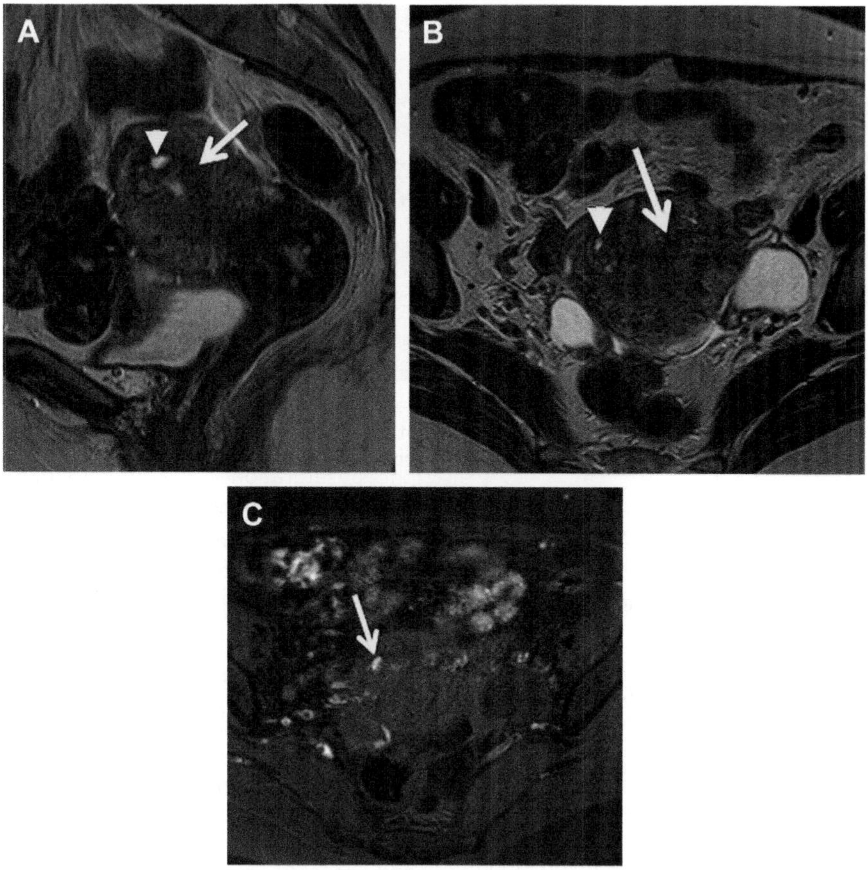

Fig. 4. Diffuse adenomyosis with hemorrhagic, submucosal microcysts. (*A*) Sagittal and (*B*) axial T2WI show diffusely thickened JZ (*arrow*) with microcysts (*arrowhead*) with intermediate to high T2 signal. Axial T1WI with fat saturation (*C*) image demonstrates corresponding high signal (hemorrhage) (*arrow*) within microcyst.

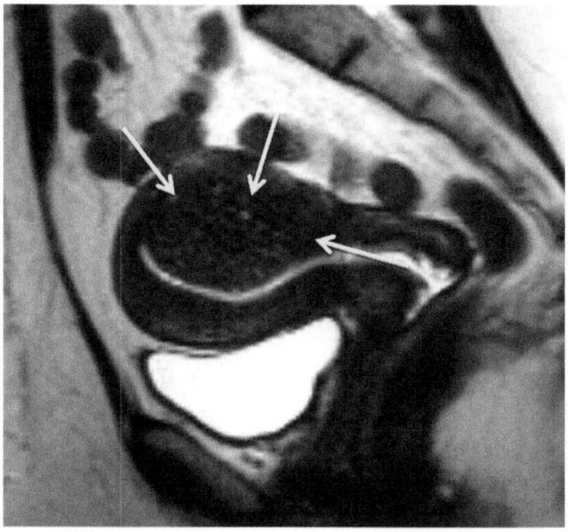

Fig. 5. A 28-year-old woman with adenomyoma who presents with pelvic pain and menorrhagia. Sagittal single shot fast spin echo T2 weighted image (a), demonstrates focal thickening of the JZ (*arrows*) of the myometrium, with multiple small cystic spaces (*arrow*). Imaging findings are classic for adenomyosis. This case demonstrates focal adenomyosis/adenomyoma. Three arrows point to the area of adenomyoma/adenomyosis.

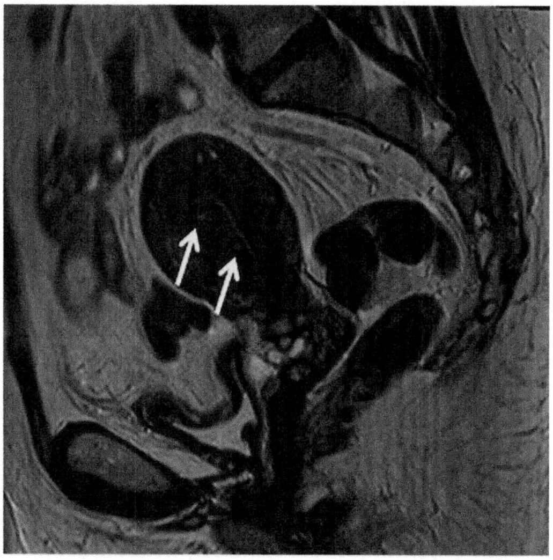

Fig. 6. Direct and indirect features of adenomyosis. Sagittal T2WI demonstrates diffuse thickening of JZ (indirect sign), with superficial cysts in submucosal myometrium (direct sign, *arrows*).

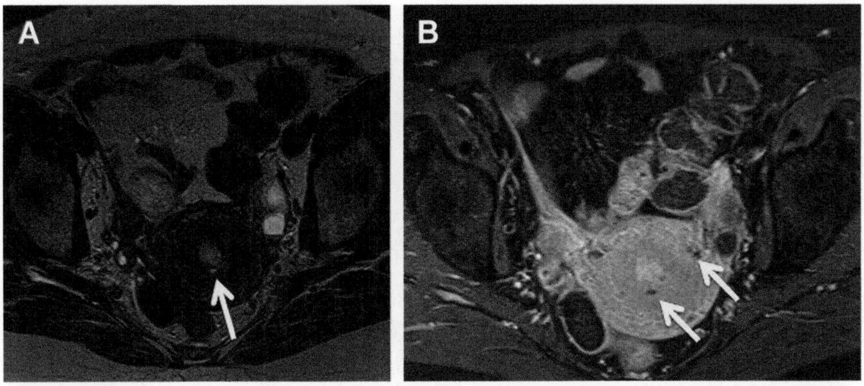

Fig. 7. Susceptibility due to hemosiderin deposition. (*A*) Axial T2WI shows diffuse JZ thickening with submucosal cyst (*arrow*). (*B*) Corresponding axial, fat-saturated gradient echo T1WI demonstrates punctate foci of susceptibility artifact (*arrows*) corresponding to submucosal cyst, indicating presence of hemosiderin.

Pitfalls and Variants

Pseudolesions

1. *Pseudothickening of the JZ*: The JZ may appear diffusely thickened during the early menstrual phase[20] and may mimic the appearance of diffuse adenomyosis. Ideally, MR imaging should be performed midcycle to avoid this pitfall.
2. *Myometrial contractions*: Focal bulging of the myometrium secondary to a uterine contraction creates poorly defined margins with the JZ and reduces the water content of the myometrium, which can mimic focal adenomyosis. Cine magnetic resonance (MR) and multiphase single-shot fast spin echo techniques may reveal the transient nature of these contractions.

Atypical lesions

1. Adenomyomatous polyp is a rare subtype of endometrial polyp, which originates from the basal layer of the endometrium. The term "adenomatous" refers to the presence of smooth muscle components within the lesion. Histologically, this lesion may be confused with an adenomyoma. MRI features are indistinguishable from routine endometrial polyps; on T2WI, the lesion typically appears as a hypointense polypoid mass, with foci on high T2 signal.[21]
2. Adenomyotic cyst, also referred to as hemorrhagic cystic adenomyosis, is a rare subtype of adenomyosis. This lesion develops following spontaneous hemorrhage of ectopic endometrial glands, with pooling of blood products. The hemorrhage is contained by a partial or complete rim of myometrial tissue, resulting in a cyst-like appearance. The cyst may be variable in size, and may be submucosal, intramyometrial, or subserosal. Patients frequently present with dysmenorrhea and menorrhagia. Hemorrhagic contents may be high signal on T1WI, with a low signal rim on T2WI (**Fig. 8**).

What Referring Physicians Need to Know: Medical Versus Surgical Management

Accurate diagnosis of adenomyosis is important in order to provide the clinician with a road map of appropriate therapeutic options. Treatment measures frequently depend on patient demographics and severity of symptoms. Hysterectomy is curative; but uterus-sparing therapies[22] offer alternative, nonsurgical options for symptomatic patients (**Table 2**). It is important to provide the clinician with the extent of disease involvement (focal vs diffuse), location of disease, and morphologic characteristics (cystic vs solid).

UTERINE LEIOMYOMAS

Discussion of Problem/Clinical Presentation

- Uterine leiomyomas, also known as fibroids or myomas, are the most common type of gynecologic tumor, affecting up to 80% of women in their lifetime,[23] with a higher incidence in black women.[24] A recent study has shown that even in women younger than 30 years, the prevalence of leiomyomas based on transvaginal ultrasound was 14.9%.[25]
- Although most patients with uterine leiomyomas are asymptomatic, between 20% and 50% can experience abnormal uterine bleeding, pelvic pain, bulky symptoms, reproductive or sexual dysfunction, or urologic symptoms, such as urinary frequency.[26–29]
- Symptomatic fibroids have a significant negative impact on women's quality of life.[30–32]

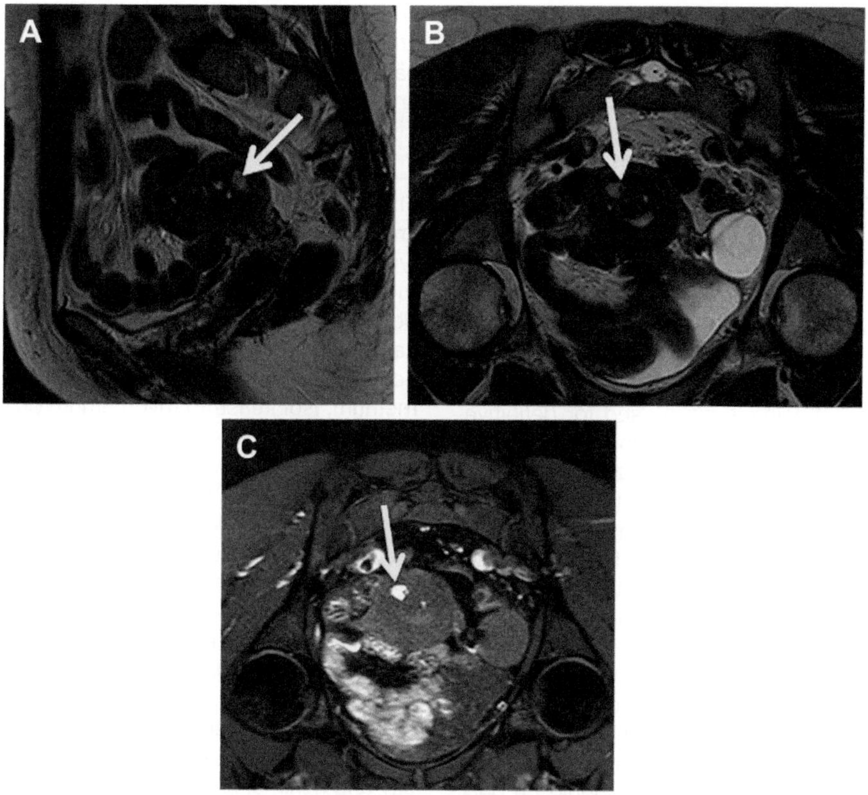

Fig. 8. Adenomyotic cyst. (*A*) Sagittal and (*B*) axial oblique T2WI reveal diffuse thickening of JZ, with focal, high-signal cyst in posterior right myometrium (*arrow*). Corresponding axial oblique T1WI with fat saturation (*C*) demonstrates T1 shortening within cyst (*arrow*), indicating hemorrhagic composition.

Anatomy

Leiomyomas are monoclonal tumors that arise from the uterine smooth muscle; 40% to 50% have a cytogenetic abnormality, most commonly involving chromosomes 6, 7, 12, and 14.[33] These disordered myofibroblasts are buried in an abundance of extracellular matrix[32] and cell proliferation; survival and extracellular matrix extension depends on progesterone and

Table 2
Adenomyosis: medical and surgical treatment options

Medical Therapies & Mechanism of Action	Surgical and Endovascular Therapies
IUD Release progesterone or danazol to reduce menorrhagia	Endometrial ablation Useful in superficial adenomyosis; usually followed by placement of progesterone IUD
GnRH agonists Bind to pituitary GnRH receptor, downregulating GnRH activity and reducing estrogen secretion, inducing atrophy of adenomyotic nodules, and reducing overall uterine size	Excision of adenomyotic nodules Useful for submucosal, intramural, and subserosal adenomyomas Uterine artery embolization Less well established than for leiomyomas, reported symptomatic relief in a subset of patients
Aromatase inhibitors Aromatase P450 expressed in endometrium, converts androgens to estrogenic steroids; aromatase inhibitors reduce local estrogen levels	Hysterectomy Definitive, curative management

Abbreviations: GnRH, gonadotropin-releasing hormone; IUD, intrauterine device.

progesterone receptor.[34] A newly published International Federation of Gynecology and Obstetrics (FIGO) leiomyoma subclassification system classifies leiomyomas based on their location as submucosal (projecting into the uterine cavity and most likely to be associated with abnormal uterine bleeding) and other (including intramural and subserosal)[35] (**Fig. 9**).

Magnetic Resonance Features and Diagnostic Criteria

Ultrasound is typically the first-line imaging modality when evaluating the uterus for leiomyomas; however, MR imaging is often used for definitive localization of leiomyomas and has the advantage of improved soft-tissue characterization. In addition, MR imaging can assess an enlarged myomatous uterus that may otherwise be challenging to assess with ultrasound because of a limited field of view.[36,37] MR imaging has reported sensitivities and specificities of 94.1% and 68.7%, respectively, for uterine leiomyomas, with a positive predictive value of 95.7%.[38]

Axial T1WI with and without fat saturation is useful to evaluate the uterine contour, lymph nodes, bone marrow, and any fat-containing lesion versus protein or hemorrhage. The T2WI should be performed in 3 orthogonal planes to better depict the zonal anatomy, and contrast enhancement should be performed to document the presence of necrosis in the uterine leiomyomas. Dynamic contrast injection should be used in women who are considering uterine artery embolization to evaluate the uterine arteries and collateral gonadal arterial supply.[39]

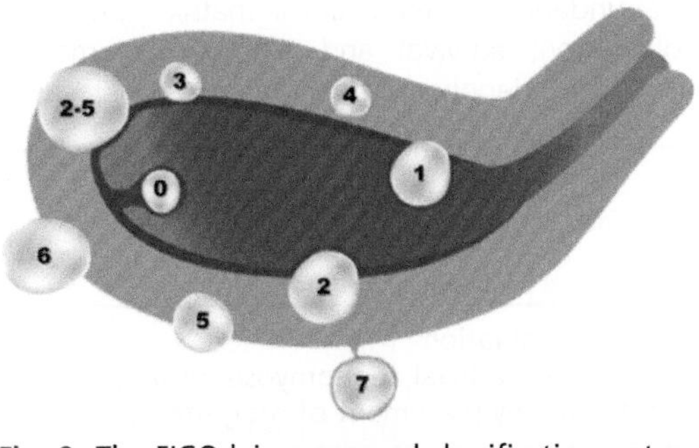

Fig. 9. The FIGO leiomyoma subclassification system. The 35 leiomyomas are classified based on location: 0: pedunculated intracavitary; 1: less than 50% intramural; 2: 50% or greater intramural; 3: contacts endometrium, 100% intramural; 4: intramural; 5: subserosal 50% or greater intramural; 6: subserosal less than 50% intramural; 7: subserosal pedunculated; 8: other (specify [eg, cervical, parasitic]). Types 0 to 2 are designated SM for submucosal, and types 3 to 7 as O for other. Combination types are indicated with 2 numbers separated by a hyphen, such as: 2-5: Submucosal and subserosal, each with less than half the diameter in the endometrial and peritoneal cavities, respectively. (*Courtesy of* Amy N. Thomas, Stanford University.)

Imaging Findings

The imaging appearance of leiomyomas on MR imaging varies depending on the degree and type of degeneration that occurs as a result of the leiomyoma outgrowing its blood supply. Nondegenerating leiomyomas on MR imaging classically appear as well-circumscribed masses of homogenous low T2 signal relative to normal myometrium, isointense to myometrium on T1WI, and enhance homogenously on postcontrast images (**Fig. 10**). Submucosal leiomyomas can also exhibit mass effect on the endometrium (**Fig. 11**).

Hypercellular leiomyomas are composed of compact smooth muscle cells with little or no collagen, demonstrate high T2 signal on MR imaging, are isointense to muscle on T1WI, and enhance similar to muscle (**Fig. 12**). Leiomyomas with cystic degeneration will demonstrate higher T2 signal intensity, and the cystic components will not enhance. Leiomyomas with myxoid degeneration will demonstrate very high T2 signal intensity and minimal enhancement (**Fig. 13**).

Necrotic leiomyomas that have not liquefied will have variable T1 signal intensity and low T2 signal intensity (**Fig. 14**). Leiomyomas with red degeneration due to hemorrhagic infarction are more commonly observed during pregnancy and can demonstrate peripheral or diffuse high T1 signal, thought to be related to either T1 shortening of methemoglobin or the proteinaceous content of the blood. On T2WI, leiomyomas are variable in signal, with or without a T2 rim of low signal[40] (**Fig. 15**).

Lipoleiomyomas with fatty degeneration are typically hyperintense on T2WI and appear hyperintense on T1WI that suppress on fat-suppression sequences. Within the lipoleiomyomas are amorphous areas of low T2 signal and low T1 signal that enhance after contrast[4] (**Fig. 16**).

Pearls, Pitfalls, and Variants

A potential pitfall in leiomyomas is a pedunculated subserosal leiomyoma, which may grow laterally and extend between the folds of the broad ligament (intraligamentous leiomyomas), simulating an ovarian mass[41] (**Fig. 17**). Conversely, ovarian fibromas and Brenner tumors, which are benign ovarian neoplasms with a significant fibrous component, can simulate a pedunculated leiomyoma. The key to distinguishing between the two entities is to identify both the continuity of

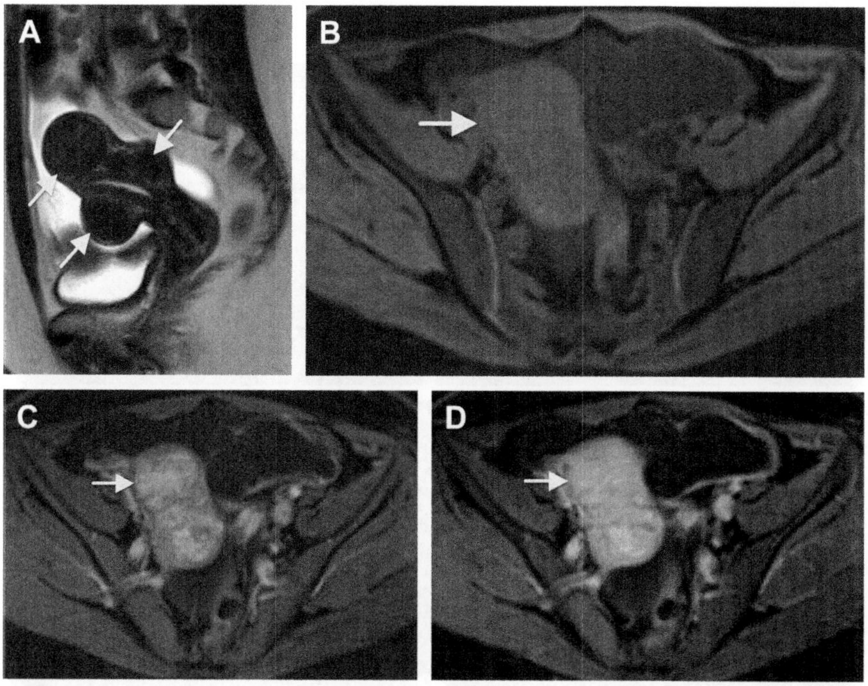

Fig. 10. Typical leiomyoma. A 25-year-old woman presented with menorrhagia. Sagittal T2WI (*A*) demonstrates multiple well-defined lesions (*white arrows*) with homogeneous T2 hypointense signal typical for leiomyomas. On axial precontrast image, the leiomyoma (*arrow*) is isointense to the background myometrium (*B*), venous phase shows the leiomyoma (*arrow*) to be isoenhancing compared to background myometrium (*C*), and delayed postcontrast T1WI demonstrate leiomyoma (*arrow*) enhancement similar to background myometrium (*D*).

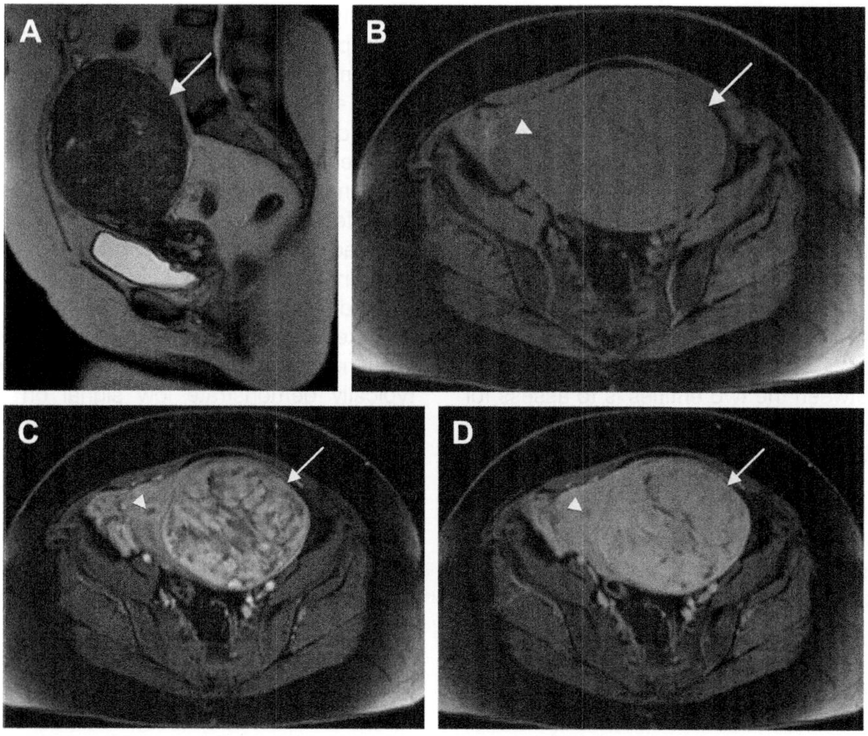

Fig. 11. A 45-year-old woman with large uterine leiomyoma. (*A*) Sagittal T2WI demonstrates a well-marginated and low-T2-signal large subserosal uterine leiomyoma (*arrow*), with foci of mild internal degeneration. (*B*) Precontrast, (*C*) venous, and (*D*) delayed postcontrast T1WI demonstrate enhancement that follows the background uterus (*arrow*). Relationship to the endometrium (*arrowhead*) is clearly delineated.

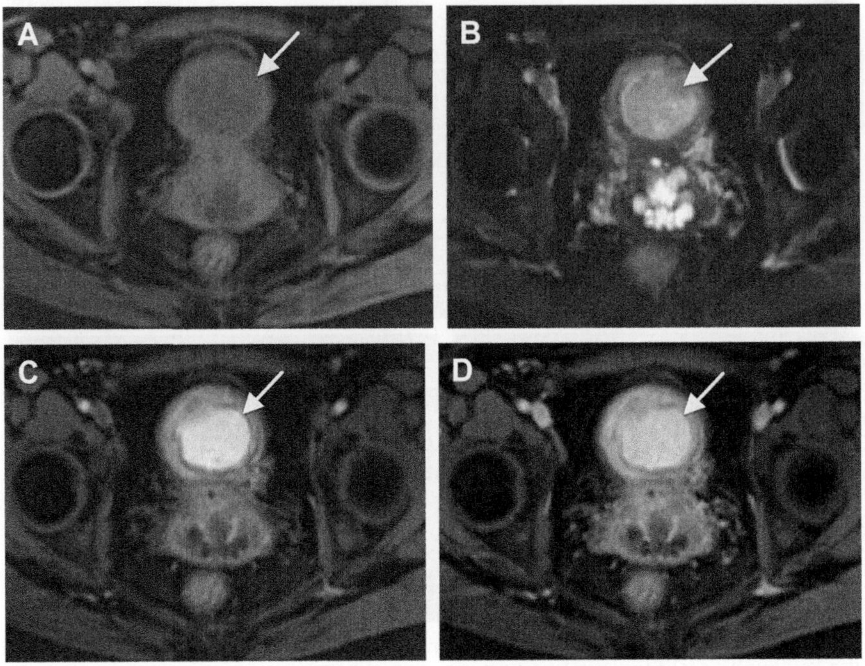

Fig. 12. Hypercellular leiomyoma. This 33-year-old woman presented with an irregular menstrual cycle. Axial precontrast T1WI (*A*) and axial postcontrast images demonstrate a well-defined lesion (*arrow*), with avid enhancement on arterial and portal venous phase (*B, C*), which follows enhancement of background myometrium on delayed phase (*D*). Imaging characteristics suggest hypercellular leiomyoma.

the adnexal mass with the adjacent myometrium via bridging vessels and a separate normal ovary.[42] Identification of ovarian tissues surrounding the mass confirms the origin of the mass as ovarian and excludes a leiomyoma. Rarely, a pedunculated subserosal leiomyoma may become parasitic by attaching to an adjacent structure, developing new blood supplies and detaching from the uterus.[43]

A second potential pitfall is in the setting of focal myometrial contractions, which can appear as low T2 signal myometrial masses and may simulate uterine leiomyomas (**Fig. 18**). The key to distinguishing between the two entities is to assess for persistence of the finding across multiple sequences: Uterine contractions are transient and usually do not persist during the entire examination or on follow-up imaging,[44] whereas leiomyomas do not change during an examination and will be present on repeat imaging.

A third potential pitfall is failure to distinguish focal adenomyomas from uterine leiomyomas. Focal adenomyomas can appear as focal low T2 signal masses in the myometrium and can mimic uterine leiomyomas (see **Fig. 5**). However, focal adenomyomas are typically more ill defined and poorly marginated than leiomyomas, which may help distinguish between the two entities. In addition, there may be small foci of high signal intensity within a focal adenomyoma on T2WI corresponding to endometrial glands.[45] Focal adenomyomas also tend to be oriented parallel to the endometrial stripe and have minimal mass effect on the endometrial canal.[39] The distinction between adenomyomas and leiomyomas is clinically important because adenomyomas cannot be effectively treated with myomectomy and may require hysterectomy.

A final potential pitfall is the submucosally located leiomyoma (**Fig. 19**), which can be mistaken for an endometrial polyp. The key distinguishing factor is that submucosal leiomyomas typically demonstrate low signal on T2WI and have a stalk that arises from the myometrium, whereas polyps tend to demonstrate more heterogeneous or high signal on T2WI[39] (**Fig. 20**).

Pathophysiology

The most common symptom for uterine leiomyomas is abnormal uterine bleeding. The exact mechanism or underlying cause is not well understood, because leiomyomas themselves are relatively avascular but seem to be surrounded by rich vasculature. Leiomyomas most commonly associated with abnormal uterine bleeding seem to be submucosal in origin, and there is suggestion that various angiogenetic and growth factors

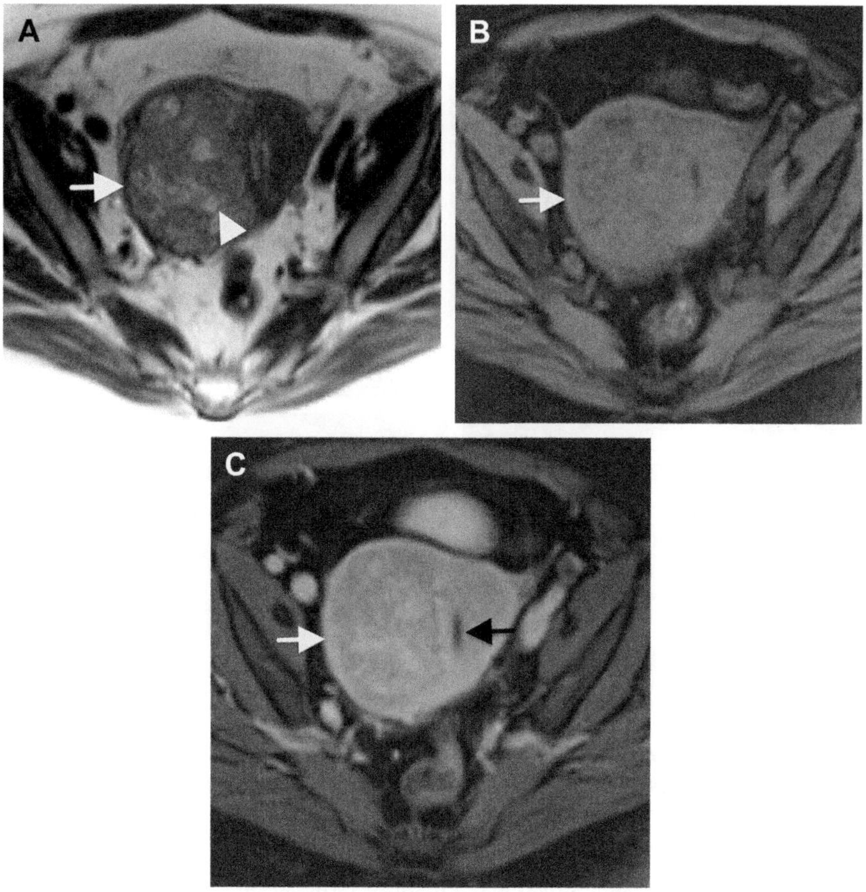

Fig. 13. A 50-year-old woman with myxoid degeneration of leiomyoma, presenting with pelvic pain. Axial T2WI (*A*), (*B*) precontrast, and (*C*) postcontrast T1WI demonstrate an enhancing mass (*arrows*) with heterogeneous signal (*arrowhead*) on T2WI. Black arrow (*C*) points to endometrium. Pathology demonstrated large leiomyoma with focal myxoid change, degenerative in nature.

secreted by the leiomyomas cause the adjacent or overlying endometrium or blood vessels surrounding the leiomyoma to bleed.[35] Hemorrhagic infarction of leiomyomas, also known as red degeneration, is most commonly associated with pregnancy.[41] Signs and symptoms of red degeneration include acute pain, low-grade fever, and leukocytosis. Red degeneration has typical MR imaging characteristics as described earlier, which can be helpful to distinguish this entity from other surgical causes of acute abdominal pain.

Uterine leiomyomas are not precursors for leiomyosarcomas. Although many leiomyosarcomas are markedly enlarged and heterogeneous in appearance, imaging alone cannot reliably distinguish between leiomyomas and leiomyosarcomas[46] (**Fig. 21**). Moreover, rapid growth of what seems to be a uterine leiomyoma may not be a good predictor of leiomyosarcoma.[47] The true incidence of occult leiomyosarcomas is contested, but the Food and Drug Administration's review of several studies estimate an aggregate incidence of approximately 1:350 for any sarcoma and 1:500 for leiomyosarcoma among women undergoing hysterectomy for leiomyomas.[48] A spectrum of morphologically abnormal uterine smooth muscle tumors spans from leiomyoma to leiomyosarcoma and may exhibit some, but not all, features of malignancy, known as smooth muscle tumors of uncertain malignant potential (STUMP)[32] (**Fig. 22**). The Society of Obstetrics and Gynecologists of Canada's guidelines suggest that postmenopausal growth of uterine leiomyomas or postmenopausal onset of symptoms should carry a higher index of suspicion for malignancy.[32]

What Referring Clinicians Need to Know

MR imaging is very helpful in the management of uterine leiomyomas because it can distinguish leiomyomas from other causes of abnormal uterine bleeding, enlarged uterus, or pelvic pain that

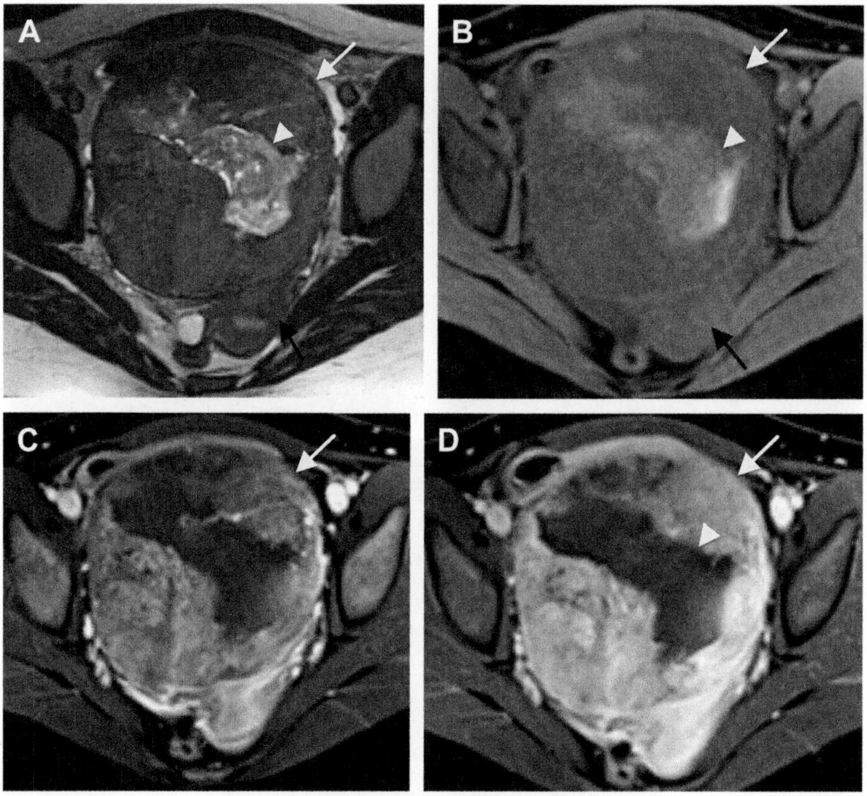

Fig. 14. A 22-year-old woman with necrotic leiomyoma, presenting with pelvic pain. Axial (*A*) T2WI, (*B*) precontrast, (*C*) venous, and (*D*) delayed postcontrast T1WI demonstrate large leiomyoma (*arrow*) inseparable from the uterus with peripheral enhancement that follows background myometrium. There is a large central area of necrosis with intrinsic proteinaceous debris and/or blood products (*arrowhead*).

may require different therapies. Additionally, MR imaging is essential in treatment planning for uterine leiomyomas, as it can accurately detect and localize individual leiomyomas. It is important for clinicians to know the exact location of the fibroids per the FIGO leiomyoma subclassification system because treatment depends on location. A detailed description of the various therapies is beyond the scope of this article.

Patients with submucosal leiomyomas less than 3 cm in size with greater than 50% of the tumor intracavitary (SM0 and SM1) are the best candidates for hysteroscopic myomectomy, whereas patients with tumors that are less than 50% intracavitary (SM2) are better suited for intra-abdominal surgery.[49] If uterine artery embolization is considered, pedunculated submucosal leiomyomas risk becoming intracavitary and superinfected. The risk for these potential complications could be assessed by reporting the relationship of the size of the leiomyoma relative to its interface with the endometrium.[50]

Pedunculated subserosal leiomyomas (O7) with a less than a 2-cm-wide stalk are relatively contraindicated for uterine artery embolization because of the risk of stalk necrosis and separation from the uterus.[51] Therefore, the stalk diameter should be included in the MR imaging report.[50] Cervical leiomyomas should be noted in the MR imaging report, as they do not tend to respond well to uterine artery embolization because of their alternate blood supply, and patients may have recurrent symptoms related to growth of the uninfarcted tissue[18,50] (**Fig. 23**).

The enhancement pattern of a leiomyoma is necessary to report for preprocedure planning for uterine artery embolization, because nonenhancing leiomyomas are unlikely to shrink and subsequently patient symptoms are unlikely to improve.[18] The addition of 3D MR angiographic imaging can also help provide a road map for evaluating the vasculature before uterine artery embolization. The relationship of the leiomyoma and the overlying myometrium is also critical to assess the amount of residual myometrium after myomectomy if fertility preservation is desired.[41]

MR imaging can also help select appropriate patients for MR-guided focused ultrasound surgery. The ideal candidate has symptomatic fibroids

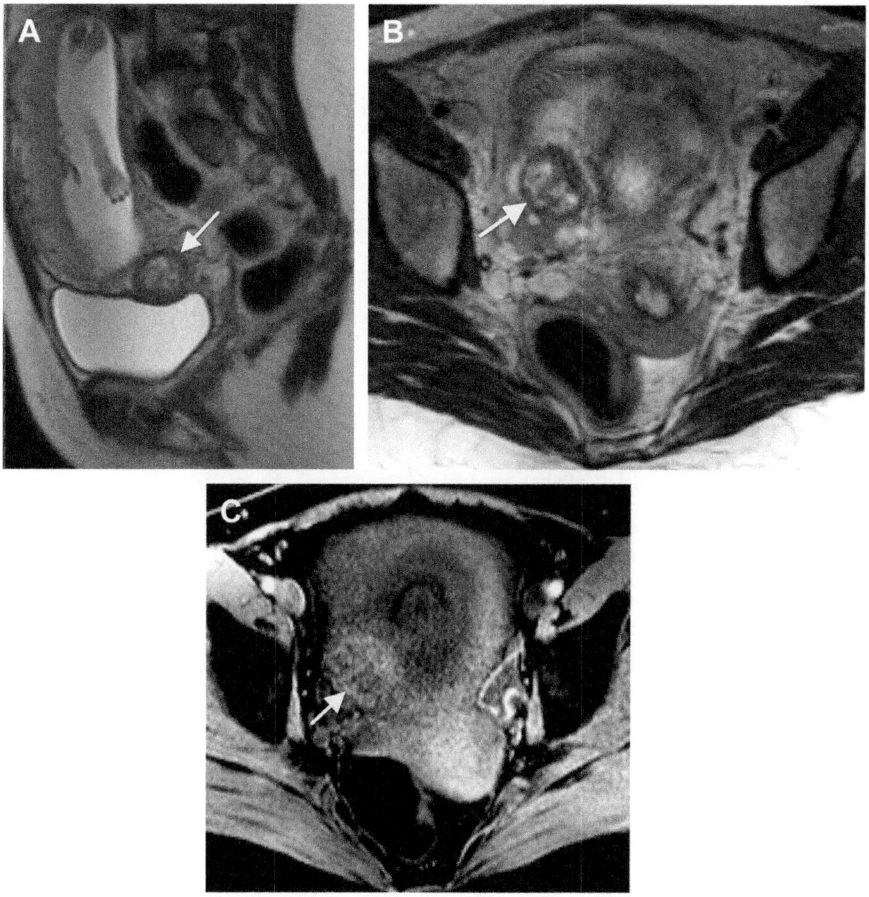

Fig. 15. A 28-year-old pregnant woman with red degeneration of leiomyoma, presenting with pelvic pain. (*A*) Sagittal and (*B*) axial T2WI and (*C*) axial precontrast T1WI demonstrate a well-defined lesion (*arrow*) with heterogeneous T2 signal and intrinsic T1 hyperintense signal to background myometrium suggesting red degeneration of leiomyoma as a cause of pain in this pregnant patient.

that are few in number and moderately sized (4–6 cm) or a single large fibroid less than 10 cm with low T2 signal on MR imaging no more than 12 cm from the abdominal wall and greater than 4 cm from the sacrum.[49]

RETAINED PRODUCTS OF CONCEPTION

Discussion of Problem/Clinical Presentation

- Retained products of conception (RPOC) complicate nearly 1% of all pregnancies and are the most common cause of postpartum bleeding,[52] frequently following termination of pregnancy[53] or second-trimester delivery.[52]
- The most common clinical presentation of RPOC is vaginal bleeding and pelvic pain.[53]
- Diagnosis and definitive treatment is important because the persistence of RPOC can lead to prolonged hemorrhage, endometritis, intrauterine adhesions, and potentially impairment of future fertility.[54]

Anatomy

The term *RPOC* refers to intracavitary uterine tissue that develops after conception and persists after delivery or termination of pregnancy.[52] The tissue is often placental trophoblastic in origin, and its connection to the endometrium provides a conduit for continued bleeding.[52]

MR Imaging Features and Diagnostic Criteria

Ultrasound is the first-line imaging modality in the diagnosis of RPOC. In cases whereby the diagnosis is not clear, MR imaging may be helpful in characterizing the size and extent of RPOC. The imaging appearance of RPOC on MR imaging depends on the degree of hemorrhage and tissue necrosis within the lesion. On MR imaging, RPOC can appear as an intracavitary soft-tissue mass with variable amounts of enhancement depending on its size and duration within the uterine cavity. The areas of enhancement suggest partially viable

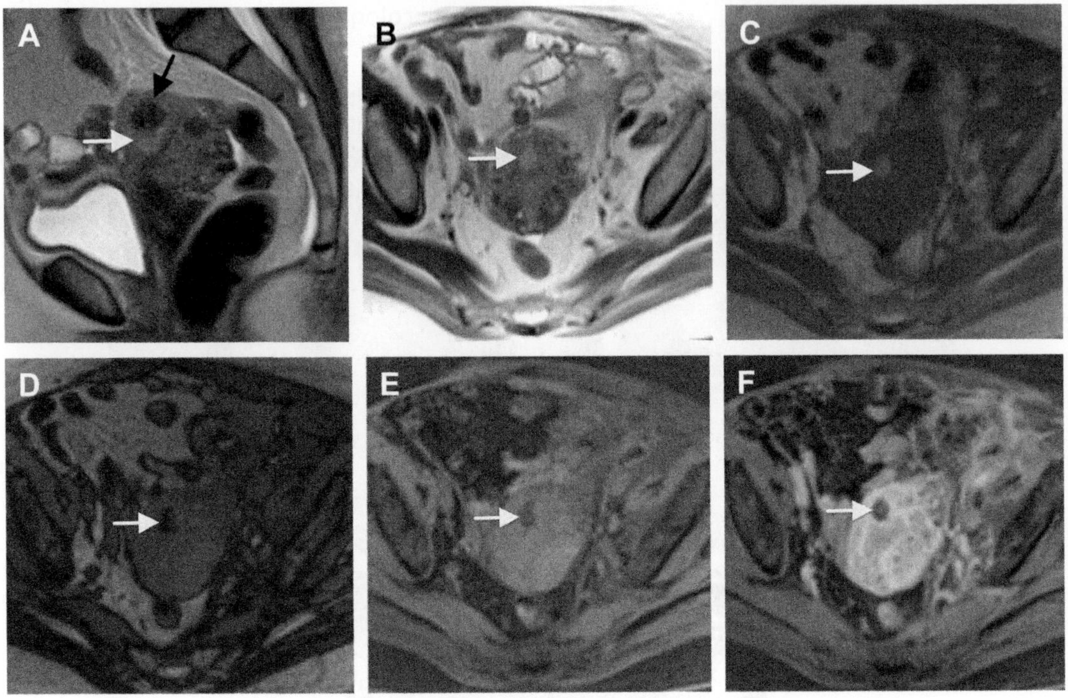

Fig. 16. A 55-year-old woman with lipoleiomyoma. (*A*) Sagittal and (*B*) axial non–fat-saturated T2WI, axial (*C*) in and (*D*) opposed phase, (*E*) precontrast and (*F*) postcontrast T1WI demonstrate a small intramural myometrial lesion (*white arrows*). Note loss of signal on opposed phase image (*D*), due to presence of fat in the lesion in keeping with lipoleiomyoma. Additional multiple typical leiomyomas in the uterus are seen (*black arrow* in *A*).

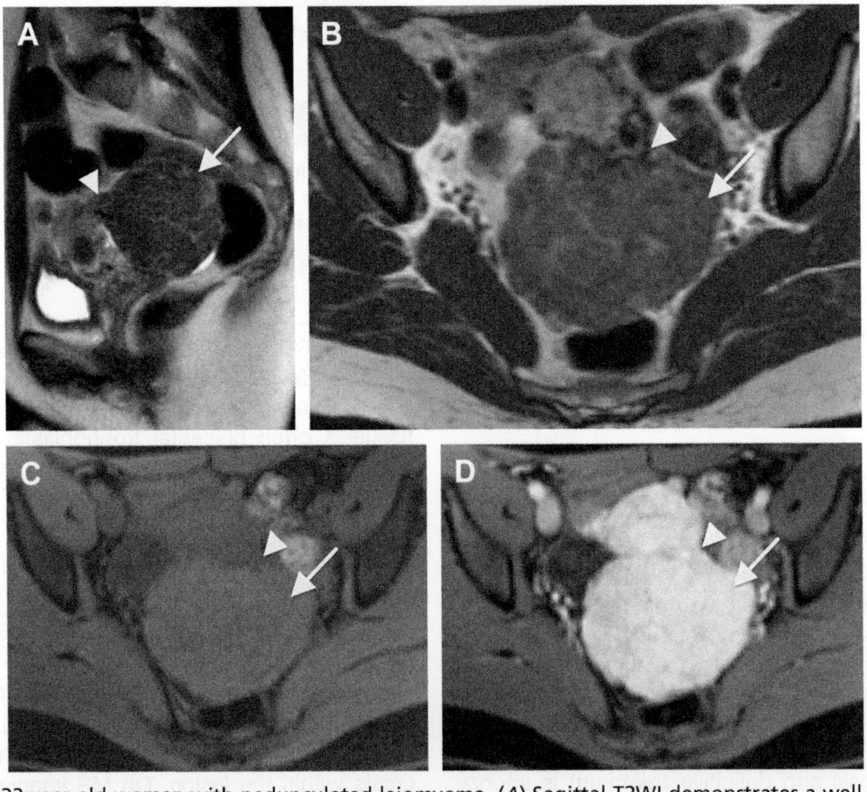

Fig. 17. A 33-year-old woman with pedunculated leiomyoma. (*A*) Sagittal T2WI demonstrates a well-defined T2 hypointense leiomyoma (*arrow*), with clear communication (*arrowhead*) with adjoining myometrium. (*B*) axial T2WI shows flow voids within bridging vessels (*arrowhead*) coursing from the uterus into adjoining leiomyoma (*arrow*) (*C*) precontrast and (*D*) venous phase postcontrast T1WI demonstrate a well-defined T2 hypointense leiomyoma (*arrow*), with clear communication (*arrowhead*) with adjoining myometrium.

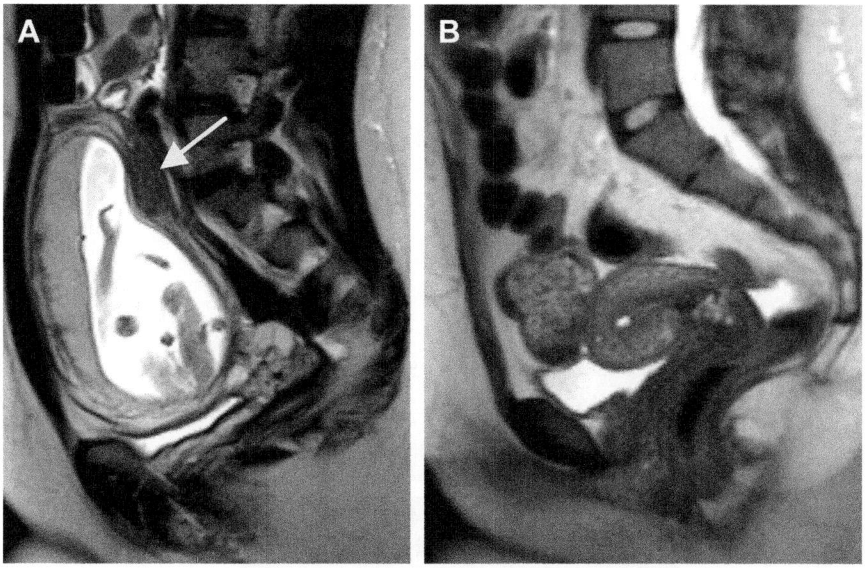

Fig. 18. A 30-year-old pregnant woman with transient uterine contraction and pelvic pain. (*A*) Sagittal T2WI demonstrates incidental T2 hypointense lesion in the myometrium (*white arrow*). In a pregnant patient, consider transient myometrial contraction, which can mimic leiomyoma. (*B*) Follow-up sagittal T2WI after delivery demonstrates no lesion in the myometrium, confirming the diagnosis of transient myometrial contraction.

chorionic tissue.[55] On T2WI, RPOC tend to have high signal intensity, similar to the intrinsic T2 signal of prepartum placental tissue (**Fig. 24**).[56]

Because vaginal bleeding is the primary clinical manifestation of RPOC, blood products are often seen in the endometrial cavity in addition to the enhancing soft-tissue mass; blood products will have varying intrinsic T1 signal depending on the acuity of the blood. If brisk bleeding is present at the time of imaging, flow voids or jets may be seen and should not be confused for an arterial venous malformation (AVM). Myometrial thinning and obliteration of the JZ on T2WI have also been reported in varying degrees in the setting of RPOC and may serve as helpful ancillary findings when endometrial soft-tissue enhancement is equivocal.[52]

Pearls, Pitfalls, and Variants

The biggest potential pitfall in the diagnosis of RPOC is in distinguishing hypervascular RPOC from AVMs (discussed later).[55] Differentiating RPOC from uterine AVM is critical when a patient presents with vaginal bleeding because dilation and curettage of a uterine AVM can aggravate hemorrhage.[57] Often, the degree of hypervascularity seen in the setting of RPOC can be so markedly robust that the vascularity obscures the underlying RPOC. Moreover, as RPOC evolves, recruitment and maintenance of vascularity may change the appearance of the retained placenta. Chronic RPOC, referred to as a placental polyp, can continue to cause postpartum bleeding and, potentially, hemorrhagic shock.[58]

Another potential pitfall is in the overlap of clinical presentation and MR findings of RPOC with gestational trophoblastic disease (GTD), particularly invasive molar pregnancies (**Fig. 25**).[59] Therefore, radiologists interpreting an intrauterine mass in postpartum patients should be cautious in making this distinction, as the treatments are very different. The serum beta–human chorionic gonadotropin (hCG) level can be helpful in distinguishing RPOC from GTD; the beta-hCG may be normal or mildly elevated in RPOC but markedly elevated in GTD. Other findings suggestive of GTD, such as abnormal uterine vasculature and ovarian theca lutein cysts, are also helpful but may not always be present.[53] Invasive molar pregnancies are characterized by growth of trophoblastic elements into the myometrium; on MR imaging, they can appear as an enhancing intracavitary mass that thins the myometrium and obliterates the JZ, similar to RPOC; however, the presence of parametrial invasion and/or extrauterine involvement (ie, lung metastases) are supportive of GTD rather than RPOC.

Pathophysiology

Often, RPOC tissue is of placental trophoblastic origin, as the placenta attaches to the uterine endometrium during fetal development. Chorionic villi are formed by the trophoblasts, which are small fingerlike processes containing fetal capillaries

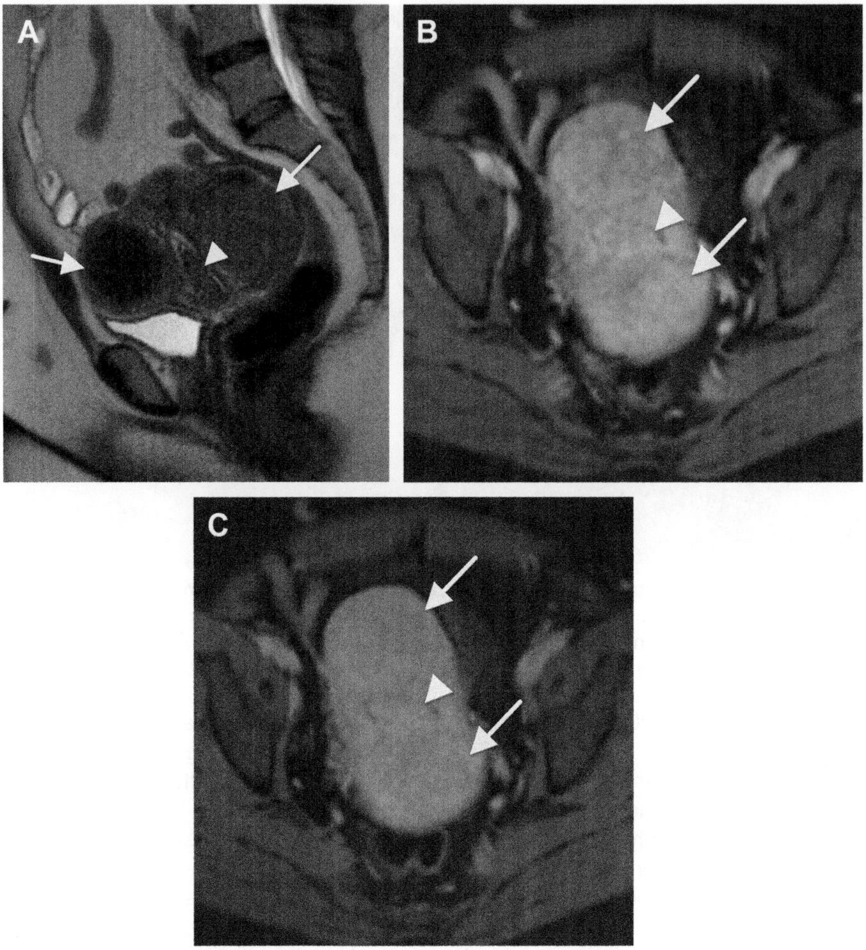

Fig. 19. A 33-year-old woman with intramural and intracavitary leiomyomas, presenting with menorrhagia. (*A*) Sagittal T2WI and axial postcontrast venous (*B*) and delayed (*C*) images demonstrate 2 intramural leiomyomas (*white arrows*) and an intracavitary leiomyoma (*arrowhead*). Postcontrast images (*B, C*) demonstrate signal intensity and enhancement that follows background myometrium.

that then invade the endometrium. Therefore, the presence of chorionic villi indicates persistent placental tissue and is key to the microscopic diagnosis of RPOC.[52]

What Referring Clinicians Need to Know

When imaging findings are suspicious for RPOC, careful correlation with relevant patient history and serum beta-hCG levels are important. The treatment of RPOC includes medical and/or surgical management, whereas GTD may require chemotherapy. The treatment approach of RPOC depends on the clinical status of patients. In patients who are hemodynamically stable, treatment options are as follows:

- Expectant management should be considered to avoid unnecessary surgery. Bleeding will eventually resolve as RPOC are naturally expelled or resorbed; however, prolonged bleeding may be bothersome for some patients, and the continued presence of retained tissue may predispose to infection/endometritis.[60]
- Medical management with uterotonics, such as misoprostol or methylergonovine, has also been shown to aid in controlling bleeding in those patients who wish to avoid additional surgery.[61]
- Surgical management with dilation and curettage or hysteroscopic removal of RPOC may be preferable for patients who present with prolonged (>3 weeks) or heavy bleeding. However, potential complications of surgery should be considered, such as infection, uterine perforation, or synechiae development. Uterine artery embolization may be considered for patients with hemorrhagic shock as

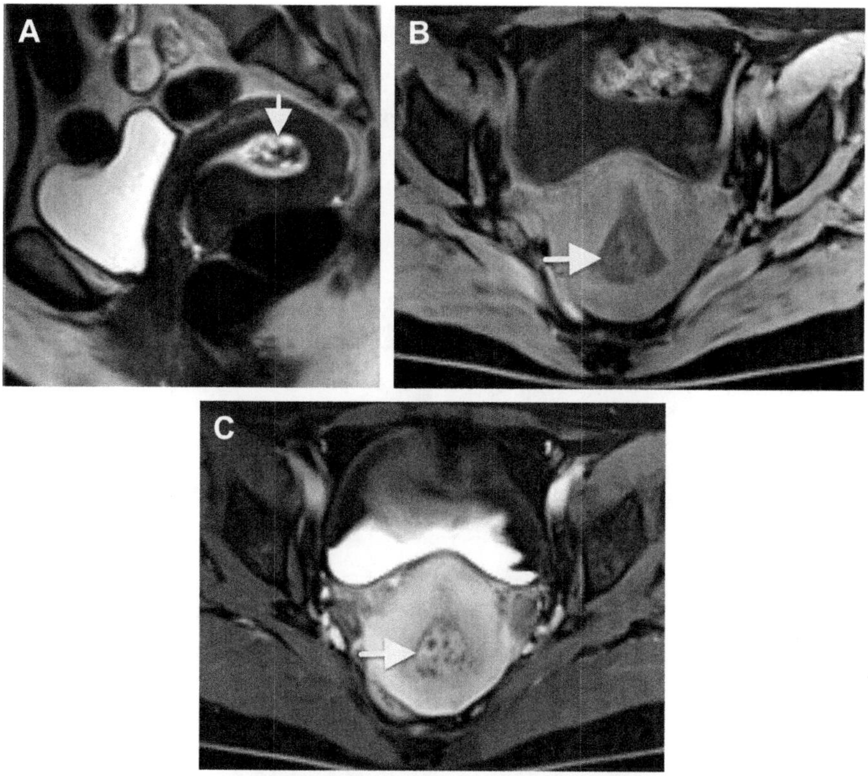

Fig. 20. A 45-year-old woman with endometrial polyp and irregular menstrual bleeding. Sagittal T2WI (*A*), axial precontrast (*B*), and postcontrast (*C*) T1WI demonstrate a heterogeneous T2 hyperintense enhancing lesion (*arrow*) in the endometrial canal, an endometrial polyp confirmed by surgical pathology. The lesion is centered within the endometrium, separate from the myometrium. This case emphasizes the difference in T2 signal from typical T2 hypointense signal seen in leiomyoma, compared with heterogeneous mainly T2 hyperintense signal in the endometrial polyp.

an alternative to surgical management.[62] In patients with life-threatening bleeding who are refractory to the aforementioned, hysterectomy as definitive treatment may ultimately be required.[62]

UTERINE ARTERIOVENOUS MALFORMATIONS

Discussion of Problem/Clinical Presentation

- Uterine AVMs are rare congenital or acquired lesions composed of abnormal communication between the uterine artery and venous plexuses of the myometrium.[63]
- Uterine AVMs are most commonly seen in women between 20 and 40 years of age presenting with menorrhagia or menometrorrhagia[64] and require blood transfusions in up to 30% of patients.[65]
- True uterine AVMs are exceedingly rare and may arise posttraumatically, usually in a setting of dilation and curettage, cesarean delivery, therapeutic abortion, endometrial carcinoma, or GTD.[66]
- The natural history is variable; some cases slowly revert to normal circulation, resolving over a period of weeks to months, whereas others will persist without regression, with increased risk of hemorrhage.[67]

Anatomy

Congenital AVMs are thought to arise from arrested vascular embryologic development resulting in anomalous differentiation and communication between arteries and veins.[66] Acquired AVMs are usually due to the development of an abnormal communication between arteries and veins following trauma or surgery, typically during the healing process.[68] Congenital AVMs generally consist of multiple small vascular connections that may invade the surrounding structures, whereas acquired AVMs tend to be communications between one artery and one vein.[68]

MR Imaging Features and Diagnostic Criteria

Ultrasound is the initial imaging modality for evaluation of abnormal vaginal bleeding. In patients with

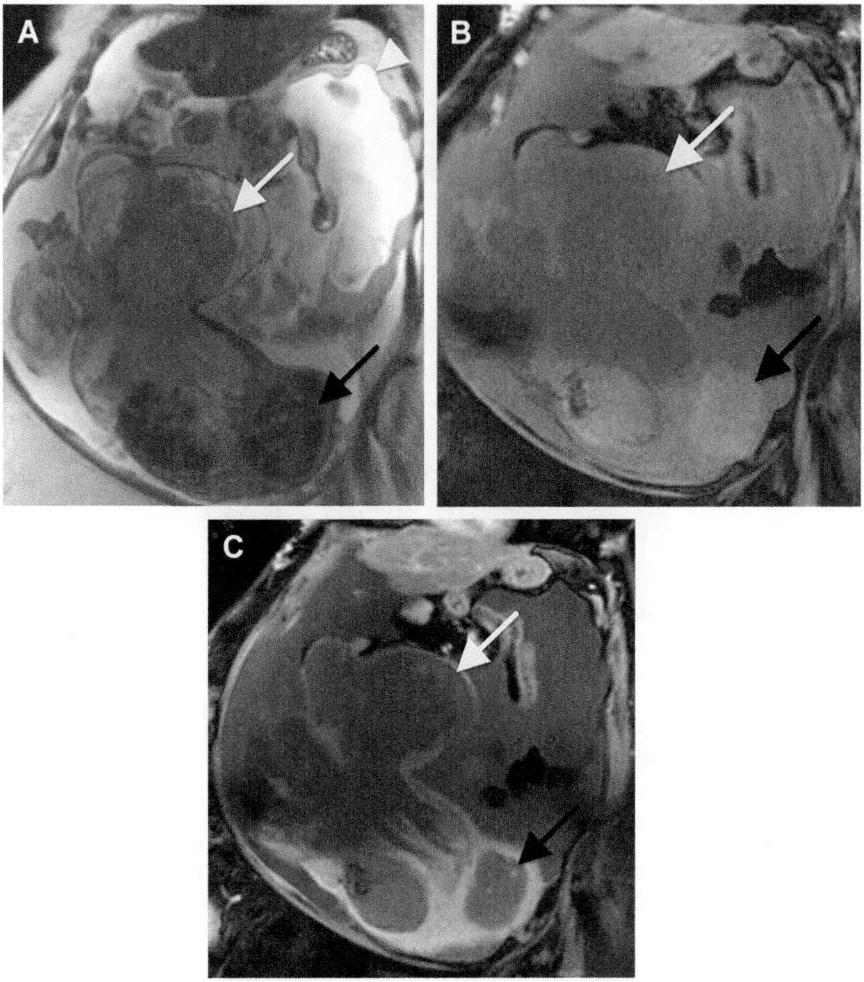

Fig. 21. A 60-year-old woman with leiomyosarcoma, presenting with pelvic pain and ascites. Coronal T2WI (*A*), coronal (*B*) precontrast, and (*C*) postcontrast T1WI demonstrate a large myometrial mass with irregular borders, central extensive necrosis, and heterogeneous peripheral enhancement in keeping with uterine sarcoma (*white arrow*). In contrast, there are 2 myometrial lesions in the lower uterine segment that demonstrate hypointense T2 signal typical for leiomyomas (*black arrow*) but no significant enhancement because of coarse calcifications. Arrowhead points to ascites.

severe vaginal bleeding and normal serum beta-hCG, the diagnosis of uterine AVM may be considered if ultrasound demonstrates multiple hypoechoic to anechoic spaces confined to the myometrium with turbulent, low-resistance, high-velocity flow on color and spectral Doppler interrogation.[66] When the diagnosis of uterine AVM is suggested on ultrasound, further characterization with MR imaging evaluation may be performed as a noninvasive modality to confirm diagnosis and delineate the extent of the AVM.[55]

MR characteristics of uterine AVM include focal bulkiness of the involved uterus with or without an underlying mass[69] exerting mass effect on surrounding structures and disrupting the JZ of the myometrium. Distinct, serpiginous, flow-related signal voids are seen within the involved area and can be associated with prominent parametrial vessels.[55] Dynamic contrast-enhanced MR angiography can be useful for both planning therapeutic embolization and monitoring the effects of treatment (**Fig. 26**). Definitive diagnosis of uterine AVM is ultimately made by angiography, in which an early draining vein is identified during arterial injection of contrast. Once diagnosis is established, embolization can be performed during angiography.

Pearls, Pitfalls, and Variants

Care should be made not to confuse physiologic arterial-venous shunting termed *transient*

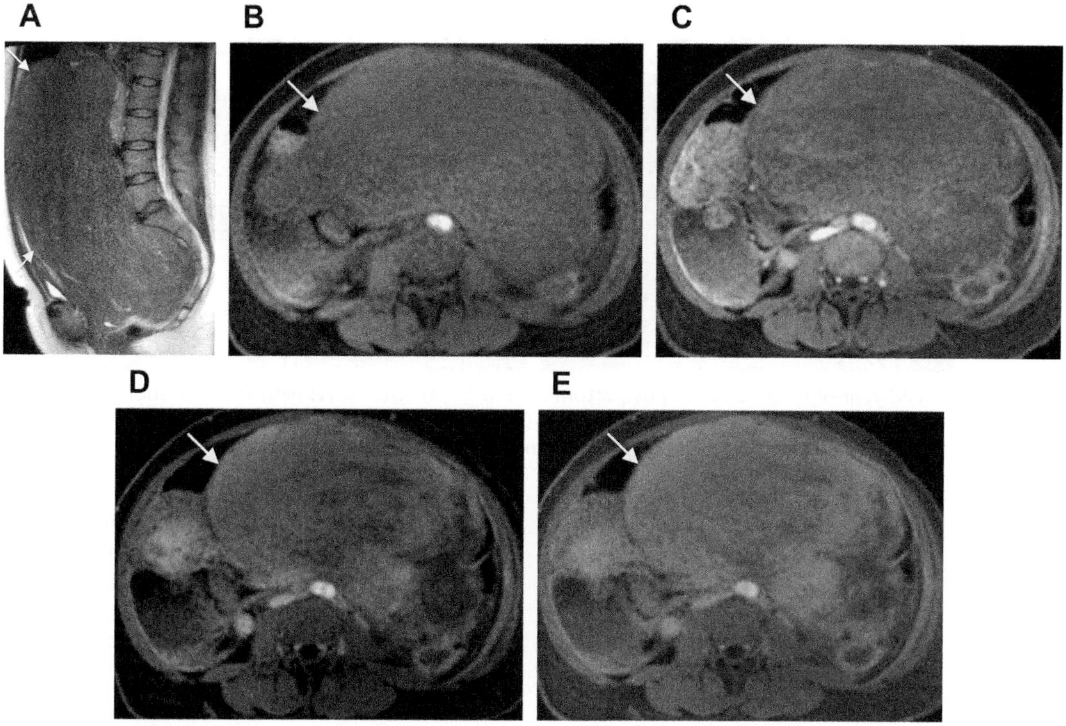

Fig. 22. A 55-year-old woman with STUMP lesion, presenting with pelvic pain. (*A*) Sagittal T2WI, axial (*B*) precontrast, (*C*) arterial, (*D*) venous, and (*E*) delayed postcontrast T1WI demonstrate a large T2 hypointense mass arising from the uterus, with slow but definite enhancement (*arrow*). Surgical pathology demonstrated STUMP. The large size of tumor is somewhat unusual.

myometrial hypervascularity for uterine AVM. Transient myometrial hypervascularity is a common finding seen in the first few weeks after pregnancy or missed abortion and will gradually involute as the myometrium and myometrial vessels contract during the normal postpartum period. Transient myometrial hypervascularity typically does not require treatment.[70]

Although uterine AVMs are often diagnosed clinically, most suspected postpartum uterine AVMs are actually RPOC with subsequent vascular remodeling such that the original RPOC are no longer visible and the vascular network associated with the RPOC is the dominant imaging finding.[71] In these cases, differentiation between the two entities can be quite challenging.

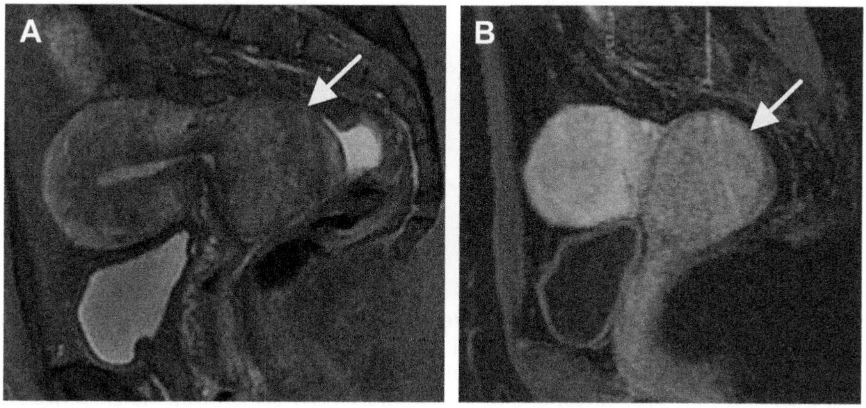

Fig. 23. A 33-year-old woman with cervical fibroid, presenting with irregular menstrual cycle. Sagittal (*A*) T2WI and (*B*) postcontrast T1WI demonstrate a well-defined lesion (*arrow*) in the cervix, with delayed enhancement as background myometrium in keeping with leiomyoma. There is mass effect on the endocervical canal.

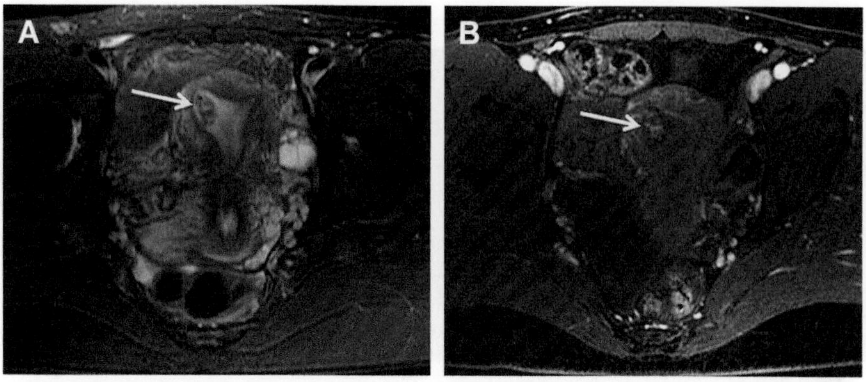

Fig. 24. RPOC. A 28-year-old woman with postpartum bleeding. (*A*) Axial T2WI with fat saturation shows a hypointense ovoid mass (*arrow*) in the right uterine cavity. (*B*) Postcontrast axial T1WI with fat saturation confirms this mass enhances. RPOC was confirmed at dilatation and curettage.

Pathophysiology

Arteriovenous malformations are composed of a tangle of vessels possessing both histologic characteristics of arteries and veins and lacking a normal intervening capillary network.[56] In the uterus, the lesions are within the myometrium and manifest as communications between the uterine arteries and myometrial venous plexuses.[63] Pathologically, the vessels are large in caliber with a muscular yet thin-walled, capillary-like network of vessels in different proportions and sizes, with areas of fibrous thickening due to high intraluminal pressure.[67]

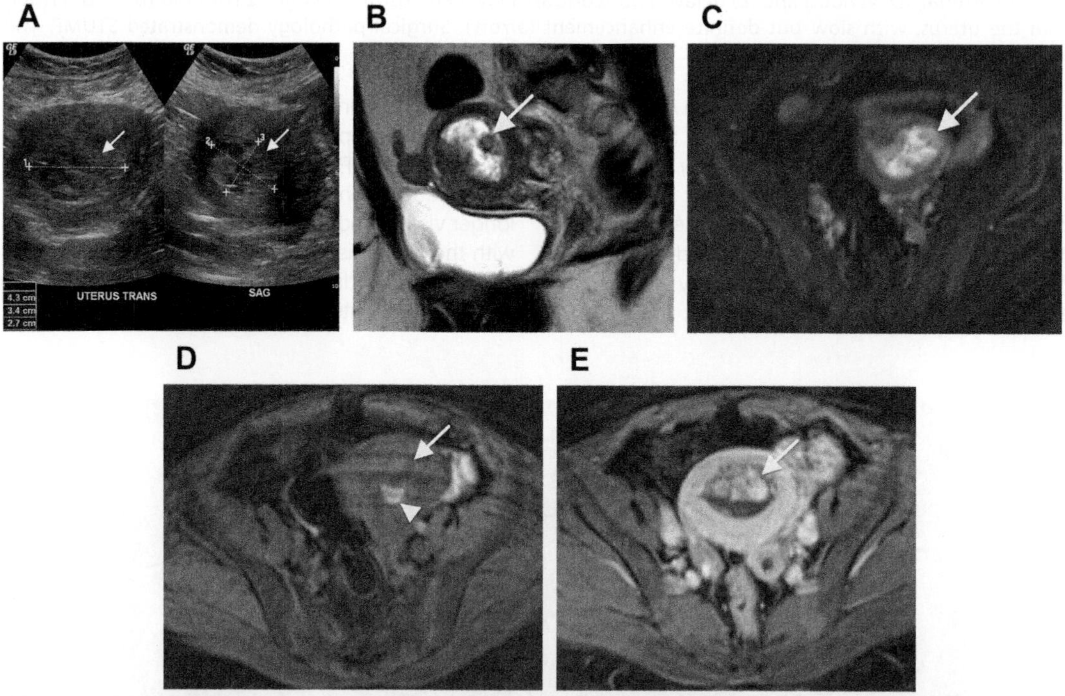

Fig. 25. A 35-year-old pregnant woman with molar pregnancy, presenting with vaginal bleeding and beta–human chorionic gonadotropin (hCG) levels greater than 100,000 mIU/mL. Gray-scale sonographic images demonstrate thickened endometrium with numerous anechoic cystic spaces (*A*) in keeping with molar pregnancy. (*B*) Sagittal and (*C*) axial T2WI, (*D*) precontrast and (*E*) postcontrast T1WI demonstrate heterogeneous enhancing soft tissue within the endometrial cavity with focal interruption of the JZ (*arrow*) raising concern for invasive molar pregnancy. There are hyperintense blood products in the endometrial cavity on T1WI (*arrowhead*). Molar pregnancy can mimic RPOC, and correlation with beta-hCG is helpful.

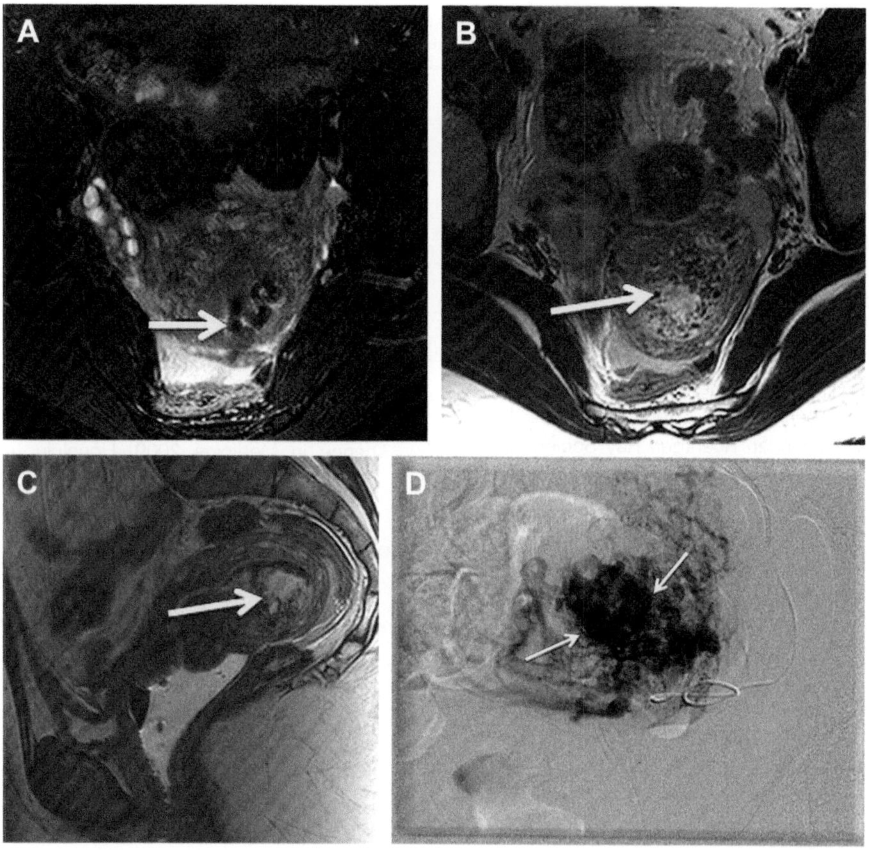

Fig. 26. Uterine arteriovenous malformation. A 29-year-old woman after dilatation and curettage for retained placenta. Axial T2WI (*A, B*) shows multiple flow voids (*arrows*) in the uterine myometrium in the region of the AVM. (*C*) Sagittal T2WI shows a heterogeneous area in the myometrium (*arrow*). (*D*) Angiogram during embolization shows a tangle of vessels (*arrows*) that were subsequently embolized.

What Referring Clinicians Need to Know

The diagnosis of uterine AVM is clinically important because curettage of an AVM may result in life-threatening hemorrhage. If patients are symptomatic and the diagnosis of uterine AVM versus RPOC is unclear, catheter angiography may be the preferred method of diagnosis and treatment via embolization, which may help avoid hysterectomy and preserve fertility.[64]

Acute management consists of hemodynamic stabilization, vaginal packing, and uterine tamponade with insertion of a Foley balloon or methylergonovine injection.[63] Intravenous estrogen has also been suggested as a treatment, because it may provide an endometrial covering over the AVM, whereas prostaglandins may aid in controlling acute bleeding.[63]

The ultimate treatment decision may depend on patients' desire for preservation of fertility. Embolization therapy has been shown to be an effective treatment of patients who want to preserve fertility.[63,67,72] If pregnancy is not desired or embolization fails, hysterectomy remains the definitive treatment of choice.[63]

SUMMARY

Adenomyosis is a common, frequently debilitating condition affecting women in their later reproductive years. Uterine leiomyomas are the most common tumor of the uterus, affecting up to 80% of women and can be a cause of abnormal uterine bleeding, pelvic pain and mass effect, and reproductive or sexual dysfunction. Differentiating RPOC, a common cause of postpartum hemorrhage, from uterine AVM is important in order to allow for optimal treatment. MR imaging has become a useful and reliable noninvasive tool in the diagnosis of all of these entities. As conservative management becomes more prevalent, it is important for the radiologist to be familiar with the relevant anatomy, histopathology, variable growth pattern, and variety of imaging appearances.

REFERENCES

1. Novellas S, Chassang M, Delotte J, et al. MRI characteristics of the uterine junctional zone: from normal to the diagnosis of adenomyosis. AJR Am J Roentgenol 2011;196:1206–13.
2. Nakai A, Reinhold C, Noel P, et al. Optimizing cine MRI for uterine peristalsis: a comparison of three different single shot fast spin echo techniques. J Magn Reson Imaging 2013;38:161–7.
3. Brosens JJ, de Souza NM, Barker FG. Uterine junctional zone: function and disease. Lancet 1995;346: 558–60.
4. Fennessy F. MRI of Benign Female Pelvis. In: Coakley F, Koenraad M, editors. Body MRI. Leesburg (VA): American Roentgen Ray Society; 2013. p. 223–30.
5. Johnson W, Taylor MB, Carrington BM, et al. The value of hyoscine butylbromide in pelvic MRI. Clin Radiol 2007;62:1087–93.
6. Kunz G, Beil D, Huppert P, et al. Adenomyosis in endometriosis–prevalence and impact on fertility. Evidence from magnetic resonance imaging. Hum Reprod 2005;20:2309–16.
7. Bergeron C, Amant F, Ferenczy A. Pathology and physiopathology of adenomyosis. Best Pract Res Clin Obstet Gynaecol 2006;20:511–21.
8. Leyendecker G, Kunz G, Kissler S, et al. Adenomyosis and reproduction. Best Pract Res Clin Obstet Gynaecol 2006;20:523–46.
9. Leyendecker G, Wildt L, Mall G. The pathophysiology of endometriosis and adenomyosis: tissue injury and repair. Arch Gynecol Obstet 2009;280:529–38.
10. Takahashi K, Nagata H, Kitao M. Clinical usefulness of determination of estradiol level in the menstrual blood for patients with endometriosis. Nihon Sanka Fujinka Gakkai Zasshi 1989;41:1849–50.
11. Mehasseb MK, Bell SC, Pringle JH, et al. Uterine adenomyosis is associated with ultrastructural features of altered contractility in the inner myometrium. Fertil Steril 2010;93:2130–6.
12. Bazot M, Cortez A, Darai E, et al. Ultrasonography compared with magnetic resonance imaging for the diagnosis of adenomyosis: correlation with histopathology. Hum Reprod 2001;16:2427–33.
13. Reinhold C, Tafazoli F, Wang L. Imaging features of adenomyosis. Hum Reprod Update 1998;4:337–49.
14. Reinhold C, Tafazoli F, Mehio A, et al. Uterine adenomyosis: endovaginal US and MR imaging features with histopathologic correlation. Radiographics 1999;19 Spec No:S147–60.
15. Dueholm M, Lundorf E, Hansen ES, et al. Magnetic resonance imaging and transvaginal ultrasonography for the diagnosis of adenomyosis. Fertil Steril 2001;76:588–94.
16. Takeuchi M, Matsuzaki K, Nishitani H. Hyperintense uterine myometrial masses on T2-weighted magnetic resonance imaging: differentiation with diffusion-weighted magnetic resonance imaging. J Comput Assist Tomogr 2009;33:834–7.
17. Koyama T, Togashi K. Functional MR imaging of the female pelvis. J Magn Reson Imaging 2007;25: 1101–12.
18. Kroencke TJ, Scheurig C, Poellinger A, et al. Uterine artery embolization for leiomyomas: percentage of infarction predicts clinical outcome. Radiology 2010;255:834–41.
19. Takeuchi M, Matsuzaki K, Nishitani H. Susceptibility-weighted imaging for the evaluation of gynecologic disease. Proceedings of the 17th meeting of the International Society for Magnetic Resonance in Medicine International Society for Magnetic Resonance in Medicine 2009. Honolulu, April 18–24, 2009.
20. Tamai K, Togashi K, Ito T, et al. MR imaging findings of adenomyosis: correlation with histopathologic features and diagnostic pitfalls. Radiographics 2005;25:21–40.
21. Yamashita Y, Torashima M, Hatanaka Y, et al. MR imaging of atypical polypoid adenomyoma. Comput Med Imaging Graph 1995;19:351–5.
22. Farquhar C, Brosens I. Medical and surgical management of adenomyosis. Best Pract Res Clin Obstet Gynaecol 2006;20:603–16.
23. Baird DD, Dunson DB, Hill MC, et al. High cumulative incidence of uterine leiomyoma in black and white women: ultrasound evidence. Am J Obstet Gynecol 2003;188:100–7.
24. Marshall LM, Spiegelman D, Barbieri RL, et al. Variation in the incidence of uterine leiomyoma among premenopausal women by age and race. Obstet Gynecol 1997;90:967–73.
25. Marsh EE, Ekpo GE, Cardozo ER, et al. Racial differences in fibroid prevalence and ultrasound findings in asymptomatic young women (18-30 years old): a pilot study. Fertil Steril 2013;99:1951–7.
26. Buttram VC Jr, Reiter RC. Uterine leiomyomata: etiology, symptomatology, and management. Fertil Steril 1981;36:433–45.
27. Cramer SF, Patel A. The frequency of uterine leiomyomas. Am J Clin Pathol 1990;94:435–8.
28. Gupta S, Jose J, Manyonda I. Clinical presentation of fibroids. Best Pract Res Clin Obstet Gynaecol 2008;22:615–26.
29. Marino JL, Eskenazi B, Warner M, et al. Uterine leiomyoma and menstrual cycle characteristics in a population-based cohort study. Hum Reprod 2004; 19:2350–5.
30. Zimmermann A, Bernuit D, Gerlinger C, et al. Prevalence, symptoms and management of uterine fibroids: an international internet-based survey of 21,746 women. BMC Womens Health 2012;12:6.
31. Downes E, Sikirica V, Gilabert-Estelles J, et al. The burden of uterine fibroids in five European

countries. Eur J obstetrics Gynecol Reprod Biol 2010;152:96–102.
32. Vilos GA, Allaire C, Laberge PY, et al. The management of uterine leiomyomas. J Obstet Gynaecol Can 2015;37:157–78.
33. Ligon AH, Morton CC. Leiomyomata: heritability and cytogenetic studies. Hum Reprod Update 2001; 7:8–14.
34. Bulun SE. Uterine fibroids. N Engl J Med 2013;369: 1344–55.
35. Munro MG, Critchley HO, Broder MS, et al. Disorders FWGoM. FIGO classification system (PALM-COEIN) for causes of abnormal uterine bleeding in nongravid women of reproductive age. Int J Gynaecol Obstet 2011;113:3–13.
36. Dudiak CM, Turner DA, Patel SK, et al. Uterine leiomyomas in the infertile patient: preoperative localization with MR imaging versus US and hysterosalpingography. Radiology 1988;167:627–30.
37. Zawin M, McCarthy S, Scoutt LM, et al. High-field MRI and US evaluation of the pelvis in women with leiomyomas. Magn Reson Imaging 1990;8:371–6.
38. Stamatopoulos CP, Mikos T, Grimbizis GF, et al. Value of magnetic resonance imaging in diagnosis of adenomyosis and myomas of the uterus. J Minimal Invasive Gynecol 2012;19:620–6.
39. Sydow B, ES S. Uterine MRI: a review of technique and diagnosis. Appl Radiol 2008;37:18–29.
40. Kawakami S, Togashi K, Konishi I, et al. Red degeneration of uterine leiomyoma: MR appearance. J Comput Assist Tomogr 1994;18:925–8.
41. Murase E, Siegelman ES, Outwater EK, et al. Uterine leiomyomas: histopathologic features, MR imaging findings, differential diagnosis, and treatment. Radiographics 1999;19:1179–97.
42. Riccio TJ, Adams HG, Munzing DE, et al. Magnetic resonance imaging as an adjunct to sonography in the evaluation of the female pelvis. Magn Reson Imaging 1990;8:699–704.
43. Gompel C, Silverberg SG. The corpus uteri. Pathology in gynecology and obstetrics. Philadelphia: Lippincott; 1994. p. 163–283.
44. Togashi K, Kawakami S, Kimura I, et al. Uterine contractions: possible diagnostic pitfall at MR imaging. J Magn Reson Imaging 1993;3:889–93.
45. Togashi K, Nishimura K, Itoh K, et al. Adenomyosis: diagnosis with MR imaging. Radiology 1988;166: 111–4.
46. Sandberg AA. Updates on the cytogenetics and molecular genetics of bone and soft tissue tumors: leiomyosarcoma. Cancer Genet Cytogenet 2005; 161:1–19.
47. Parker WH, Fu YS, Berek JS. Uterine sarcoma in patients operated on for presumed leiomyoma and rapidly growing leiomyoma. Obstet Gynecol 1994; 83:414–8.
48. Siedhoff MT, Kim KH. Morcellation and myomas: balancing decisions around minimally invasive treatments for fibroids. J Surg Oncol 2015;112: 769–71.
49. Owen C, Armstrong AY. Clinical management of leiomyoma. Obstet Gynecol Clin North Am 2015; 42:67–85.
50. Deshmukh SP, Gonsalves CF, Guglielmo FF, et al. Role of MR imaging of uterine leiomyomas before and after embolization. Radiographics 2012;32: E251–81.
51. Katsumori T, Akazawa K, Mihara T. Uterine artery embolization for pedunculated subserosal fibroids. AJR Am J Roentgenol 2005;184:399–402.
52. Sellmyer MA, Desser TS, Maturen KE, et al. Physiologic, histologic, and imaging features of retained products of conception. Radiographics 2013;33: 781–96.
53. Noonan JB, Coakley FV, Qayyum A, et al. MR imaging of retained products of conception. AJR Am J Roentgenol 2003;181:435–9.
54. Abbasi S, Jamal A, Eslamian L, et al. Role of clinical and ultrasound findings in the diagnosis of retained products of conception. Ultrasound Obstet Gynecol 2008;32:704–7.
55. Lee NK, Kim S, Lee JW, et al. Postpartum hemorrhage: clinical and radiologic aspects. Eur J Radiol 2010;74:50–9.
56. Kido A, Togashi K, Koyama T, et al. Retained products of conception masquerading as acquired arteriovenous malformation. J Comput Assist Tomogr 2003;27:88–92.
57. Masselli G, Gualdi G. MR imaging of the placenta: what a radiologist should know. Abdom Imaging 2013;38:573–87.
58. Kanaoka Y, Maeda T, Nakai Y, et al. Placental polyp: power Doppler imaging and conservative resection. Ultrasound Obstet Gynecol 1998;11:225–6.
59. Leyendecker JR, Gorengaut V, Brown JJ. MR imaging of maternal diseases of the abdomen and pelvis during pregnancy and the immediate postpartum period. Radiographics 2004;24:1301–16.
60. Nanda K, Lopez LM, Grimes DA, et al. Expectant care versus surgical treatment for miscarriage. Cochrane Database Syst Rev 2012;(3):CD003518.
61. Chambers DG, Mulligan EC. Treatment of suction termination of pregnancy-retained products with misoprostol markedly reduces the repeat operation rate. Aust N Z J Obstet Gynaecol 2009;49: 551–3.
62. Miyahara Y, Makihara N, Yamasaki Y, et al. In vitro fertilization-embryo transfer pregnancy was a risk factor for hemorrhagic shock in women with placental polyp. Gynecol Endocrinol 2014; 30:502–4.
63. Hoffman MK, Meilstrup JW, Shackelford DP, et al. Arteriovenous malformations of the uterus: an

uncommon cause of vaginal bleeding. Obstet Gynecol Surv 1997;52:736–40.

64. Livermore J, Adusumilli S. MRI of benign uterine conditions. Appl Radiol 2007. Available at: http://appliedradiology.com/articles/mri-of-benign-uterine-conditions. Accessed April 9, 2017.

65. Manolitsas T, Hurley V, Gilford E. Uterine arteriovenous malformation–a rare cause of uterine haemorrhage. Aust N Z J Obstet Gynaecol 1994;34:197–9.

66. Polat P, Suma S, Kantarcy M, et al. Color Doppler US in the evaluation of uterine vascular abnormalities. Radiographics 2002;22:47–53.

67. Timor-Tritsch IE, Haynes MC, Monteagudo A, et al. Ultrasound diagnosis and management of acquired uterine enhanced myometrial vascularity/arteriovenous malformations. Am J Obstet Gynecol 2016;214:731.e1-10.

68. Hashim H, Nawawi O. Uterine arteriovenous malformation. Malays J Med Sci 2013;20:76–80.

69. Huang MW, Muradali D, Thurston WA, et al. Uterine arteriovenous malformations: gray-scale and Doppler US features with MR imaging correlation. Radiology 1998;206:115–23.

70. Van Schoubroeck D, Van den Bosch T, Scharpe K, et al. Prospective evaluation of blood flow in the myometrium and uterine arteries in the puerperium. Ultrasound Obstet Gynecol 2004;23:378–81.

71. Kamaya A, Ro K, Benedetti NJ, et al. Imaging and diagnosis of postpartum complications: sonography and other imaging modalities. Ultrasound Q 2009;25:151–62.

72. Vogelzang RL, Nemcek AA Jr, Skrtic Z, et al. Uterine arteriovenous malformations: primary treatment with therapeutic embolization. J Vasc Interv Radiol 1991;2:517–22.

MR Imaging of Abnormal Placentation

Manjiri Dighe, MD

KEYWORDS

• Accreta • Placenta • Morbidly adherent placenta • Placental invasion

KEY POINTS

- Incidence of morbidly adherent placenta (MAP) is increasing with the incidence of cesarean sections.
- Ultrasound is the primary screening technique for evaluation of MAP, and MR imaging is used if ultrasound is limited or equivocal for high-risk patients and for delivery planning.
- MR imaging should be performed between 24 and 32 weeks of gestational age to avoid common pitfalls.

INTRODUCTION

Morbidly adherent placenta (MAP) encompasses a spectrum of conditions characterized by abnormal adherence of the placenta to the implantation site.[1] Classification of MAP is based on the degree of trophoblastic invasion through myometrium and uterine serosa and includes accreta, when the villi are attached to the myometrium but do not invade the muscle; increta, when the placenta invades partially through the myometrium; and percreta, when it invades up to and beyond the uterine serosa.[2]

Clinically, MAP becomes a problem during delivery when the placenta does not completely separate from the uterus, which can be followed by a cascade of events, including massive hemorrhage leading to disseminated intravascular coagulation, the need for hysterectomy, surgical injury to the bladder, uterus, bowel, or neurovascular structures, adult respiratory distress syndrome, acute transfusion reaction, electrolyte imbalance, and renal failure.[3–6] MAP is associated with up to one-half of emergency peripartum hysterectomies.[3–6]

The incidence of MAP is increasing and seems to parallel the increase in cesarean delivery rate. The frequency of MAP has increased by more than 10-fold in the past 30 years to approximately 3 cases per 1000 deliveries.[7,8] Other risk factors for MAP include any myometrial damage from previous myomectomy, endometrial defects due to vigorous curettage resulting in Asherman syndrome,[9] submucous leiomyomas, thermal ablation,[10] and uterine artery embolization.[11] Placenta previa is also a risk factor for MAP; however, this may be due to the increased incidence of placenta previa in patients with prior cesarean sections. Silver and colleagues[7] found that in the presence of placenta previa the risk of MAP was 3%, 11%, 40%, 61%, and 67% for the first, second, third, fourth, and fifth or greater repeat cesarean deliveries, respectively. This is hypothesized to be due to the increased risk of incomplete reapproximation of the incised edges as the incidence of repeat cesarean sections increases. Garmi and colleagues[12] were able to show in vitro that an induced sharp decidual incision, which would imitate the in vivo process of a cesarean section, increased the invasion potential of trophoblastic cells. Placenta previa without prior cesarean delivery confers a very low risk of MAP, of about 1% to 5%.

Disclosure Statement: Dr M. Dighe has received research funding support from Philips Healthcare.
Radiology, UWMC, University of Washington, 1959 Northeast Pacific Street, Box 357115, Seattle, WA 98195, USA
E-mail address: dighe@uw.edu

Magn Reson Imaging Clin N Am 25 (2017) 601–610
http://dx.doi.org/10.1016/j.mric.2017.03.002

Maternal mortality with MAP has been reported to be as high as 7%.[13] The average blood loss at delivery in women with MAP is estimated to be 3 to 5 L[14]; as many as 90% of patients with MAP require blood transfusion, with 40% requiring more than 10 units of packed red blood cells.[2] A multidisciplinary team including individuals with special expertise in high-risk obstetrics, gynecologic surgery, urology, radiology, obstetric anesthesia, and blood banking has been shown to reduce mortality.[15–18]

WHY MR IMAGING?

Ultrasound (US) is the primary diagnostic tool for MAP and is performed as the initial screening examination. In patients with a placenta previa or a low-lying placenta after the initial screening examination performed at 18 to 20 weeks, a repeat examination at 32 weeks is recommended to evaluate the placental location.[19] US has been reported to have a sensitivity of 91% and a specificity of 97% for the diagnosis of MAP in a recent meta-analysis[20] and is able to evaluate for MAP in most cases. MR imaging is indicated when the US evaluation is limited or equivocal for patients with high clinical risk factors for MAP. In cases where US has provided a definitive diagnosis, MR imaging is usually performed for delivery planning because it is able to outline the anatomy of the invasion, relate it to regional vascular system, and confirm parametrial invasion and possible ureteral involvement.[21]

HOW TO DO IT?

MR imaging sequences with high temporal resolution and good contrast-to-noise ratios are used for placental imaging. MR imaging is typically performed on a 1.5-T system; however, recently 3 T has been used by some institutions to perform their fetal imaging as well. A study by Victoria and colleagues[22] comparing 1.5 T and 3 T for fetal imaging found that although some structures like spine and cartilage were better seen on 3 T and their imaging scores improved with increasing gestational age, overall, more imaging artifacts were seen on the 3-T MR imaging. No specific articles exist to date evaluating the usefulness of 3-T MR imaging in placental imaging. The American College of Radiology (ACR)–Society for Pediatric Radiology Practice Parameter for safe and optimal performance of fetal MR imaging suggests absence of any reported adverse effects to the mother or developing fetus at 3 T or weaker magnetic fields; however, the investigators acknowledge that most of their data were from research involving 1.5 T or less.[23] A multichannel phased array coil is typically used, and the examination typically takes about 15 to 30 minutes to complete. If the patient cannot tolerate a supine position, especially in the later part of pregnancy, a left lateral decubitus or oblique position may be better tolerated. This position decreases the risk of impaired venous return from caval compression by the uterus. Ideally, the bladder is only partially distended both for patient comfort and to be able to evaluate bladder wall invasion if present. Breath-hold techniques can be used to minimize breathing motion artifacts.

Single-shot T2-weighted (T2W) echo-planar fast spin-echo sequences in multiple planes are used to image the placenta. Acquisitions in axial, sagittal, and coronal plane with respect to the uterus are performed to image all regions of the placenta. True fast imaging with steady state precession (FISP) can also be used to help eliminate artifacts caused by maternal and fetal motion. At the author's institution, they acquire True FISP images in all 3 planes as well. T1-weighted images can be acquired to evaluate for areas of hemorrhage if placental abruption is of concern; however, T1-weighted images need not be performed as routine. Gadolinium-based contrast agents (GBCA) can add to the diagnostic value of T2-weighted imaging (T2WI) for the diagnosis of placenta accreta; however, they are rarely used in pregnant women due to persistent uncertainty regarding fetal risks posed by GBCA crossing the placenta. Millischer and colleagues[24] found an increase in the accuracy of diagnosis in both the senior and the junior radiologist on addition of gadolinium to their examinations. The Contrast Media Safety Committee of the European Society of Urogenital Radiology reviewed the literature and determined that no effect on the fetus has been reported following the use of gadolinium contrast media[25]; however, the ACR guidelines recommend that intravenous gadolinium should be avoided during pregnancy and should be only used if absolutely essential.[26] The protocol used at the author's institution is shown in **Table 1**. In addition, a radiologist is always available to review the images before the patient is taken off the gantry table and to suggest any additional or oblique images if necessary.

Recently, the utility of diffusion-weighted imaging (DWI) in defining placental invasion was evaluated by Morita and colleagues.[27] DWI at a b value of 1000 s/mm^2 clearly defined the border between the placenta and myometrium because only the placenta showed very high signal intensity at this high b value. The corresponding image at a b value of 0 s/mm^2 showed the myometrium with high

Table 1
MR imaging parameters for imaging the placenta

Sequence	Planes	TR (ms)	TE (ms)	FOV (cm)	Slice Thickness (mm)	Matrix	ETL	Flip Angle (°)
Ultra-fast spin-echo T2 half-Fourier	Axial, coronal sagittal	1800	64	32–40	5	256 × 160	256	160
True FISP/BFFE	Axial, coronal, sagittal	411	1.8	32–40	5	256 × 182	1	62
T1-weighted TSE	Axial	684	10	32–40	6	320 × 240	3	180
T2-weighted TSE	Sagittal	4650	79	32–40	5	256 × 256	19	144
DWI (b values = 0, 400, 800 s/mm^2)	Axial	6800	60	38	7	140 × 140	1	90

Abbreviations: ETL, Echo train length; FOV, Field of View; TE, Echo Time; TR, Repetition time; TSE, Turbo spine echo.

signal intensity compared with the surrounding fat. They postulate that the fusion of these 2 images would be able to provide better diagnosis of placenta accreta.

WHEN TO DO IT?

Horowitz and colleagues[28] found that placental MR imaging examinations performed before 24 weeks showed an unacceptable accuracy, sensitivity, positive predictive value, and likelihood ratio for the detection of abnormal placentation. They recommend waiting to perform the placental MR imaging after 24 weeks even if the 20-week screening US is suspicious for abnormal placentation. Placental MR imaging examinations performed at or after 24 weeks in their study had a very high positive predictive value of 96%, good sensitivity of 79%, and specificity of 94%, which was better than those examinations performed before 24 weeks. D'Antonio and colleagues[29] suggest that serial follow-up scans in the third trimester, starting from 28 weeks of gestation, are needed in order to predict accurately the extent of the invaded area and to plan the best surgical treatment.

IMAGING FEATURES

Several signs have been described on MR imaging to help diagnose MAP or placenta accreta, with some of the common ones listed in **Box 1**.

Normal Myometrium and Placenta

On T2WI, placenta appears predominantly homogenous with intermediate signal intensity in the second trimester with increasing heterogeneity seen in the later gestational ages and is usually clearly distinct from the underlying myometrium (**Fig. 1**). Regularly spaced, uniformly thin, linear areas of decreased signal intensity are seen in the myometrium, likely due to the areas of normal placental septal attachment (**Fig. 2**). These are more commonly seen when imaged with a 3-T system and are distinct from the thicker septae seen with MAP. Normal retroplacental vascularity is seen as a thin layer of numerous flow voids just under the placenta. Myometrial thickness varies with the gestational age with progressive thinning seen later in pregnancy.[30] The gravid uterus is pear shaped with the fundus and body being wider than the lower uterine segment (LUS), and the contour is smooth with no areas of focal bulging seen (**Fig. 3**).[31]

Placenta Previa

Patients with placenta previa are at increased risk of developing MAP (**Fig. 4**). With placenta previa and one previous cesarean section, the risk of MAP was found to be 24% by Clark and colleagues[32] and increased to 67% with a

Box 1
Signs suggesting morbidly adherent placenta

Placenta previa

Uterine bulging

Heterogenous signal intensity within the placenta

Dark intraplacental bands on T2-weighted images

Focal interruptions in the myometrial wall

Direct visualization of the invasion of pelvic structures by placental tissue

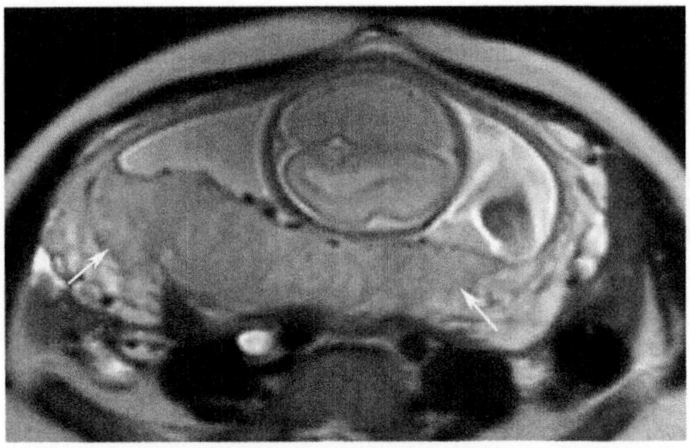

Fig. 1. Normal placenta on MR imaging. Axial T2WI from a 25-week fetus shows a normal homogenous appearance of the placenta (*arrows*).

placenta previa and 4 or more cesarean sections. Another study by Silver and colleagues[7] found that the risk of MAP increases from 0.03% to 3% in first pregnancy in the presence of placenta previa and from 4.7% to 40% or more after greater than 3 cesarean sections. However, patients with placenta previa and no history of prior cesarean section had a very low risk of MAP at 0.26%.[32] A normally positioned placenta should be 2 cm or more away from the internal cervical os. A low-lying placenta is defined as a placenta with its lower edge less than 2 cm from the internal os. Placenta previa is defined as any degree of placenta covering the internal os (**Fig. 5**). A recent executive summary of a multisociety meeting on fetal and placental imaging discouraged the use of the terms complete, partial, or marginal previa and recommended providing a description of the findings in the body of the report.[33]

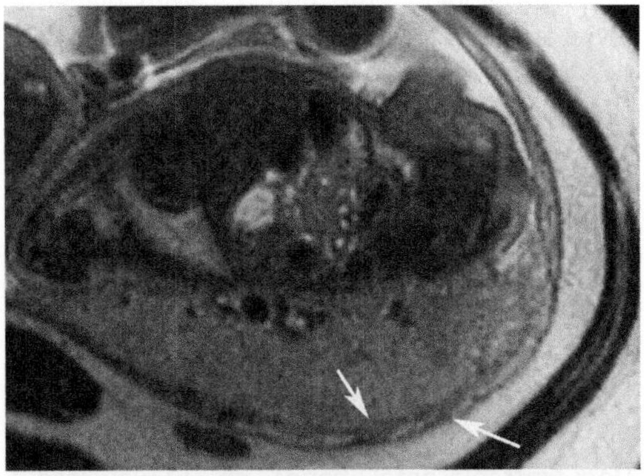

Fig. 2. Normal appearance of the myometrium with thin septae seen in it. A 28-week-old fetus with a normal-appearing placenta. Note the thin regularly spaced uniform septations (*arrows*) seen in the myometrium, likely from placental attachment to the myometrium.

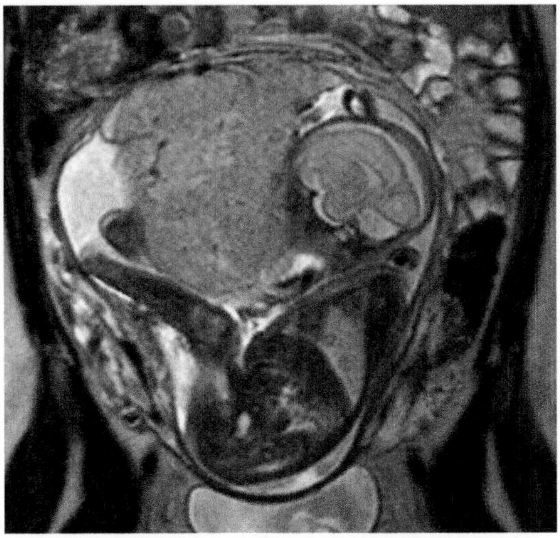

Fig. 3. Normal pear shape of gravid uterus. A pregnant patient at 30 weeks' gestational age showing a normal pear shape of the uterus, larger at the fundus and narrower at the lower uterine segment.

Uterine Bulging

Abnormal uterine bulging has been found to be significantly associated with MAP with a sensitivity and a specificity of 79.1% and 90.2%,

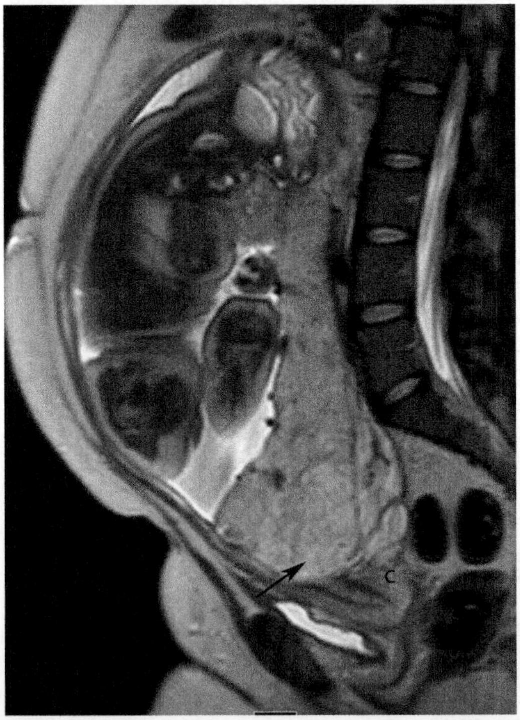

Fig. 4. Placenta previa. Sagittal T2WI showing the bulk of the placenta (*arrow*) overlying the internal os suggesting a placenta previa. This patient has a uniform thickness to her myometrium with no other features seen to suggest MAP. c = cervix.

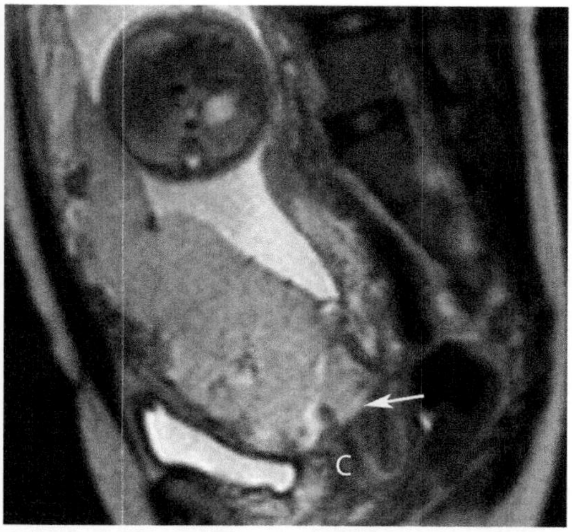

Fig. 5. Placenta previa. A 27-week-old fetus with placenta previa. Note the placenta (*arrow*) overlying the internal os of the cervix (C).

respectively.[34–39] Uterine bulging is seen due to mass effect of the placenta on the myometrium and may occur anywhere along the disruption. It might lead to loss of the normal pear shape of the gravid uterus, leading to an hourglass shape on coronal and/or sagittal images (**Fig. 6**).[40]

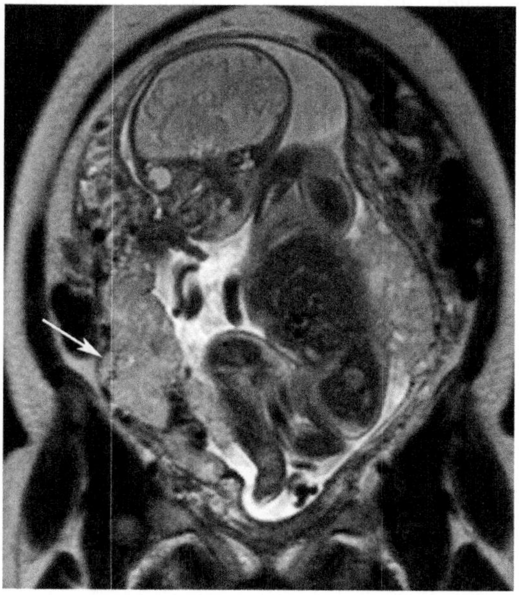

Fig. 6. Loss of uterine shape. A 34-week pregnant patient with known placenta percreta. Note the loss of normal pear shape of the uterus with bulging seen in the right lateral part of the uterus (*arrow*).

Heterogenous Signal Intensity Within the Placenta

Heterogeneity in the placenta may correspond to areas of hemorrhage and is a subjective sign, depending on the gestational age of the placenta and the presence of T2 dark bands (**Fig. 7**). However, this sign has not been clearly defined in terms of imaging parameters and remains qualitative and largely based on thick intraplacental bands and intraplacental flow voids.[36] Placental infarcts may also contribute to the heterogeneity and can be seen in 25% of normal placentas (**Fig. 8**).[41] Although placental heterogeneity was not found to be significantly associated with MAP by Bour and colleagues,[36] other studies have shown a sensitivity of 78.6% and specificity of 87.7% in the detection of MAP.[37]

Dark Intraplacental Bands on T2-Weighted Imaging

Dark intraplacental bands on T2WI have been shown to be an important feature of MAP with a sensitivity of 87.9% and specificity of 71.9%.[37] These bands originate from the basilar plate at the maternal side of the placenta (**Fig. 9**) and show decreased signal on True FISP/FIESTA/bFFE images, whereas vascular lacunae show increased signal on these images.[34] They have been shown to correspond to areas of fibrin deposition on histopathology[42,43] and a sequela of hemorrhage.[44] They can be seen in normal mature placenta after 30 weeks of gestation, or in the setting of preeclampsia and intrauterine growth restriction (IUGR) (**Fig. 10**).[41,44]

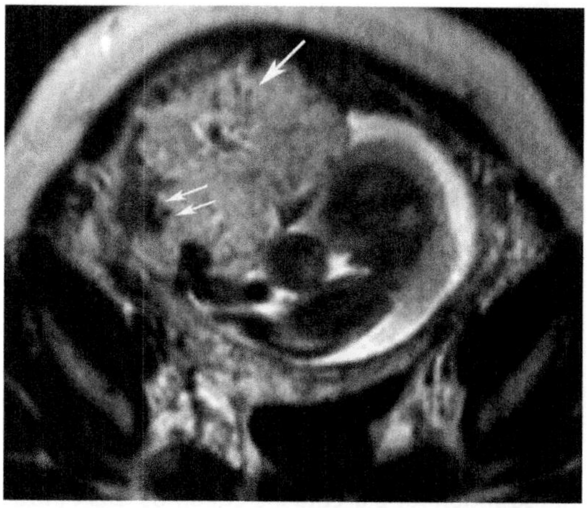

Fig. 7. Heterogeneity in the placenta. A 32-week-old fetus with known placenta increta. The placenta showed areas of heterogeneity (*arrow*) along with dark intraplacental bands (*double arrows*).

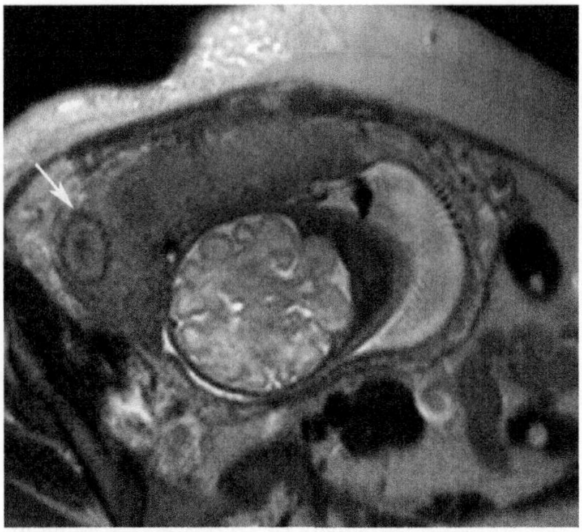

Fig. 8. Heterogeneity in the placenta due to infarction. A 34-week-old fetus with a suspicion for placenta increta on US. An area of heterogeneity was seen in the placenta in the right lower quadrant (*arrow*) with no other features of MAP. This was called normal with no evidence of MAP, and the area of heterogeneity was suspected to be due to infarction. This was confirmed on histopathology.

Focal Interruptions of Myometrium by Placenta

Focal interruptions of myometrium by placenta may be present without other imaging signs. If the interruption borders the serosa and if the myometrium has "split" beneath the attaching placenta (**Fig. 11**), this corresponds to placenta percreta on histopathology.[29] This finding has high sensitivity and specificity, 83.8% and 82.4%, for MAP among experienced readers.[45]

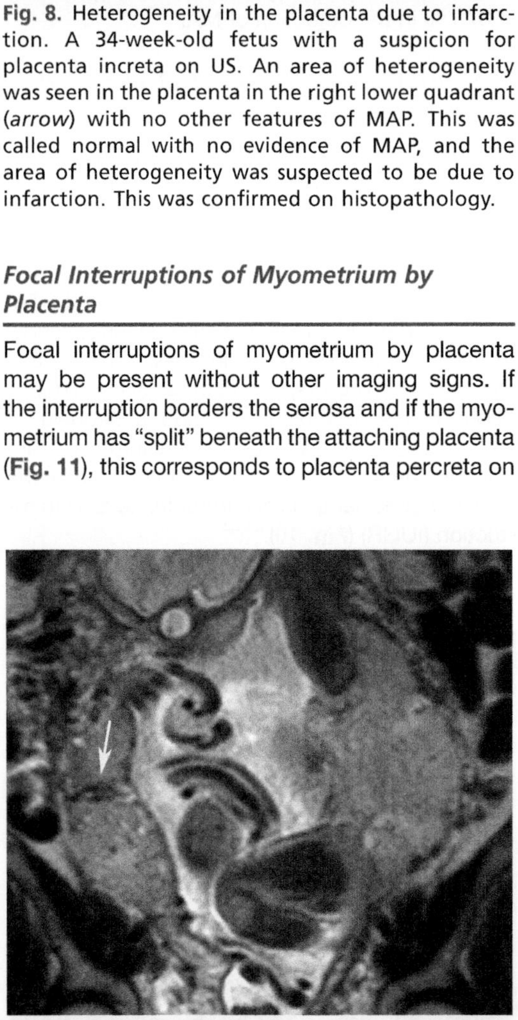

Fig. 9. Dark intraplacental bands. A 33-week-old fetus with suspicion for placenta increta on US. Dark intraplacental bands (*arrow*) were seen on MR imaging along with areas of uterine bulging (not shown); hence, this was suggested to be placenta increta. This was confirmed on histopathology.

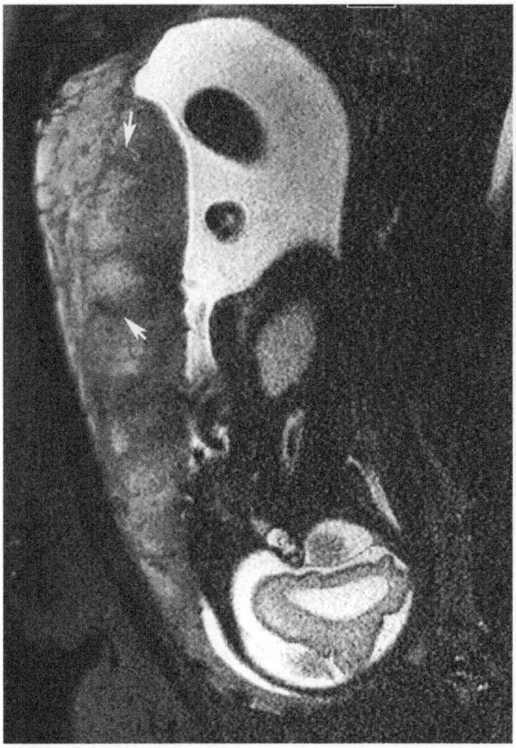

Fig. 10. Normal placental heterogeneity and bands. A 35-week-old fetus with mild ventriculomegaly seen on US. MR imaging was performed on a 3-T machine to evaluate cause of ventriculomegaly. The image illustrates heterogeneity and dark bands in the placenta (*arrows*); however, this was due to the imaging at high field strength in an older fetus and not to MAP.

Direct Visualization of the Invasion of Pelvic Structures by Placental Tissue

By definition, extension of the placental tissue outside the uterus is seen in placenta percreta only (**Fig. 12**). External structures involved include bladder, bowel, anterior abdominal wall, and lateral parametrium. Thiravit and colleagues[46] have reported a sensitivity of 41.7% and a specificity of 100% for this finding.

ACCURACY AND INTEROBSERVER VARIABILITY

A recent meta-analysis by D'Antonio and colleagues[37] found that MR imaging had a sensitivity, specificity, positive likelihood ratio, negative likelihood ratio, and diagnostic odds ratio of 94.4%, 84%, 5.91, 0.07, and 89, respectively, for detection of MAP, 92.9%, 97.6%, 6.24, 0.18, and 44.2,

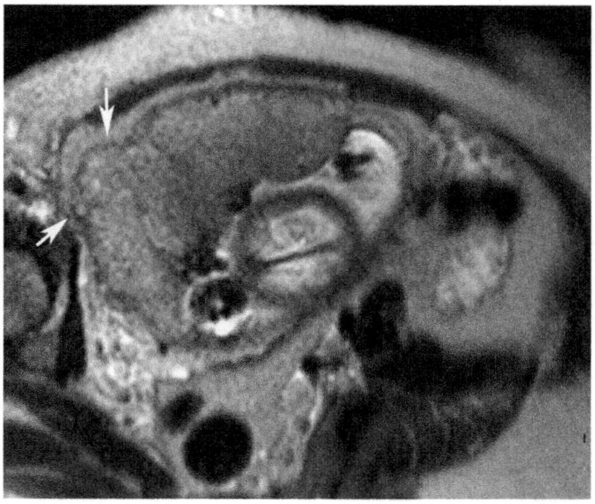

Fig. 11. Uterine myometrial interruption. A 30-week-old fetus with suspected placenta increta. MR imaging showed an area of focal interruption in the myometrium (*arrows*) along the right lateral wall. This was suggested to be an area of focal placenta percreta, which was confirmed on histopathology.

respectively, for evaluation of depth of invasion, and 99.6%, 95%, 15.8, 0.02, and 803, respectively, for the evaluation of topography of the invasion. Hence, MR is considered to be accurate for the diagnosis of MAP; however, there is significant variability in clinical practice.

Alamo and colleagues[45] found that overall sensitivity and specificity for placental invasion were 90.9% and 75.0% for more experienced reviewers versus 81.8% and 61.8% for less experienced reviewers, respectively. However, Ueno and colleagues[47] found that when they developed a radiologic score based on the imaging findings on MR imaging, their less experienced reviewers attained equally good diagnostic performance as their more experienced reviewers.

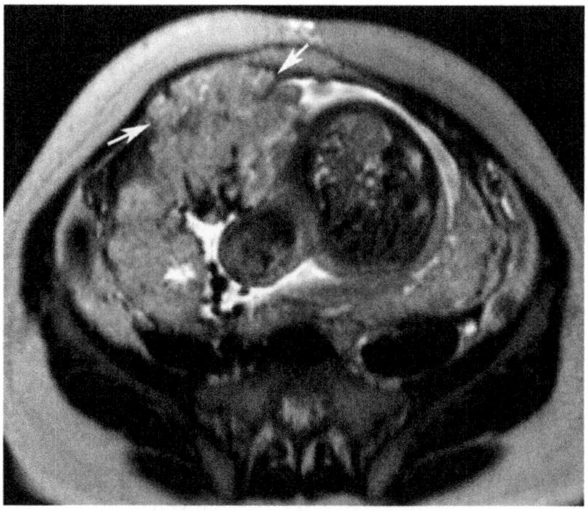

Fig. 12. Involvement of surrounding structures. A 35-week-old fetus with suspicion for placenta percreta on US. MR imaging showed an area of focal myometrial interruption with extension of placenta into the anterior abdominal wall (*arrows*). This was consistent with percreta on surgery and histopathology.

DIAGNOSTIC PITFALLS

Several pitfalls have been described in interpretation of placental MR imaging and are shown in **Box 2**.

Thinning or Loss of Retroplacental T2 Dark Zone

Thinning or loss of retroplacental T2 dark zone has been described on US in normal pregnancies as a retroplacental hypoechoic line, which corresponds to the retroplacental clear space. Absence of this line has been described in cases of MAP on US and MR imaging; however, it is often absent in normal pregnancies as well and therefore not considered to be specific for this diagnosis. Because the myometrium thins as the pregnancy progresses and can be difficult to visualize, relying on this sign alone can lead to false positive interpretations.[30]

Bladder Varices

Bladder varices are common and can mimic a uterine bulge or area of increased vascularity due to placental invasion. Correlation with US and diffusion-weighted MR imaging (DWI) sequences can help avoid this pitfall (**Fig. 13**). Bladder varices can lead to significant hemorrhage during cesarean section surgery, and their presence should be noted in the report.[48]

Uterine Dehiscence

Uterine dehiscence can cause uterine bulging due to the absence of the myometrium in the site of the dehiscence, leading to a false positive diagnosis of

Box 2
Diagnostic pitfalls in MR evaluation of morbidly adherent placenta

Overreliance on thinning or loss of retroplacental T2 dark zone

Bladder varices mimic MAP

Uterine dehiscence causing myometrial defect (rather than primary placental process)

Focal physiologic uterine bulge in the region of maternal umbilicus

Dark intraplacental areas from other causes

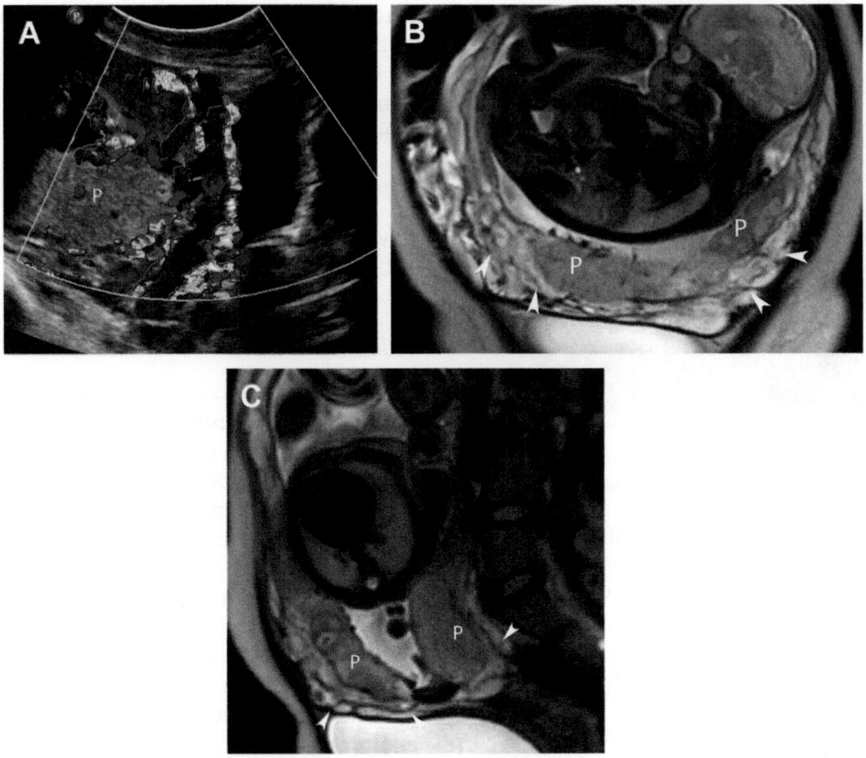

Fig. 13. Pitfall due to uterine vascularity. A 34-week-old pregnant patient with placenta previa (P) and increased vascularity seen in the lower uterine segment and along the interface with the bladder seen on a sagittal image on US (*A*). MR was performed to evaluate for MAP. Coronal (*B*) and sagittal (*C*) images through the lower uterine segment on MR showed no evidence of MAP. There was increased vascularity seen in the LUS, likely from multiple uterine varices (*arrowheads*). These vessels were seen to be bright on T2WIs due to the slow flow in them and not seen to be dark on T2WI as is typically seen with flow voids.

placenta percreta.[48] The placenta in the case of uterine dehiscence would not be adherent. Management in uterine dehiscence is close follow-up and evaluation for signs of uterine rupture, because uterine dehiscence could progress to uterine rupture, which is associated with a poor fetal outcome and high maternal morbidity.[49]

Focal Bulge in the Area of the Maternal Umbilicus

Cuthbert and colleagues[48] have suggested that because the rectus sheath separates as the pregnancy progresses, a focal bulge can be seen in the underlying anterior myometrium in the region of the maternal umbilicus.

Dark Intraplacental Areas

Dark intraplacental areas can be seen in placental infarction and intervillous thrombus in normal, preeclamptic, or IUGR patients and are imperfectly specific for MAP. Heterogeneity of the placenta is also a subjective finding and varies with gestational age, with increased heterogeneity seen in later gestational ages as described above.[50]

CLINICAL IMPACT

Patients with MAP commonly require a cesarean-hysterectomy because significant hemorrhage is quite common. Patients do not require additional fetal surveillance because MAP is not associated with increased risk of fetal death or IUGR.[51] In the absence of bleeding or other antepartum complications, planned late preterm delivery (after 36 weeks) is preferred to avoid the risks associated with emergency delivery for hemorrhage.[52] Depending on the organs and structures involved, additional surgical services like gynecologic oncology, urology, general surgery, and/or vascular surgery may be required to provide additional surgical expertise if needed. If the diagnosis of MAP is uncertain or if only placenta accreta is suspected, a period of observation for placental separation without excessive bleeding can be considered. If placenta increta or percreta is suspected, in most cases cesarean-hysterectomy is performed. In rare instances when removal of the uterus is not possible or is deemed too dangerous due to extensive invasion into surrounding tissues, conservative therapy is considered in which placenta and uterus are left in situ and a delayed hysterectomy is performed at a later date.[53] Presurgical information about the depth of invasion and location of the invasion in cases with MAP is hence essential for accurate surgical planning.

SUMMARY

The incidence of MAP is increasing, predominantly due to an increase in the number of cesarean sections. Knowledge of the common findings of MAP on MR imaging is important to be able to provide an accurate diagnosis. MR imaging should supplement US in patients with posterior placenta or equivocal findings on US, and for surgical planning. MR imaging should be performed between 24 and 32 weeks of gestational age in order to avoid pitfalls. Imaging assessment with MR imaging can help in adequate delivery planning and management in order to minimize perinatal morbidity and mortality.

REFERENCES

1. Oyelese Y, Smulian JC. Placenta previa, placenta accreta, and vasa previa. Obstet Gynecol 2006;107:927.
2. Committee on Obstetric Practice. Committee opinion no. 529: placenta accreta. Obstet Gynecol 2012;120:207.
3. Habek D, Becareviç R. Emergency peripartum hysterectomy in a tertiary obstetric center: 8-year evaluation. Fetal Diagn Ther 2007;22:139.
4. Rahman J, Al-Ali M, Qutub HO, et al. Emergency obstetric hysterectomy in a university hospital: a 25-year review. J Obstet Gynaecol 2008;28:69.
5. Glaze S, Ekwalanga P, Roberts G, et al. Peripartum hysterectomy: 1999 to 2006. Obstet Gynecol 2008;111:732.
6. Zelop CM, Harlow BL, Frigoletto FD, et al. Emergency peripartum hysterectomy. Am J Obstet Gynecol 1993;168:1443.
7. Silver RM, Landon MB, Rouse DJ, et al. Maternal morbidity associated with multiple repeat cesarean deliveries. Obstet Gynecol 2006;107:1226.
8. Belfort MA. Publications Committee ScfM-FM. Placenta accreta. Am J Obstet Gynecol 2010;203:430.
9. Al-Serehi A, Mhoyan A, Brown M, et al. Placenta accreta: an association with fibroids and Asherman syndrome. J Ultrasound Med 2008;27:1623.
10. Hamar BD, Wolff EF, Kodaman PH, et al. Premature rupture of membranes, placenta increta, and hysterectomy in a pregnancy following endometrial ablation. J Perinatol 2006;26:135.
11. Pron G, Mocarski E, Bennett J, et al. Pregnancy after uterine artery embolization for leiomyomata: the Ontario multicenter trial. Obstet Gynecol 2005;105:67.
12. Garmi G, Goldman S, Shalev E, et al. The effects of decidual injury on the invasion potential of trophoblastic cells. Obstet Gynecol 2011;117:55.
13. O'Brien JM, Barton JR, Donaldson ES. The management of placenta percreta: conservative and operative strategies. Am J Obstet Gynecol 1996;175:1632.
14. Hudon L, Belfort MA, Broome DR. Diagnosis and management of placenta percreta: a review. Obstet Gynecol Surv 1998;53:509.
15. Ng MK, Jack GS, Bolton DM, et al. Placenta percreta with urinary tract involvement: the case for a multidisciplinary approach. Urology 2009;74:778.
16. Hull AD, Moore TR. Multiple repeat cesareans and the threat of placenta accreta: incidence, diagnosis, management. Clin Perinatol 2011;38:285.
17. Eller AG, Bennett MA, Sharshiner M, et al. Maternal morbidity in cases of placenta accreta managed by a multidisciplinary care team compared with standard obstetric care. Obstet Gynecol 2011;117:331.
18. Allahdin S, Voigt S, Htwe TT. Management of placenta praevia and accreta. J Obstet Gynaecol 2011;31:1.
19. Dashe JS, McIntire DD, Ramus RM, et al. Persistence of placenta previa according to gestational age at ultrasound detection. Obstet Gynecol 2002;99:692.
20. D'Antonio F, Iacovella C, Bhide A. Prenatal identification of invasive placentation using ultrasound: systematic review and meta-analysis. Ultrasound Obstet Gynecol 2013;42:509.
21. Palacios Jaraquemada JM, Bruno CH. Magnetic resonance imaging in 300 cases of placenta accreta: surgical correlation of new findings. Acta Obstet Gynecol Scand 2005;84:716.
22. Victoria T, Johnson AM, Edgar JC, et al. Comparison between 1.5-T and 3-T MRI for fetal imaging: is there an advantage to imaging with a higher field strength? AJR Am J Roentgenol 2016;206:195.
23. ACR–SPR practice parameter for the safe and optimal performance of fetal magnetic resonance imaging (MRI). American College of Radiology; 2015. Available at: https://www.acr.org/~/media/CB384A65345F402083639E6756CE513F.pdf. Accessed April 5, 2017.
24. Millischer AE, Salomon LJ, Porcher R, et al. Magnetic resonance imaging for abnormally invasive placenta: the added value of intravenous gadolinium injection. BJOG 2017;124(1):88–95.
25. Webb JA, Thomsen HS, Morcos SK, et al. The use of iodinated and gadolinium contrast media during pregnancy and lactation. Eur Radiol 2005;15:1234.

26. Kanal E, Barkovich AJ, Bell C, et al. ACR guidance document on MR safe practices: 2013. J Magn Reson Imaging 2013;37:501.
27. Morita S, Ueno E, Fujimura M, et al. Feasibility of diffusion-weighted MRI for defining placental invasion. J Magn Reson Imaging 2009;30:666.
28. Horowitz JM, Berggruen S, McCarthy RJ, et al. When timing is everything: are placental MRI examinations performed before 24 weeks' gestational age reliable? AJR Am J Roentgenol 2015;205:685.
29. D'Antonio F, Palacios-Jaraquemada J, Lim PS, et al. Counseling in fetal medicine: evidence-based answers to clinical questions on morbidly adherent placenta. Ultrasound Obstet Gynecol 2016;47:290.
30. Baughman WC, Corteville JE, Shah RR. Placenta accreta: spectrum of US and MR imaging findings. Radiographics 2008;28:1905.
31. Kim JA, Narra VR. Magnetic resonance imaging with true fast imaging with steady-state precession and half-Fourier acquisition single-shot turbo spin-echo sequences in cases of suspected placenta accreta. Acta Radiol 2004;45:692.
32. Clark SL, Koonings PP, Phelan JP. Placenta previa/accreta and prior cesarean section. Obstet Gynecol 1985;66:89.
33. Reddy UM, Abuhamad AZ, Levine D, et al. Fetal imaging: executive summary of a joint Eunice Kennedy Shriver National Institute of Child Health and Human Development, Society for Maternal-Fetal Medicine, American Institute of Ultrasound in Medicine, American College of Obstetricians and Gynecologists, American College of Radiology, Society for Pediatric Radiology, and Society of Radiologists in Ultrasound Fetal Imaging workshop. Obstet Gynecol 2014;123:1070.
34. Lax A, Prince MR, Mennitt KW, et al. The value of specific MRI features in the evaluation of suspected placental invasion. Magn Reson Imaging 2007;25:87.
35. Riteau AS, Tassin M, Chambon G, et al. Accuracy of ultrasonography and magnetic resonance imaging in the diagnosis of placenta accreta. PLoS One 2014;9:e94866.
36. Bour L, Placé V, Bendavid S, et al. Suspected invasive placenta: evaluation with magnetic resonance imaging. Eur Radiol 2014;24:3150.
37. D'Antonio F, Iacovella C, Palacios-Jaraquemada J, et al. Prenatal identification of invasive placentation using magnetic resonance imaging: systematic review and meta-analysis. Ultrasound Obstet Gynecol 2014;44:8.
38. Teo TH, Law YM, Tay KH, et al. Use of magnetic resonance imaging in evaluation of placental invasion. Clin Radiol 2009;64:511.
39. Noda Y, Kanematsu M, Goshima S, et al. Prenatal MR imaging diagnosis of placental invasion. Abdom Imaging 2015;40:1273.
40. Leyendecker JR, DuBose M, Hosseinzadeh K, et al. MRI of pregnancy-related issues: abnormal placentation. AJR Am J Roentgenol 2012;198:311.
41. Blaicher W, Brugger PC, Mittermayer C, et al. Magnetic resonance imaging of the normal placenta. Eur J Radiol 2006;57:256.
42. Derman AY, Nikac V, Haberman S, et al. MRI of placenta accreta: a new imaging perspective. AJR Am J Roentgenol 2011;197:1514.
43. Ueno Y, Kitajima K, Kawakami F, et al. Novel MRI finding for diagnosis of invasive placenta praevia: evaluation of findings for 65 patients using clinical and histopathological correlations. Eur Radiol 2014;24:881.
44. Lim PS, Greenberg M, Edelson MI, et al. Utility of ultrasound and MRI in prenatal diagnosis of placenta accreta: a pilot study. AJR Am J Roentgenol 2011; 197:1506.
45. Alamo L, Anaye A, Rey J, et al. Detection of suspected placental invasion by MRI: do the results depend on observer' experience? Eur J Radiol 2013;82:e51.
46. Thiravit S, Lapatikarn S, Muangsomboon K, et al. MRI of placenta percreta: differentiation from other entities of placental adhesive disorder. Radiol Med 2017;122(1):61–8.
47. Ueno Y, Maeda T, Tanaka U, et al. Evaluation of interobserver variability and diagnostic performance of developed MRI-based radiological scoring system for invasive placenta previa. J Magn Reson Imaging 2016;44:573.
48. Cuthbert F, Teixidor Vinas M, Whitby E. The MRI features of placental adhesion disorder-a pictorial review. Br J Radiol 2016;89:20160284.
49. Sinha M, Gupta R, Gupta P, et al. Uterine rupture: a seven year review at a tertiary care hospital in New Delhi, India. Indian J Community Med 2016;41:45.
50. Varghese B, Singh N, George RA, et al. Magnetic resonance imaging of placenta accreta. Indian J Radiol Imaging 2013;23:379.
51. Usta IM, Hobeika EM, Musa AA, et al. Placenta previa-accreta: risk factors and complications. Am J Obstet Gynecol 2005;193:1045.
52. Warshak CR, Ramos GA, Eskander R, et al. Effect of predelivery diagnosis in 99 consecutive cases of placenta accreta. Obstet Gynecol 2010;115:65.
53. Alkazaleh F, Geary M, Kingdom J, et al. Elective nonremoval of the placenta and prophylactic uterine artery embolization postpartum as a diagnostic imaging approach for the management of placenta percreta: a case report. J Obstet Gynaecol Can 2004;26:743.

From Staging to Prognostication

Achievements and Challenges of MR Imaging in the Assessment of Endometrial Cancer

Stephanie Nougaret, MD, PhD[a,b,*], Yulia Lakhman, MD[c], Hebert Alberto Vargas, MD[c], Pierre Emmanuel Colombo, MD, PhD[d], Shinya Fujii, MD, PhD[e], Caroline Reinhold, MD, MSc[f], Evis Sala, MD, PhD[c]

KEYWORDS

• Endometrial cancer • MR Imaging • DWI • DCE • Staging

KEY POINTS

- Endometrial cancer incidence is increasing owing mostly to Western lifestyle.
- Preoperative MR imaging helps in the selection of patients who may benefit from minimally invasive surgery.
- The combination of T2-weighted, diffusion-weighted, and dynamic contrast-enhanced MR imaging provides a "one-stop shop" approach for the accurate staging of patients with endometrial cancer.
- Sequences angled perpendicularly to the endometrial cavity are critical to accurately assess the depth of myometrial invasion.

INTRODUCTION

Endometrial cancer is the fourth most common malignancy in women, with more than 60,000 newly diagnosed cases in the United States in 2016.[1] Its incidence is increasing, mainly owing to increased life expectancy and obesity rates.[1,2] Approximately 75% of cases occur in postmenopausal women, with a mean age at presentation of 63 years.[3] Most endometrial cancers are diagnosed at an early stage (80% stage I), with 5-year survival rates of more than 95%.[3]

Endometrial cancer is staged surgically using the International Federation of Gynecology and Obstetrics (FIGO) system. The standard surgical staging procedure consists of hysterectomy, bilateral salpingo-oophorectomy, lymph node dissection, peritoneal washing, and omental biopsies.[4] However, although the FIGO stage correlates with prognosis, preoperative staging is essential

The authors have nothing to disclose.
Drs Y. Lakhman, H.A. Vargas, and E. Sala were funded in part through the NIH/NCI Cancer Center Support Grant P30 CA008748.
[a] IRCM, Montpellier Cancer Research institute, 208 Ave des Apothicaires, Montpellier 34295, France; [b] Department of Radiology, Montpellier Cancer institute, INSERM, U1194, University of Montpellier, 208 Ave des Apothicaires, Montpellier 34295, France; [c] Department of Radiology, Memorial Sloan Kettering Cancer Center, 1275 York Avenue, New York, NY 10065, USA; [d] Department of Surgery, Montpellier Cancer institute, 208 Ave des Apothicaires, Montpellier 34295, France; [e] Department of Radiology, Tottori University, 683-8503 86 Nishi-cho, Yonago-shi, Tottori-ken, Tottori, Japan; [f] Department of Radiology, McGill University, 845 rue Sherbrroke Ouest, Montreal H3G 1A3, Canada
* Corresponding author. Radiology Department, Montpellier Cancer Institute (ICM), 31 rue de la Croix verte, Montpellier cedex 5 34298, France.
E-mail address: stephanienougaret@free.fr

Magn Reson Imaging Clin N Am 25 (2017) 611–633
http://dx.doi.org/10.1016/j.mric.2017.03.010

to tailor treatment. Indeed, early stage patients may be treated appropriately with minimally invasive surgery and without lymphadenectomy.[5,6] This approach leads to reduced morbidity and shorter duration of hospital stay, with an outcome comparable to the standard, more extensive staging procedure.[7–9] The effective implementation of this management approach relies on accurate preoperative staging.

MR imaging is the imaging modality of choice to determine the depth of myometrial invasion preoperatively, which in turn correlates with tumor grade, presence of lymph node metastases, and overall survival.[10,11] MR imaging is recommended by the American College of Radiologists[12] and the European Society of Radiology for preoperative endometrial cancer staging.[10] The combination of T2-weighted imaging (T2WI), dynamic contrast-enhanced (DCE) MR imaging, and diffusion-weighted imaging (DWI) offers the best diagnostic accuracy in staging of endometrial cancer.[13]

In this review, we emphasize the advantages and challenges of MR imaging staging of endometrial cancer, especially focusing on the MR imaging acquisition protocol and the role of DWI and DCE MR imaging.

PATIENT POPULATION AND TUMOR TYPE

Incidence and Risk Factors

Endometrial cancer is the most common gynecologic cancer in North America (**Box 1**).[1] Furthermore, the number of cases is projected to increase by 55% in the United States between 2010 and 2030.[14] The increasing incidence is thought to be mainly related to the Western lifestyle and obesity in particular.[15,16] Obesity increases estrogen production via its aromatization in adipose tissues.[16,17] Diabetes mellitus is associated with an increased risk, probably related to concurrent obesity, although an independent association between diabetes and endometrial cancer has been reported.[18,19] Nulliparity and infertility are additional risk factors, including polycystic ovarian syndrome.[20] Other risk factors for endometrial cancer include unopposed estrogen therapy such as tamoxifen, estrogen-producing tumors, and early menarche/late menopause.[15,21,22] Most cases of endometrial cancer are sporadic; however, 5% have an hereditary basis related to the Lynch syndrome.[23] This syndrome is due to germ-line mutations of one of the DNA repair genes MSH2, MLH1, and MSH6.

Box 1
Risk factors for endometrial cancer

Excess estrogen exposure

Exogenous estrogen or estrogen agonists

- Unopposed estrogen therapy
- Tamoxifen
- Estrogen–progestin postmenopausal hormone therapy
- Phytoestrogens

Endogenous estrogen

- Obesity
- Chronic anovulation
- Early menarche and late menopause
- Estrogen secreting tumors

Age

Family history of Lynch syndrome

Associated factors

Nulliparity and infertility

Diabetes

Breast cancer

Tubal ligation

Protective factors

Hormonal contraceptives

Increased maternal age

Smoking

Diet and exercise

- Physical activity
- Tea
- Coffee

Pathogenesis

Endometrial carcinomas have been traditionally divided into 2 subtypes based on prognosis (**Table 1**). Type 1 endometrial carcinomas are estrogen-dependent tumors and include FIGO grades 1 and 2 endometrioid adenocarcinomas. Type 2 endometrial carcinomas include serous papillary, clear cell adenocarcinomas, carcinosarcomas, and FIGO grade 3 endometrioid adenocarcinomas. Type II tumors are not driven by estrogen and tend to present at a higher stage and behave more aggressively. Several genomic and molecular characteristics support this dichotomous classification and have become an integral component of the pathologic evaluation. Type I tumors are associated preferentially with genetic alterations in PTEN, KRAS, CTNNB1, and PIK3CA, whereas serous carcinomas usually harbor TP53 mutations. The Cancer Genome Atlas Research Network has improved the evaluation of the molecular landscape of endometrial cancer

Table 1
Endometrial cancer types

	Type I Endometrial Carcinoma	Type II Endometrial Carcinoma
Hormone dependency	Estrogen dependent	Non estrogen dependent
Percentage	80–85	10–15
Age at diagnosis	Younger patient (premenopausal to perimenopausal)	Older (postmenopausal)
Risk factors	Obesity Unopposed estrogen exposure Nulliparity and infertility (polycystic ovary syndrome)	None
Histologic features	Low-grade tumor Endometrioid grades 1–2 Endometrioid with squamous differentiation Mucinous	High-grade tumor Endometrioid grade 3 Clear cell Serous Undifferentiated Carcinosarcoma
Precursor	Arising from endometrial hyperplasia	Endometrial intraepithelial carcinoma
Associated genetic factor	PTEN or KRAS gene mutation Microsatellite instability	P53 mutation
Clinical course	Early initial stage (70%) Slow growing Local recurrence	Advanced initial stage (60%) Rapid progression Aggressive behavior with poor prognosis Abdominal and lymphatic recurrence
5-year overall survival	80%	40%

significantly by describing 4 molecular subtypes, including[1] POLE, the smallest group with an excellent prognosis[2]; microsatellite unstable tumors[3]; copy number low microsatellite stable tumors and[4]; copy number high tumors with mostly TP53 mutations. This latter group includes serous carcinomas and is associated with a poor prognosis.

Diagnosis

Abnormal vaginal bleeding is the most common initial presentation of endometrial cancer. The standard diagnostic evaluation includes pelvic ultrasound and pipelle endometrial biopsy or dilatation and curettage. Thresholds of endometrial thickness of 4 or 5 mm have been proposed to detect endometrial cancer with a sensitivity of up to 95% and specificity of 77%[24] in postmenopausal women. A recent metaanalysis suggested a more stringent threshold of 3 mm to achieve a higher sensitivity (97.5%).[25]

MR IMAGING PROTOCOL

Patient Preparation

- To diminish artifacts owing to peristalsis, patients are typically instructed to fast for 4 to 6 hours before MR imaging. An antiperistaltic agent, such as butylscopolamine bromide or glucagon, is usually administered intramuscularly or intravenously at the beginning of the examination.
- Patients are also instructed to empty their urinary bladder to decrease phase ghost artifacts related to bladder motion and filling.
- Imaging is performed with the patient in the supine position using a multichannel phase array surface coil. Saturation bands placed along the subcutaneous fat of the anterior and posterior body wall are useful to diminish near-field artifact.
- Endometrial cancer is often diagnosed after dilation and curettage. MR imaging interpretation is usually not affected adversely by uterus changes after this procedure and MR imaging can be performed after vaginal bleeding has stopped.

MR Imaging Protocol

The combination of conventional (T2WI) and functional sequences (DWI and DCE MR imaging) provides a "one-stop shop" approach for the staging of patients with endometrial cancer (**Table 2**).

Table 2
MR imaging endometrial cancer protocol

	Coronal T2	Axial T1	Axial T2	Sagittal T2	Axial Oblique T2	Sagittal DWI	Axial Oblique DWI	Sagittal DCE	Axial Oblique DCE
FOV (cm)	36–44	32–36	20–24	20–24	20–24	20–24	20–24	20–24	20–24
Thickness (mm)	6	5	4	4	4	4	4	4 /–2	4 /–2
Gap (mm)	1	1	0.4	0.4	0.3	0	0	0	0
Echo time (ms)	104	Min	120	120	120	Min	Min	2.1	2.1
Relaxation time (ms)	500–1600	Min	3500–4000	3500–4000	4000–4500	5000	5000	6.4	6.4
Flip angle	90	90	90	90	90	N/A	N/A	80	80
Bandwidth (kHz)	32	32	32	32	32	N/A	N/A	83	83
ETL	200	3–4	28	28	28	N/A	N/A	N/A	N/A
NEX	1	2	3	3	3	6	6	1	1
Frequency steps	300	448	384	384	384	90	90	320	320
Phase encoding steps	200	224	256	256	256	192	192	280	280

Abbreviations: DCE, dynamic contrast enhanced; DWI, diffusion-weighted imaging; ETL, echo-train length; FOV, field of view; NEX, number of excitations.

Conventional sequences

The conventional protocol includes small field of view (FOV) high-resolution axial, and sagittal, T2WI within the pelvis and large FOV axial T1-weighted imaging or T2WI of the abdomen and pelvis. A large FOV coronal T2 on the whole abdomen and pelvis may be added optionally.

In addition, a high-resolution, small FOV, axial oblique T2WI angled perpendicularly to the endometrial cavity is critical to assess the depth of myometrial invasion.

Image acquisition optimization for T2WI angled perpendicularly to the endometrium

- Thin section (3–4 mm).
- Small FOV (20–24 cm).
- The uterus can have a variable position within the pelvis and it may be tilted to the left or right of the midline. If oblique axial images are prescribed using only sagittal images, this may not yield an imaging plane that is precisely perpendicular to the endometrial cavity. A "double oblique images" angled both in the sagittal and coronal planes create a " true oblique" that is exactly orthogonal to the endometrial cavity[26] (**Figs. 1** and **2**).

Functional MR imaging

Diffusion-weighted imaging An imaging protocol should also include DWI in at least 1 but preferably in 2 planes (axial oblique along the uterus with the same orientation as axial oblique T2WI and sagittal) with a minimum of 2 b values (eg, b = 400, b = 800). Acquiring T2WI and DWI on the same plane allows images fusion and optimizes anatomic correlation.

DWI is traditionally implemented as an echoplanar imaging sequence. However, echoplanar imaging is highly prone to susceptibility artifacts and image blurring owing to the relatively long gradient echo train used for image acquisition. Parallel imaging is now widely used to reduce the echo train length and, thus, geometric distortions inherent to echoplanar imaging. Recently, FOCUS imaging (FOV optimized and constrained undistorted single-shot DWI) has been investigated in prostate and endometrial cancer.[27,28] This new acquisition technique uses a 2-dimensional, spatially selective echoplanar radiofrequency excitation pulse and a 180° refocusing pulse reducing the FOV in the phase-encoding direction. Reduced phase direction FOV technique improves the spatial resolution, without associated phase

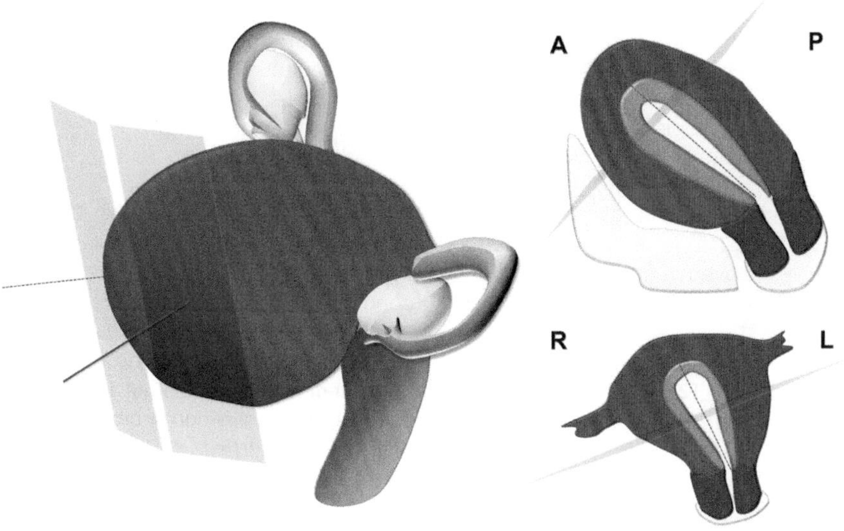

Fig. 1. The "double oblique T2": Drawing showing a 3-dimensional anteverted and right-sided uterus. To get a true axial acquisition to uterine body, a double axial oblique sequence perpendicular to both the sagittal and coronal axis of the uterus must be acquired. A, anterior; L, left; P, posterior; R, right.

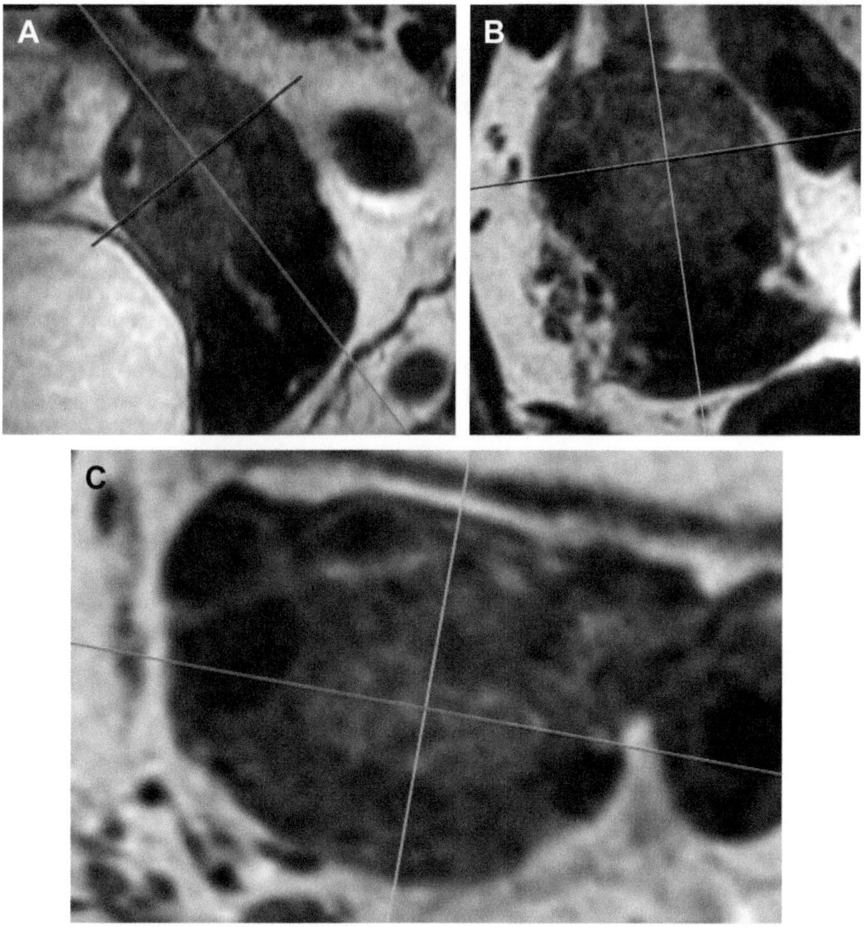

Fig. 2. Sagittal (*A*) and coronal (*B*) T2-weighted imaging sequences showing an anteverted (*A*) and right tilted (*B*) uterus. Angling the axis along the sagittal and coronal orientation of the uterus enables a true double oblique sequence (*C*) with an accurate evaluation of the depth of myometrial invasion.

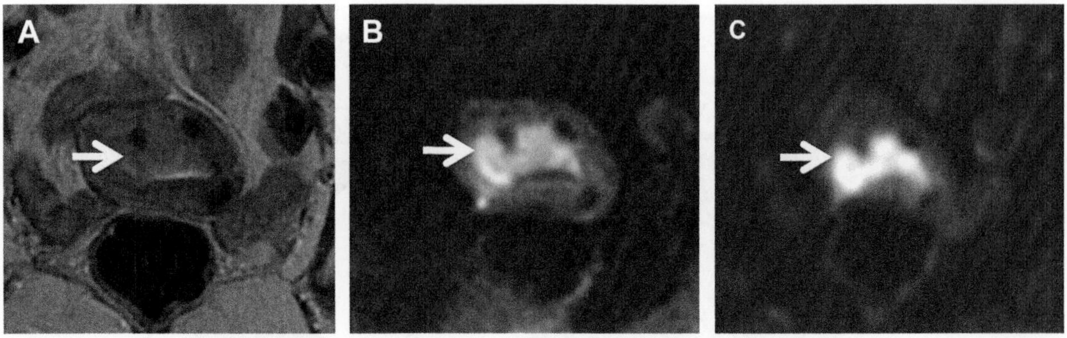

Fig. 3. Field of view optimized and constrained undistorted single-shot diffusion-weighted imaging (DWI) (FOCUS). (*A*) Axial oblique T2-weighted imaging showing an ill-defined endometrial lesion; note the poor tumor-to-myometrium contrast at the interface (*arrow*). (*B*) FOCUS DWI acquisition demonstrates increased resolution with better tumor delineation compared with standard DWI (*C*) (*arrow*).

wrapround artifact and with decreased artifacts related to motion and susceptibility, which are common with a large FOV[28] (**Fig. 3**).

Dynamic Multiphase Contrast-Enhanced MR Imaging

DCE MR images are obtained with a 3-dimensional gradient echo T1WI, fat-saturated sequence after the administration of 0.1 mmol/kg of gadolinium at a rate of 2 mL/s. The most commonly used sequences are LAVA (GE, Fairfield, CT), VIBE (Siemens, Munich, Germany), and THRIVE (Philips, Amsterdam, the Netherlands). Images are traditionally acquired before contrast injection and then during multiple phases of enhancement in sagittal planes at 25 seconds, 1 minutes, and 2 minutes after injection; a delayed sequence is acquired on axial oblique 4 minutes after injection.

- Early phase images (25 seconds to 1 minute after contrast administration) are optimal for the detection of subendometrial enhancement that corresponds with the inner junctional zone, which enhances earlier than the rest of the myometrium. Uninterrupted subendometrial linear enhancement nearly excludes superficial myometrium invasion.
- Equilibrium phase images (2–3 minutes after injection) are best for the evaluation of deep myometrium invasion.
- Recently, an imaging delay of approximately 90 seconds has been reported as the optimal timing delay for best tumor–myometrium contrast.[29]
- Delayed phase images (4–5 minutes after injection) are optimal for the detection of cervical stroma invasion.

DYNAMIC CONTRAST-ENHANCED MR IMAGING CANCER DETECTION AND DIAGNOSIS

Endometrial cancer is typically diagnosed by endometrial sampling. However, in some cases endometrial sampling is not possible, owing to cervical stenosis for instance, or its results are inconclusive. In these situations, MR imaging is helpful in cancer depiction.

Classic Tumor Appearance on MR Imaging

Three distinct zones are apparent on T2WI of the uterus: (1) the high signal intensity of endometrium surrounded by (2) the low signal intensity junctional zone (inner myometrium), which in turn is surrounded by (3) the intermediate signal intensity outer myometrium.

- On T2WI, the tumor usually demonstrates intermediate to low T2 signal intensity relative to the hyperintense normal endometrium (**Fig. 4**). However, small tumors may not be associated with endometrial thickening or can have a signal intensity similar to that of the normal endometrium. In those cases, functional sequences may be particularly helpful.
- On DCE MR imaging, small tumors may enhance early compared with the normal endometrium. In the later phases of enhancement, these tumors may appear hypointense relative to the myometrium.
- On DWI, tumors appear hyperintense on the high B-value DWI image with corresponding hypointense signal on the apparent diffusion coefficient (ADC) map (see **Fig. 4**).

Data are accumulating to support the use of DWI as a tool to differentiate endometrial cancer from

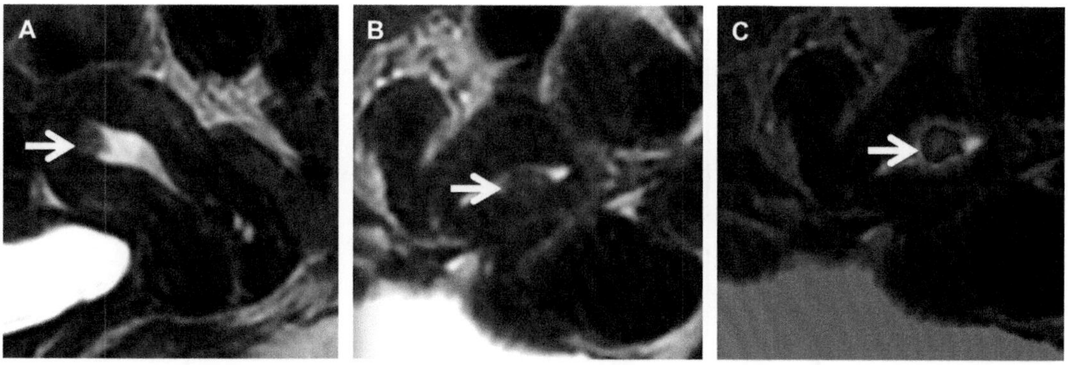

Fig. 4. Stage IA endometrial cancer. (*A*) Sagittal and (*B*) axial oblique T2-weighted imaging (T2WI) shows relative small distention of the endometrial cavity by an intermediate signal intensity tumor (*arrow*) within the fundus. (*C*) Fused axial obliqueT2WI–diffusion-weighted imaging (DWI) shows a small focus of hyperintense DWI signal within the endometrial cavity (*arrow*) in keeping with stage IA tumor invading less than 50% of the myometrium.

normal endometrium or benign uterine disorders.[30–34] Multiples studies have shown that ADC values of endometrial cancers are significantly lower than those of endometrial polyps and normal endometrium.[30–34] In a cohort, of 70 cancer patients and 36 control subjects, Rechichi and colleagues[31] found that there was no overlap in ADC values between endometrial cancer and normal endometrium. The authors were able to define using 2b values (b = 0, b = 1000) and an ADC value threshold of 1.05×10^{-3} mm^2/s to distinguish endometrial cancer from normal endometrial tissue. Others have proposed cutoffs ranging from 1.05 to 1.28 to distinguish malignant from benign lesions with a range of sensitivities of 60.1% to 87% and specificity of 100%.[30,32,35,36] This information might be of particular relevance when endometrial biopsy is not possible or inconclusive.

DYNAMIC CONTRAST-ENHANCED MR IMAGING CANCER STAGING

Stage I

Stage IA tumors invade less than 50% of the myometrial thickness and stage IB tumors involve more than 50% of the myometrial thickness (**Tables 3** and **4**).

Why is it important to assess deep myometrial invasion?

It is important to distinguish stage IA from stage IB disease because stage IB is associated with a high risk of lymphovascular space invasion (LVSI), which directly correlates with the risk for lymph node metastases and relapse.

How to differentiate stage IA and stage IB?

Measuring the depth of tumor extension within the myometrium A line must be drawn along the expected inner edge of the myometrium (endometrium–myometrium junction) on axial oblique images acquired perpendicular to the endometrium (**Fig. 5**). Then, 2 lines are drawn: one measuring the thickness of the entire myometrium and another measuring the maximum tumor extent within the myometrium. The ratio of the 2 lines detailed represent the percentage of myometrial invasion.

Pearls An intact, low signal intensity junctional zone on T2WI and a smooth uninterrupted band of early subendometrial enhancement on DCE MR imaging almost completely excludes myometrial invasion (**Fig. 6**).

Pitfalls

- Tumor evaluation on T2WI may be limited when the tumor is isointense to the myometrium, or when the zonal anatomy of the uterus is less well-defined, as is often seen after menopause. DCE MR imaging and DWI can help to overcome these pitfalls by improving tumor delineation (**Fig. 7**).
- Occasionally, a large tumor can distend the endometrial cavity and compress the surrounding myometrium; deep myometrial invasion should not be overcalled in these situations. Symmetry and smooth tumor contours favor stage IA (**Fig. 8**).
- Cornual regions of the uterus demonstrate a thinner myometrium compared with other areas of the uterine corpus and the depth of myometrial invasion at this level is frequently overestimated. The addition of DCE MR imaging and DWI to T2WI can improve preoperative staging accuracy (**Fig. 9**).

Table 3
FIGO Staging with MR imaging correspondence

FIGO Stage	Description	MR imaging	
I	Tumor confined to corpus uteri		
IA	≤50% of myometrial depth	Abnormal signal intensity extends into the ≤50% of myometrium.	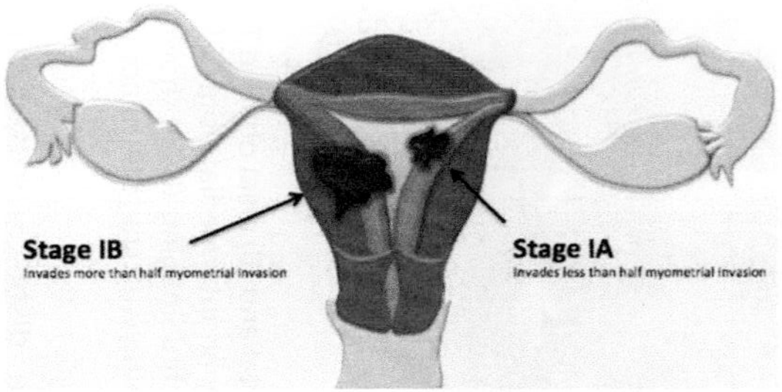Stage IB Invades more than half myometrial invasion Stage IA Invades less than half myometrial invasion
IB	>50% of myometrial depth	Abnormal signal intensity extends into >50% of myometrium	
II	Tumor invades cervical stroma but does not extend beyond uterus	Disruption of hypointense stroma by tumor	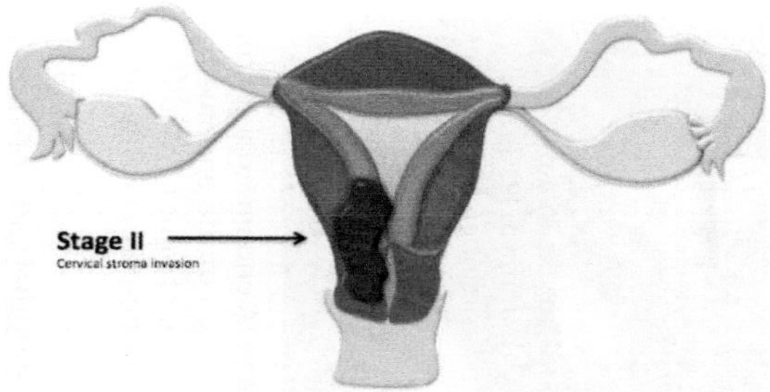Stage II Cervical stroma invasion

III	Local and/or regional spread of tumor		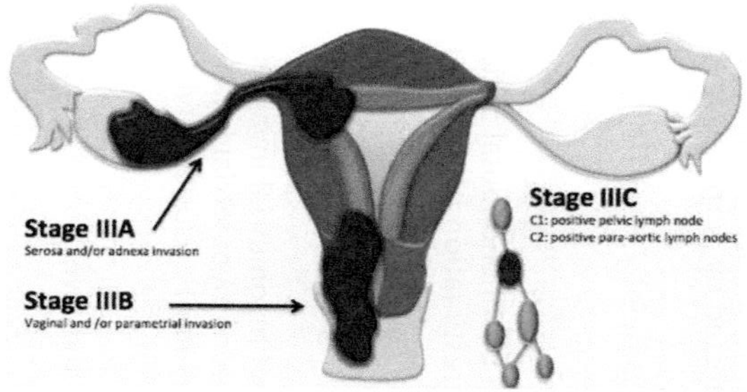
IIIA	Tumor invades serosa of corpus uteri and/or adnexa	Disruption of continuity of outer myometrium	
IIIB	Vaginal and/or parametrial involvement	Segmental loss of hypointense vaginal wall	
IIIC	Metastases to pelvic and/or paraaortic lymph nodes	Regional or paraaortic nodes	
IIIC1	Positive pelvic nodes	Node size $\geq$10 mm, irregular contour, similar signal intensity to that of primary tumor	
IIIC2	Positive paraaortic lymph nodes		
IV	Tumor invades bladder and/or bowel mucosa; distant metastases may be present		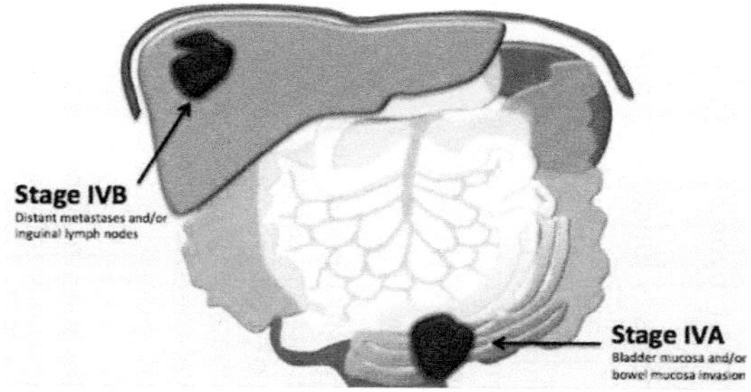
IVA	Tumor invasion of bladder and/or bowel mucosa (biopsy proven)	Abnormal signal intensity disrupts normal hypointense muscle and invades bladder and/or rectal mucosa; Bullous edema does not indicate stage IVA	
IVB	Distant metastases, including intraabdominal metastases and/or inguinal lymph nodes	Tumor in distant sites or organs	

Table 4
Pearls and pitfalls of MR imaging of endometrial carcinoma

T2	Pearls Assessment of the depth of myometrial invasion is optimized by perpendicular plane to endometrium An intact low-signal intensity junctional zone on T2WI excludes myometrial invasion Pitfalls Small tumor may be undetectable on T2WI Poor tumor-to-myometrium interface may be present in postmenopausal patient Adenomyosis and leiomyomas can lead to under or overestimation of depth of myometrial invasion
DCE MR imaging	Pearls Improves detection of small tumors and delineation of large necrotic tumor Maximum tumor/myometrium contrast at 90 s Increases the accuracy of T2WI for evaluation of depth of myometrial invasion Contiguous band of subendometrial enhancement excludes myometrial invasion Enhancement of cervical mucosa on delayed images (4–5 min) excludes cervical stromal invasion Pitfalls Depth of myometrial invasion may be overestimated at the level of the cornua because the myometrium is thin at this level
DWI	Pearls Can detect small tumors Lesion characterization if hysteroscopy is not possible (eg, cervical canal stenosis) Increases the accuracy of T2WI for evaluation of depth of myometrial invasion and cervical stromal invasion. Assessment of extrauterine disease in advanced cancer (small vaginal implants, peritoneal implants) Diagnosis of tumor recurrence Pitfalls Should always be read in conjunction with T2WI More prone to susceptibility artifact

Abbreviations: DCE, dynamic contrast enhanced; DWI, diffusion-weighted imaging; T2WI, T2-weighted imaging.

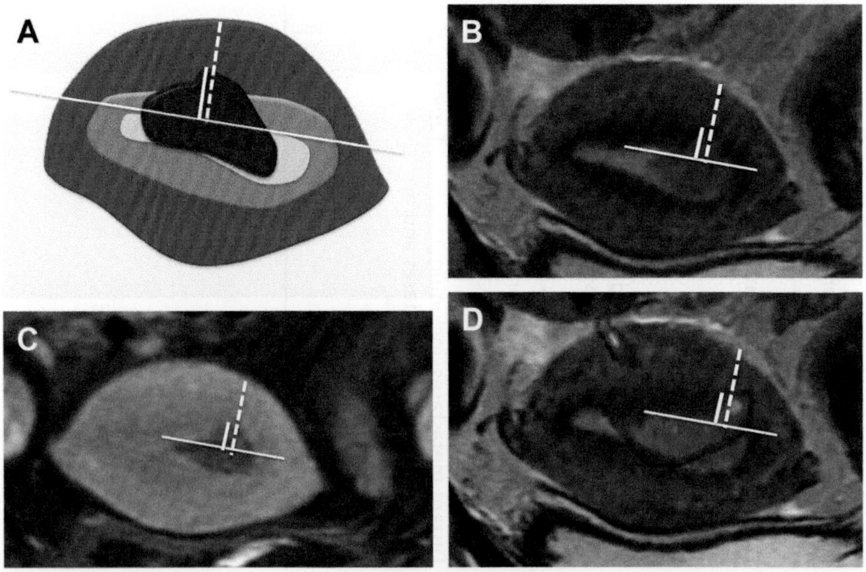

Fig. 5. Measuring the depth of tumor extension within the myometrium. (*A*) How to measure accurately the depth of tumor extension within the myometrium. A line must be drawn along the expected inner edge of the myometrium on a plane strictly perpendicular to the endometrium. Then, 2 lines are drawn, one measuring the thickness of the entire myometrium and another measuring the maximum tumor extent within the myometrium. The ratio of the 2 lines detailed represents the percentage of myometrial invasion. (*B–D*) Corresponding measurement images on T2-weighted imaging, dynamic contrast-enhanced imaging, and diffusion-weighted imaging axial oblique sequences.

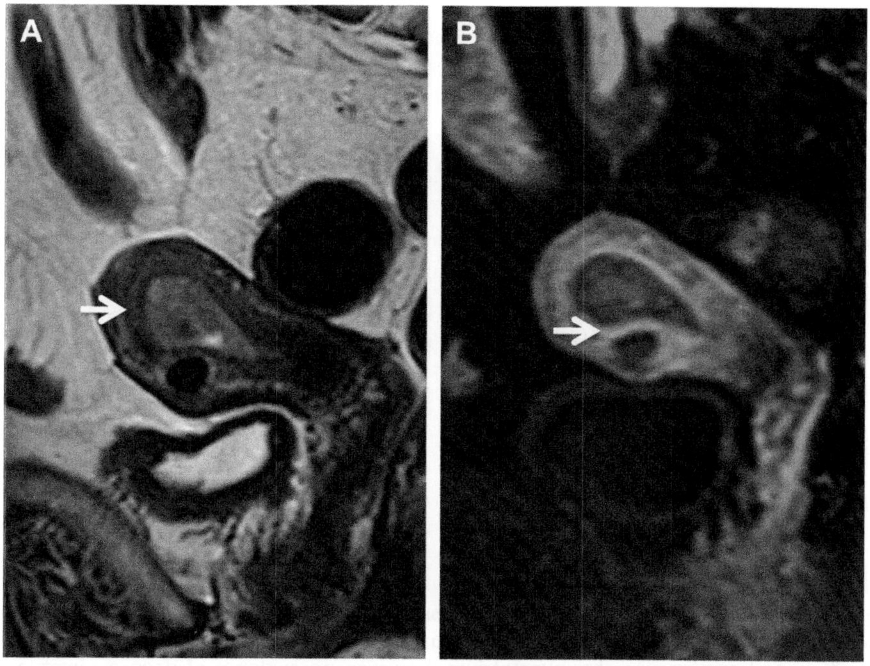

Fig. 6. Stage IA endometrial cancer. (*A*) Sagittal T2-weighted imaging (T2WI) and (*B*) dynamic contrast-enhanced (DCE) MR imaging demonstrate a tumor distending the endometrial cavity. The junctional zone shows an intact low-signal intensity (*arrow, A*) on T2WI and a smooth band of early subendometrial enhancement is seen on DCE MR imaging (*arrow, B*). Those 2 features exclude myometrial invasion, which is particularly important if fertility preservation is an option.

- Other pitfalls in assessing the depth of myometrial invasion in endometrial carcinoma are related to the presence of leiomyomas and/or adenomyosis. On MR imaging, adenomyosis is usually seen as areas of poorly defined T2WI hypointense signal intensity with an obscure junctional zone (**Fig. 10**). This presentation may make it difficult to determine the extent of endometrial cancers and lead to errors in staging. DCE MR

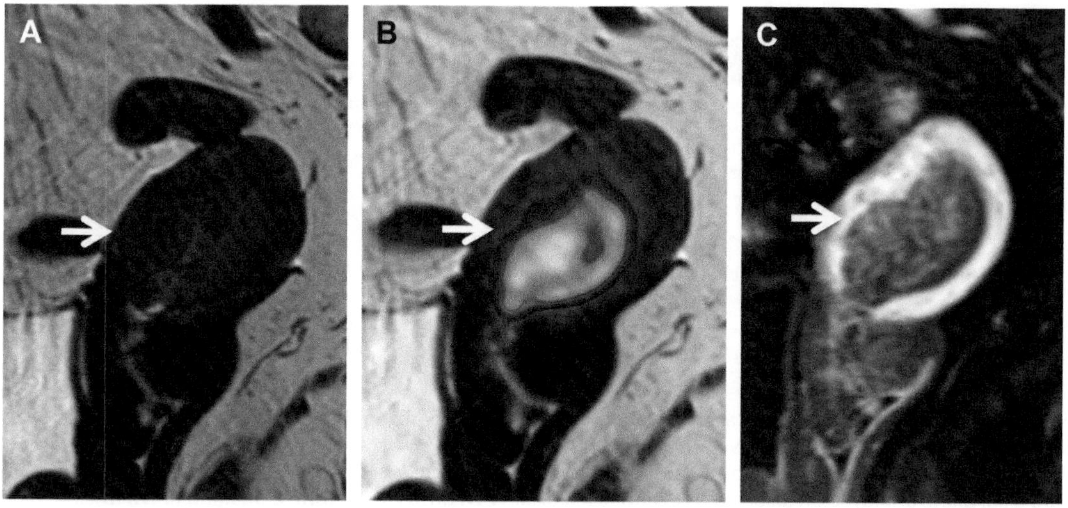

Fig. 7. Stage IA endometrial cancer with poor tumor-to-myometrium contrast at the interface on T2-weighted imaging (T2WI). (*A*) Sagittal T2WI shows an endometrial cancer with poor tumor delineation on T2WI and questionable deep myometrial invasion (*arrow*). (*B*) Fused sagittal T2WI–diffusion-weighted imaging and dynamic contrast-enhanced MR imaging (*C*) do not demonstrate deep myometrial invasion (*arrows*).

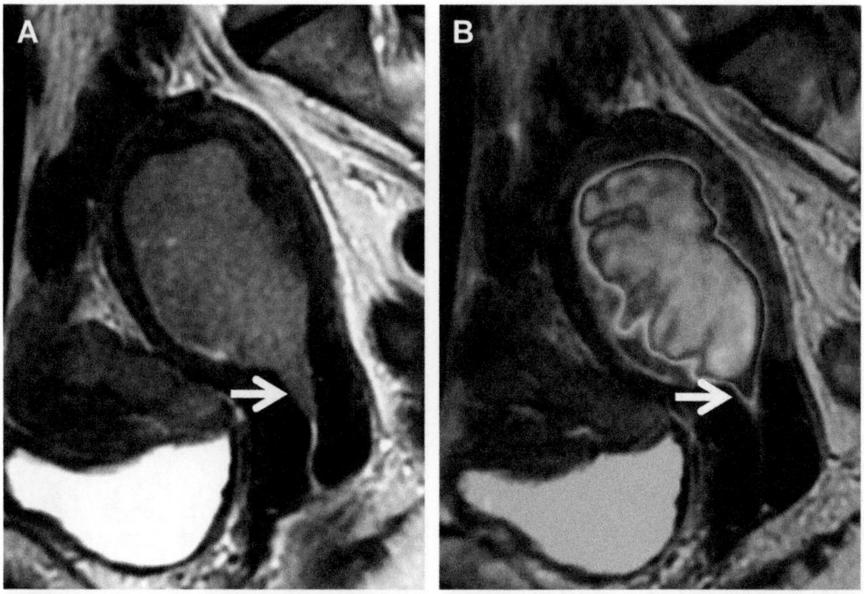

Fig. 8. Stage IA endometrial cancer distending the endometrial cavity. (*A*) Sagittal T2-weighted imaging (T2WI) and (*B*) fused sagittal T2WI-diffusion-weighted imaging show an endometrial tumor markedly distending the endometrial cavity and compressing the myometrium; however, no evidence of deep myometrial invasion is seen. Note the tumor extension within the internal os without extension to the cervical stroma (*arrows*).

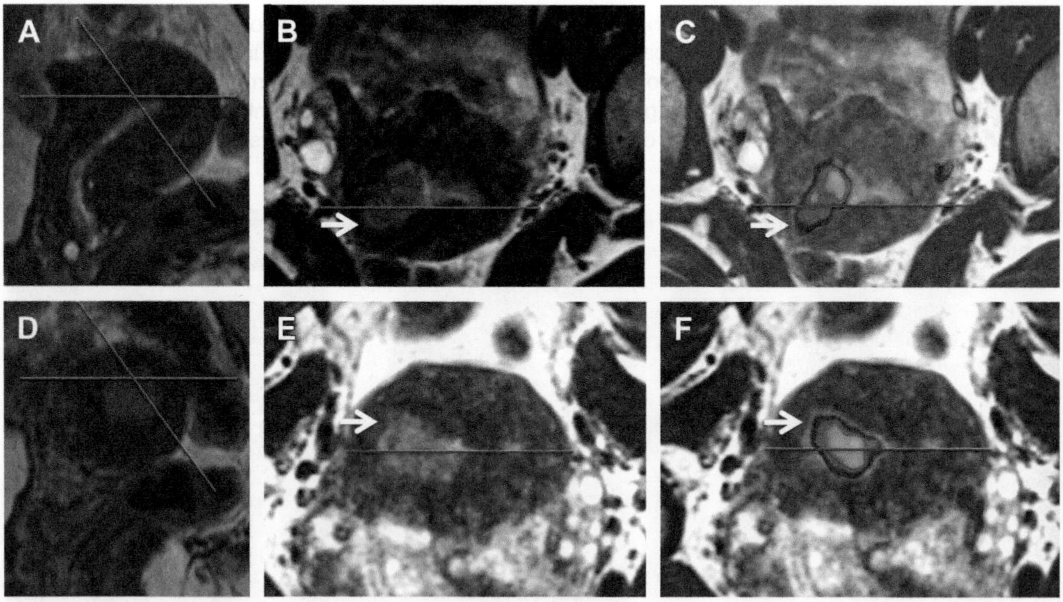

Fig. 9. Stage IA endometrial cancer at the level of the cornua, emphasizing the importance of correct selection of the imaging plane. (*A*) Sagittal T2-weighted imaging (T2WI) shows a retroverted uterus and an endometrial cavity distended by tumor at the level of the right cornua (*B*). The *purple line* on (*A*) and (*B*) corresponds to the standard axial plane displayed on axial T2WI (*C*) and fused axial T2WI diffusion-weighted imaging (DWI) (*D*). The *pink line* on (*A*) and (*B*) corresponds to axial oblique images perpendicular to the endometrial axis displayed on axial oblique T2WI (*E*) and axial oblique fused T2WI–DWI (*F*). On standard axial images (*C*) and (*D*) deep myometrial invasion is suspected (*arrow*); however, using the correct axis, as shown on (*E*) and (*F*), no deep myometrial invasion is seen. Uncorrected axis images resulted in tumor overstaging.

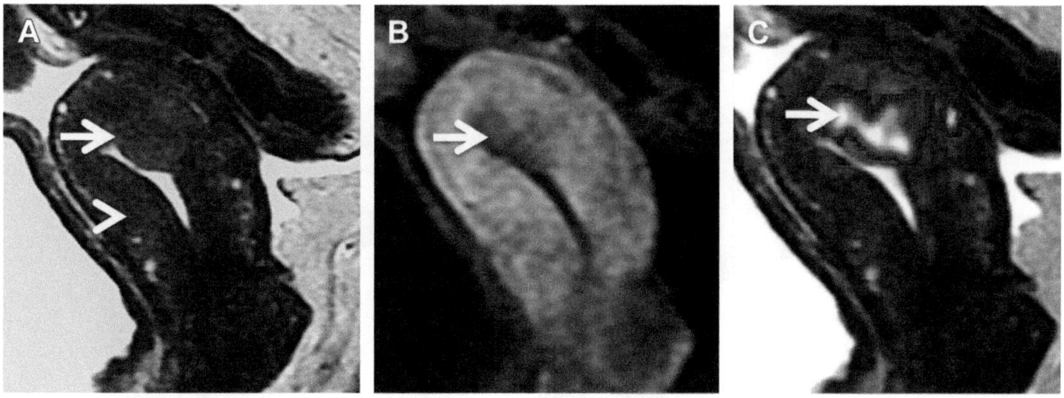

Fig. 10. Stage IB endometrial cancer with adenomyosis obscuring margins on T2-weighted imaging (T2WI). (*A*) Sagittal T2WI demonstrates a thick junctional zone (*arrowhead*) and a poorly delineated tumor to myometrium interface (*arrow*). The tumor extent is difficult to assess on T2WI. (*B*) Dynamic contrast-enhanced MR imaging demonstrates a vague ill-defined hypoenhancing area (*arrow*). (*C*) Fused T2WI–diffusion-weighted imaging (DWI) demonstrates deep myometrial invasion (*arrow*). DWI helps tumor staging in case of adenomyosis.

imaging[37] and DWI[38] have been shown to improve tumor delineation and increase accuracy of tumor staging in this setting.

What does the literature say regarding this?

In routine clinical practice, the combination of T2WI, DWI, and DCE MR imaging offers a "one-stop shop" imaging approach to assess deep myometrial invasion with a high accuracy.

The combination of DCE MR imaging and T2WI has been used traditionally in routine clinical practice to evaluate the depth of myometrial invasion. A metaanalysis including 11 articles and 548 patients demonstrated that DCE MR imaging has a higher specificity than T2WI to predict deep myometrial invasion (specificity DCE MR imaging, 72%; specificity T2WI, 58%; $P<.05$) but similar sensitivity (sensitivity DCE MR imaging, 81%; sensitivity T2WI, 87%; $P>.05$).[39] Because DCE MR imaging improves tumor delineation, it is particularly useful in postmenopausal patients when the T2 tumor signal intensity may be isointense to the normal myometrium. In young women, who want to preserve their fertility and may be treated nonoperatively, it is essential to rule out myometrial invasion. DCE MR imaging has shown an added value as a continuous subendometrial enhancement band almost completely excludes myometrial invasion.[40]

In recent years, multiple publications have demonstrated the added value of DWI for the evaluation of myometrial invasion.[31,38,41–47] As a result, DWI is now widely used as an adjunct to T2WI and DCE MR imaging in routine clinical practice.[13] It remains to be determined whether combined T2WI and DWI is superior to DCE MR. In a metaanalysis including 9 studies (442 patients) comparing the diagnostic accuracy of DCE MR imaging and DWI to predict deep myometrial invasion, the pooled sensitivities of DWI and DCE MR imaging were the same (0.86). Similarly, pooled specificities did not significantly differ ($P = .16$) between the 2 sequences (DWI = 0.86 and DCE MR imaging = 0.82). However, in a more recent metaanalysis including 15 studies and 849 patients, the specificity of T2WI plus DWI was superior to that of DCE MR imaging (specificity DCE MR imaging, 0.86; specificity T2WI + DWI, 0.947; $P = .0035$).[43] The potential superiority of DWI in assessing myometrial invasion might be explained by its increased accuracy in challenging cases, that is, in the presence of leiomyomas, adenomyosis, poor tumor-to-myometrium contrast, loss of the junctional zonal anatomy, and cornual tumor extension.[38]

Stage II

Stage II endometrial cancer is defined by the presence of cervical stromal invasion.

Why is it important to detect cervical stromal invasion?

Stages I and II display different prognoses. Cervical stroma invasion is associated with an higher risk of LVSI, which is directly correlated with the risk of lymph nodes metastases.

How to look for the presence of cervical stroma invasion on MR imaging?

Pearls

- Cervical stroma invasion is best depicted on sagittal and axial oblique T2WI.
- On T2WI, cervical stroma invasion is defined as the disruption of the normal low signal intensity of the cervical stroma by the intermediate tumor signal (**Fig. 11**).

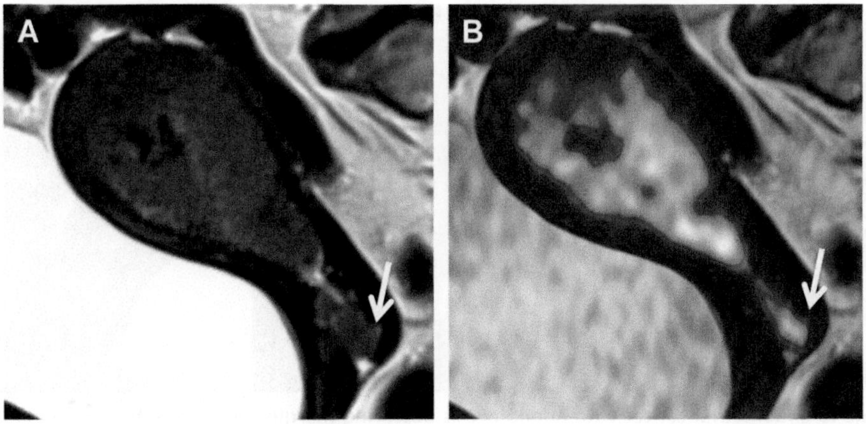

Fig. 11. Stage II tumor. (*A*) Sagittal T2-weighted imaging (T2WI) and (*B*) fused sagittal T2WI diffusion-weighted imaging demonstrate distention of the endometrial cavity by a tumor that extends into the cervix. Invasion of the cervical stroma is present (*arrows*).

- On DCE MR imaging, cervical stroma invasion is defined as an interruption of the normal enhancement of the cervical stroma.
- On DWI, the presence of high signal intensity on high b-value and lower signal intensity on ADC maps disrupting the cervical stroma suggest cervical stroma invasion.

Pitfalls

- A tumor protruding into the internal os does not always indicate cervical stroma invasion. Cervical stroma must be disrupted to diagnose invasion (**Fig. 12**).
- Cervical stromal invasion may be present without invasion of the endocervical mucosa because of adjacent contiguous myometrial invasion.
- Nabothian cysts in the cervix may result in focal high signal intensity on DWI because of the T2 shine-through effect. The lack of restriction on ADC map in case of Nabothian cysts enables differentiation from tumor extension within the cervix.

What does the literature say about MR imaging and cervical stromal invasion?

Several studies have suggested that DCE MR imaging is superior to T2WI in detecting cervical stromal invasion[48,49]; however, others have found a relative low sensitivity (33%–57%) but high specificity of DCE MR imaging (95%–97%) to identify cervical stromal invasion.[50,51]

Recently, DWI has been evaluated in cervical stromal invasion.[45,52] Lin and colleagues[51] demonstrated a higher diagnostic performance

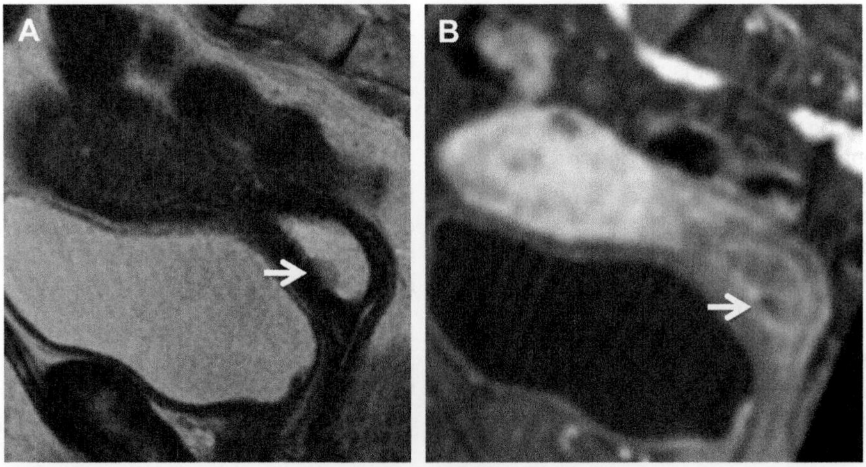

Fig. 12. Widening of the cervical canal. (*A*) Sagittal T2-weighted imaging shows widening of the cervical canal. The preservation of a normal hypointense cervical stroma interface with the tumor excludes stroma invasion (*arrow*). (*B*) Dynamic contrast-enhanced MR imaging delayed images (3 minutes) show smooth, linear enhancement of the cervical mucosa, excluding cervical stromal invasion (*arrow*).

of DWI compared with DCE MR imaging (DWI R1/R2 AUC values = 0.98/0.97; DCE MR imaging R1/R2 AUC values = 0.94/0.88). Interestingly, the authors pointed out that cervical canal widening was a cause of false negative on DCE MR imaging and T2WI but not on DWI.

Stage III

When should we look more carefully for stage III disease?

Type 2 tumors are associated with more advanced stages and, hence, higher rates of direct spread to the adnexa or vaginal metastases, a finding that can easily be missed if not assessed carefully.[53–56]

How should we look for stage III on MR imaging?

Stage IIIA Stage IIIA tumors invade the uterine serosa and appear as an area of intermediate to high signal intensity disrupting the normal smooth contour of the outer myometrium (**Fig. 13**). On DCE MR imaging, the loss of normal rim of enhancement of the outer myometrium indicates serosal involvement.

Direct spread to the adnexa (**Fig. 14**) or ovarian metastases are considered stage IIIA disease. In patients with endometrial cancer, care should be taken to exclude the presence of an ovarian mass. Indeed, synchronous primary ovarian carcinoma coexists with endometrial cancer in 5% to 8% of cases.[57,58] Although not always possible on imaging or pathologic analysis, it is important to distinguish synchronous primary ovarian cancer from endometrial cancer ovarian metastasis because they do not share the same prognosis.[58,59] In a recent study including 72 patients, the 10-year overall survival rates of patients with synchronous primary cancers of endometrium and ovary was 61.3%, significantly higher than the overall survival of the patient group with ovarian metastasis from endometrial cancer (36.6%; $P = .029$).[59]

Signs favoring synchronous ovarian and endometrial cancer on MR imaging (Fig. 15)

- Uterus: early stage endometrial cancer with minimal or no myometrial invasion.
- Ovary: unilateral, large mass in the background of endometriosis or borderline tumor.

Signs favoring ovarian metastasis from endometrial cancer on MR imaging (Fig. 16)

- Uterus: deep myometrial invasion and/or tubal invasion.
- Ovary: smaller mass, bilateral ovarian involvement.

Stage IIIB Stage IIIB tumors involve the vagina either by direct invasion or metastatic spread. DWI is particularly helpful to detect small cervical and vaginal implants.

Stage IIIC Stage IIIC disease is characterized by lymph node metastases, and is subdivided into pelvic (stage IIIC1) and paraaortic (stage IIIC2) nodal involvement. Risk factors for lymph nodes metastases include type 2 tumors, grade 3 tumors, LVSI, and deep myometrial invasion.[60,61]

The distribution of lymph node metastases is influenced by tumor location. The middle and lower parts of the uterus drain to the parametrium, and the paracervical and obturator nodes. The upper part of the uterus drains to common iliac and paraaortic lymph nodes. Inguinal nodes are not in the regional lymphatic drainage pathway for endometrial carcinoma and, if present, they signify stage IV disease.

What does the literature say about MR imaging and lymph node metastases?

Lymph node short axis size greater than 1 cm has been reported to be highly specific for lymph nodes metastases, albeit with a very poor

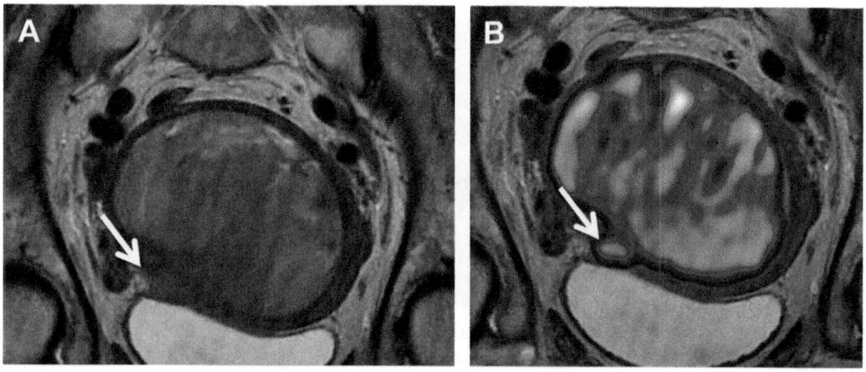

Fig. 13. Stage IIIA tumor. (*A*) Axial oblique T2-weighted imaging (T2WI) and (*B*) fused axial oblique T2WI-diffusion-weighted imaging show tumor extension beyond the uterine serosa (*arrows*).

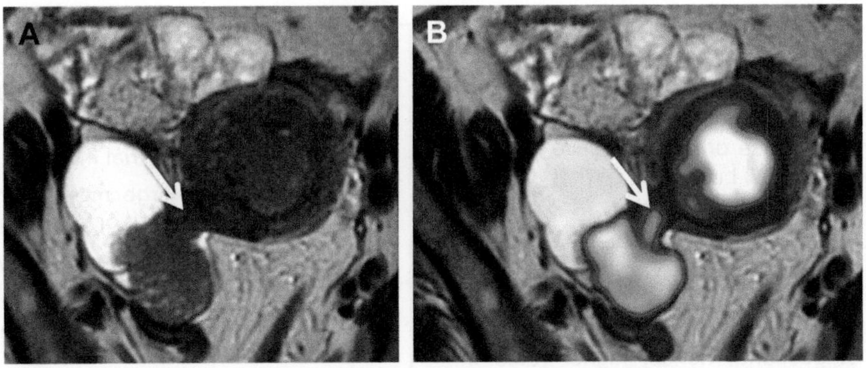

Fig. 14. Stage IIIA tumor. (*A*) Axial oblique T2-weighted imaging (T2WI) and (*B*) fused axial oblique T2WI-diffusion-weighted imaging (DWI) show direct tumor spread to the right adnexa (*arrows*). Note the added value of DWI, which helps to confirm the tumor's direct extension to the ovary.

sensitivity (range, 36%–89.5%).[62–64] In contradistinction to rectal cancer staging,[65] attempts to increase sensitivity using nodal shape and margins have not been successful.[64] Recently, DWI has been investigated in lymph node metastases,[66–70] because nodes can be detected easily on DWI.[69,70] However, to date, none of the studies were able to distinguish benign from malignant lymph nodes owing to an overlap in ADC values. Hope has been raised by the use of ultrasmall paramagnetic iron oxide particles. In a study including 768 lymph nodes where 335 were correlated with MR imaging, Rockall and colleagues[71] demonstrated an increase in sensitivity using ultrasmall paramagnetic iron oxide particles (reader 1, 93%; reader 2, 82%) compared with size criteria (29%). Unfortunately, ultrasmall paramagnetic iron oxide particles are not available commercially at present. Other alternatives are eagerly sought for improving lymph node staging with MR imaging. Extrauterine disease may be well-evaluated by PET imaging with fluorodeoxyglucose

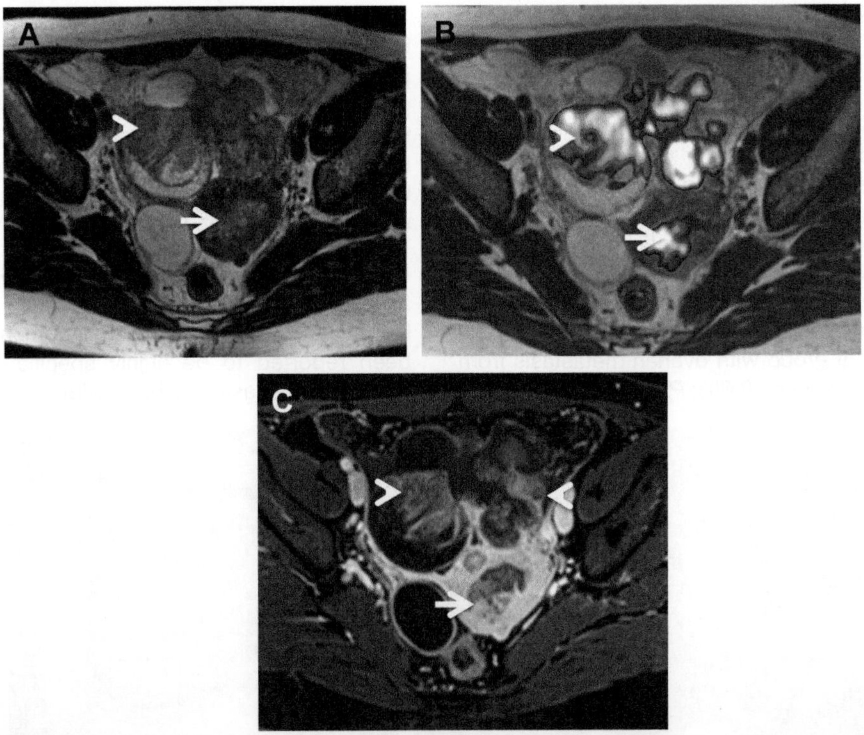

Fig. 15. Synchronous primary endometrioid endometrial and endometrioid ovarian carcinoma. (*A*) Axial oblique T2-weighted imaging (T2WI), (*B*) fused axial oblique T2WI and (*C*) dynamic contrast-enhanced MR imaging demonstrate an endometrial tumor (*arrows*) associated with a large left complex solid and cystic mass in keeping with a primary ovarian tumor (*arrowheads*).

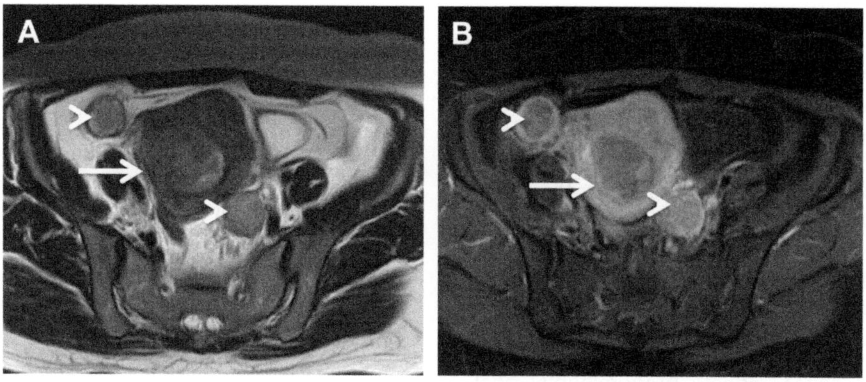

Fig. 16. Stage IIIA endometrial cancer with ovarian involvement: (*A*) Axial oblique T2-weighted imaging and (*B*) Dynamic contrast-enhanced MR imaging demonstrate 2 small hypointense (*A, arrowheads*) hypo enhancing (*B, arrowhead*) masses within the ovaries in keeping with metastases from a primary endometrial cancer (*arrows*).

F 18[72,73]; thus, the development of PET/MR imaging has the potential to improve endometrial cancer assessment.

Stage IV

Stage IV disease is defined as direct invasion of the bladder or rectal mucosa (stage IVA) or the presence of distant metastases (stage IVB).

Assessment of stage IVA on MR imaging

- Rectum or bladder wall invasion is best evaluated in the sagittal plane.
- Preservation of the fat plane between tumor and bladder or rectum exclude stage IVA. On T2WI, transmural tumor extension into the bladder or rectum must be seen to indicate bladder or rectal invasion. In inconclusive cases, cystoscopy or rectosigmoidoscopy is indicated. The presence of bladder mucosal edema is not indicative of mucosal invasion (**Fig. 17**).

Assessment of stage IVB on MR imaging

In stage IVB disease, distant metastases, including suprarenal paraaortic lymphadenopathy

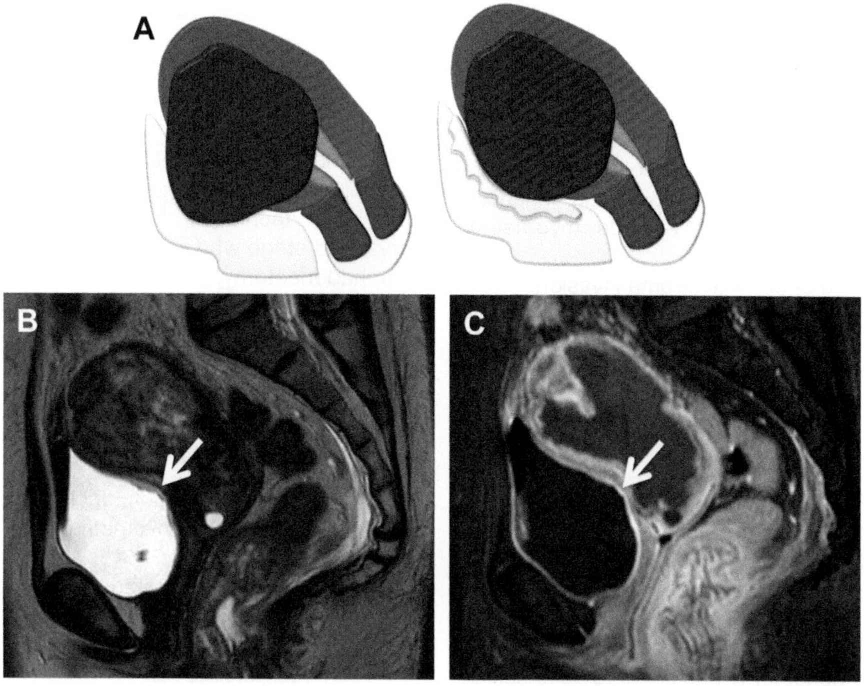

Fig. 17. (*A*) Bladder involvement. Submucosal bullous edema is not equivalent to bladder invasion; tumor must be seen within the bladder to suggest bladder invasion. (*B*) Sagittal T2-weighted imaging shows a large endometrial mass associated with bullous edema of the bladder (*arrow*). (*C*) On dynamic contrast-enhanced MR imaging, no intraluminal extension within the bladder is seen (*arrow*).

and inguinal lymph node metastases, are seen.[54] Malignant ascites and peritoneal implants are more common with type 2 endometrial tumors. DWI can help to detect small serosal/peritoneal deposits, which otherwise may be easily missed on T2WI.[74] Pelvic wall invasion should be suspected when the distance between the tumor and the pelvic wall is less than 3 mm.

MR IMAGING CANCER PROGNOSTICATION AND MANAGEMENT

Conservative, Fertility-Sparing Management

Endometrial cancer affects predominantly postmenopausal women, but 15% to 25% of patients are diagnosed before menopause.[1] The use of progestogen may be an alternative for women who want to preserve their fertility and have low-grade disease limited to the endometrium. Response evaluation is performed at 6 to 9 months with repeat dilatation and curettage and imaging. The response rate to conservative management is 75%, but the rate of recurrence is high at 30% to 40%. After completion of family, surgery is advised owing to the high risk of recurrence.

Eligibility criteria for fertility-sparing treatment

- Patients must have a well-differentiated (FIGO grade 1) endometrioid adenocarcinoma proven on dilatation and curettage, as this approach is more accurate than pipelle biopsy.
- MR imaging assessment should demonstrate
  - No myometrial invasion: Presence of both intact low signal intensity junctional zone on T2WI and smooth continuous band of early subendometrial enhancement are useful to exclude myometrial invasion.[40]
  - Absence of cervical stroma invasion.
  - Absence of metastases to the ovary or synchronous primary ovarian neoplasm.
  - Absence of nodal metastasis.

Surgical Treatment of Early Stage Disease: Stage I Endometrial Cancer

The standard therapy for endometrial cancer includes total hysterectomy and bilateral salpingo-oophorectomy with peritoneal washings and pelvic plus paraaortic lymph node dissection. However, performing systematic lymphadenectomy in all patients remains controversial. Lymphadenectomy has a 7% to 10% risk of lymphocele and increases anesthesia and operative time.[75] In addition, lymphadenectomy has a 23% risk of lower extremity lymphedema.[76] Two large clinical trials showed no survival benefit of lymph node dissection in patients with FIGO grade 1 or 2 stage IA endometrial cancer. In the ASTEC trial (Adjuvant External Beam Radiotherapy in the Treatment of Endometrial Cancer) including 1408 women with malignancies confined to the uterus, there was no difference in overall survival or recurrence-free survival in patients without or with pelvic lymphadenectomy.[9] The SEPAL study (Survival Effect of Para-aortic Lymphadenectomy in Endometrial Cancer) compared systematic pelvic lymphadenectomy with systematic pelvic and paraaortic lymphadenectomy and suggested that only high-risk patients may benefit from aggressive surgery.[77] A Cochrane metaanalysis based on 2 randomized clinical trials, the ASTEC trial[9] and the PACINI trial,[78] including 1945 patients, showed no evidence that lymphadenectomy decreases risk of death or disease recurrence compared with no lymphadenectomy in women with early stage disease.[8] Therefore, some surgical groups propose sentinel lymph node mapping before lymphadenectomy to select patients who would benefit from lymph nodes dissection.[79–84] The role of sentinel lymph node mapping is currently being evaluated, but has already been included in the National Comprehensive Cancer Network guidelines for uterine cancer.[85] The National Comprehensive Cancer Network guidelines recommend sentinel lymph node mapping for the surgical staging of "apparent uterine-confined malignancy when there is no metastasis demonstrated by imaging studies or no obvious extrauterine disease at exploration." Therefore, MR imaging plays a critical role in distinguish patient who may benefit from this technique from those with more advanced stage who should undergo systematic lymphadenectomy.

In the meantime, risk stratification algorithms that aggregate multiple prognostic factors of recurrence risk have been evaluated.[8,86–89] In this regard, European Society for Medical Oncology guidelines propose to subdivide stage I cancer into risk categories[6,90]:

- Low risk: stage I endometrioid, grades 1 and 2, less than 50% myometrial invasion, LVSI negative.
- Intermediate risk: stage I endometrioid, grades 1 and 2, 50% or greater myometrial invasion, LVSI negative.
- High-intermediate risk
  1. Stage I endometrioid, grade 3, less than 50% myometrial invasion, regardless of LVSI status.

  2. Stage I endometrioid, grades 1 and 2, LVSI positive, regardless of depth of myometrial invasion.
- High risk
  1. Stage I endometrioid, grade 3, 50% or greater myometrial invasion, regardless of LVSI status
  2. Stage II
  3. Stage III, no residual disease
  4. Nonendometrioid (serous, clear cell, or undifferentiated carcinoma or carcinosarcoma)

The European Society for Medical Oncology guidelines do not recommend lymphadenectomy in the low-risk group.[6,90] Consequently, preoperative information about depth of myometrial invasion and histologic grade are essential to tailor the surgical approach for these patients.

As described, MR imaging can accurately predict the depth of myometrial invasion, whereas histologic grade can be determined with endometrial sampling. However, the histologic grade and subtype of endometrial carcinoma from biopsy are subject to sampling error.[91–93] Multiple studies have tried to evaluate the potential role of DWI in predicting tumor grade, but the results are inconclusive.[31,32,34,35,47,94–98] Several studies have demonstrated an association between low ADC values and high-grade tumor,[34,47,95,98] although others did not find the difference.[31,32] Indeed, there is considerable overlap between ADC values, which limits a precise estimation of histologic grade based on ADC values alone. Recently, Fukunaga and colleagues,[99] demonstrated the role of DCE MR imaging in predicting tumor histology. In a relative large cohort of 77 patients, the investigators demonstrated that type 2 tumors were associated with a higher maximum signal intensity and wash in rate compared with type 1 tumors.

Surgical Treatment: Stage II

Stage II cancer necessitates hysterectomy, bilateral salpingo-oophorectomy, and lymphadenectomy. Radical hysterectomy is not generally recommended, but should be considered in cases of obvious involvement of the parametria. Preoperative MR imaging evaluation enables accurate evaluation of the cervical stroma and parametria and helps to guide surgical management.

Surgical Treatment: Stage III and Up

Maximal surgical debulking is imperative in patients with stage III and IV endometrial cancer. In this setting, MR imaging can map the locations of peritoneal tumor implants especially using DWI and detect invasion of the bladder and rectum.

SUMMARY

As we enter the era of personalized medicine with therapies stratified according to the risk of local and distant recurrence, imaging has become an essential tool in preoperative decision making, to avoid both undertreatment and overtreatment. Although highly accurate in the assessment of myometrial invasion, MR imaging has not yet been widely accepted by gynecologists, despite the trend toward minimally invasive surgery for the low-risk patient. For now, MR imaging enables patient risk stratification by helping the surgeon to better identify those women who will most likely benefit from thorough lymphadenectomy and who should be referred to a dedicated oncology center. However, the upcoming challenge of MR imaging will be to better evaluate nodal involvement; the introduction of PET/MR imaging in the clinical arena is likely to contribute to this critical challenge. Ongoing development of dedicated molecular probes is likely to make PET/MR imaging a very important tool in the preoperative staging and surveillance of patients with endometrial cancer.

ACKNOWLEDGMENTS

We thanks Dr Nougaret who performed all the drawing.

REFERENCES

1. Siegel RL, Miller KD, Jemal A. Cancer statistics, 2016. CA Cancer J Clin 2016;66(1):7–30.
2. Chen X, Xiang YB, Long JR, et al. Genetic polymorphisms in obesity-related genes and endometrial cancer risk. Cancer 2012;118(13):3356–64.
3. Cramer DW. The epidemiology of endometrial and ovarian cancer. Hematol Oncol Clin North Am 2012;26(1):1–12.
4. Pecorelli S. Revised FIGO staging for carcinoma of the vulva, cervix, and endometrium. Int J Gynaecol Obstet 2009;105(2):103–4.
5. Colombo N, Creutzberg C, Amant F, et al. ESMO-ESGO-ESTRO consensus conference on endometrial cancer: diagnosis, treatment and follow-up. Radiother Oncol 2015;117(3):559–81.
6. Colombo N, Preti E, Landoni F, et al. Endometrial cancer: ESMO clinical practice Guidelines for diagnosis, treatment and follow-up. Ann Oncol 2013;24(Suppl 6):vi33–8.
7. Wright JD, Huang Y, Burke WM, et al. Influence of Lymphadenectomy on Survival for Early-Stage Endometrial Cancer. Obstet Gynecol 2016;127(1):109–18.
8. Frost JA, Webster KE, Bryant A, et al. Lymphadenectomy for the management of endometrial cancer. Cochrane Database Syst Rev 2015;(9):CD007585.

9. ASCET study group, Kitchener H, Swart AM, Qian Q, et al. Efficacy of systematic pelvic lymphadenectomy in endometrial cancer (MRC ASTEC trial): a randomised study. Lancet 2009;373(9658):125–36.
10. Kinkel K, Forstner R, Danza FM, et al. Staging of endometrial cancer with MRI: guidelines of the European Society of Urogenital Imaging. Eur Radiol 2009;19(7):1565–74.
11. Ben-Shachar I, Vitellas KM, Cohn DE. The role of MRI in the conservative management of endometrial cancer. Gynecol Oncol 2004;93(1):233–7.
12. Lalwani N, Dubinsky T, Javitt MC, et al. ACR appropriateness criteria(R) pretreatment evaluation and follow-up of endometrial cancer. Ultrasound Q 2014;30(1):21–8.
13. Sala E, Rockall AG, Freeman SJ, et al. The added role of MR imaging in treatment stratification of patients with gynecologic malignancies: what the radiologist needs to know. Radiology 2013;266(3): 717–40.
14. Sheikh MA, Althouse AD, Freese KE, et al. USA endometrial cancer projections to 2030: should we be concerned? Future Oncol 2014;10(16): 2561–8.
15. Crosbie EJ, Zwahlen M, Kitchener HC, et al. Body mass index, hormone replacement therapy, and endometrial cancer risk: a meta-analysis. Cancer Epidemiol Biomarkers Prev 2010;19(12):3119–30.
16. Reeves KW, Carter GC, Rodabough RJ, et al. Obesity in relation to endometrial cancer risk and disease characteristics in the Women's Health Initiative. Gynecol Oncol 2011;121(2):376–82.
17. Painter JN, O'Mara TA, Marquart L, et al. Genetic risk score Mendelian randomization shows that obesity measured as body mass index, but not waist:hip ratio, is causal for endometrial cancer. Cancer Epidemiol Biomarkers Prev 2016;25(11): 1503–10.
18. Luo J, Beresford S, Chen C, et al. Association between diabetes, diabetes treatment and risk of developing endometrial cancer. Br J Cancer 2014; 111(7):1432–9.
19. Zhang ZH, Su PY, Hao JH, et al. The role of preexisting diabetes mellitus on incidence and mortality of endometrial cancer: a meta-analysis of prospective cohort studies. Int J Gynecol Cancer 2013;23(2): 294–303.
20. Barry JA, Azizia MM, Hardiman PJ. Risk of endometrial, ovarian and breast cancer in women with polycystic ovary syndrome: a systematic review and meta-analysis. Hum Reprod Update 2014;20(5): 748–58.
21. Allen NE, Tsilidis KK, Key TJ, et al. Menopausal hormone therapy and risk of endometrial carcinoma among postmenopausal women in the European Prospective Investigation Into Cancer and Nutrition. Am J Epidemiol 2010;172(12):1394–403.
22. Karageorgi S, Hankinson SE, Kraft P, et al. Reproductive factors and postmenopausal hormone use in relation to endometrial cancer risk in the Nurses' Health Study cohort 1976-2004. Int J Cancer 2010; 126(1):208–16.
23. Lynch HT, Snyder CL, Shaw TG, et al. Milestones of Lynch syndrome: 1895-2015. Nat Rev Cancer 2015; 15(3):181–94.
24. Smith-Bindman R, Kerlikowske K, Feldstein VA, et al. Endovaginal ultrasound to exclude endometrial cancer and other endometrial abnormalities. JAMA 1998;280(17):1510–7.
25. Timmermans A, Opmeer BC, Khan KS, et al. Endometrial thickness measurement for detecting endometrial cancer in women with postmenopausal bleeding: a systematic review and meta-analysis. Obstet Gynecol 2010;116(1):160–7.
26. Rauch GM, Kaur H, Choi H, et al. Optimization of MR imaging for pretreatment evaluation of patients with endometrial and cervical cancer. Radiographics 2014;34(4):1082–98.
27. Feng Z, Min X, Sah VK, et al. Comparison of field-of-view (FOV) optimized and constrained undistorted single shot (FOCUS) with conventional DWI for the evaluation of prostate cancer. Clin Imaging 2015; 39(5):851–5.
28. Bhosale P, Ma J, Iyer R, et al. Feasibility of a reduced field-of-view diffusion-weighted (rFOV) sequence in assessment of myometrial invasion in patients with clinical FIGO stage I endometrial cancer. J Magn Reson Imaging 2016;43(2):316–24.
29. Park SB, Moon MH, Sung CK, et al. Dynamic contrast-enhanced MR imaging of endometrial cancer: optimizing the imaging delay for tumour-myometrium contrast. Eur Radiol 2014;24(11): 2795–9.
30. Takeuchi M, Matsuzaki K, Nishitani H. Diffusion-weighted magnetic resonance imaging of endometrial cancer: differentiation from benign endometrial lesions and preoperative assessment of myometrial invasion. Acta Radiol 2009;50(8):947–53.
31. Rechichi G, Galimberti S, Signorelli M, et al. Endometrial cancer: correlation of apparent diffusion coefficient with tumor grade, depth of myometrial invasion, and presence of lymph node metastases. AJR Am J Roentgenol 2011;197(1):256–62.
32. Bharwani N, Miquel ME, Sahdev A, et al. Diffusion-weighted imaging in the assessment of tumour grade in endometrial cancer. Br J Radiol 2011; 84(1007):997–1004.
33. Inada Y, Matsuki M, Nakai G, et al. Body diffusion-weighted MR imaging of uterine endometrial cancer: is it helpful in the detection of cancer in nonenhanced MR imaging? Eur J Radiol 2009;70(1):122–7.
34. Tamai K, Koyama T, Saga T, et al. Diffusion-weighted MR imaging of uterine endometrial cancer. J Magn Reson Imaging 2007;26(3):682–7.

35. Fujii S, Matsusue E, Kigawa J, et al. Diagnostic accuracy of the apparent diffusion coefficient in differentiating benign from malignant uterine endometrial cavity lesions: initial results. Eur Radiol 2008;18(2): 384–9.
36. Kilickesmez O, Bayramoglu S, Inci E, et al. Quantitative diffusion-weighted magnetic resonance imaging of normal and diseased uterine zones. Acta Radiol 2009;50(3):340–7.
37. Utsunomiya D, Notsute S, Hayashida Y, et al. Endometrial carcinoma in adenomyosis: assessment of myometrial invasion on T2-weighted spin-echo and gadolinium-enhanced T1-weighted images. AJR Am J Roentgenol 2004;182(2): 399–404.
38. Beddy P, Moyle P, Kataoka M, et al. Evaluation of depth of myometrial invasion and overall staging in endometrial cancer: comparison of diffusion-weighted and dynamic contrast-enhanced MR imaging. Radiology 2012;262(2):530–7.
39. Wu LM, Xu JR, Gu HY, et al. Predictive value of T2-weighted imaging and contrast-enhanced MR imaging in assessing myometrial invasion in endometrial cancer: a pooled analysis of prospective studies. Eur Radiol 2013;23(2):435–49.
40. Fujii S, Kido A, Baba T, et al. Subendometrial enhancement and peritumoral enhancement for assessing endometrial cancer on dynamic contrast enhanced MR imaging. Eur J Radiol 2015;84(4): 581–9.
41. An Q, Ynag J, Zhu Y. Diffusion weighted imaging and contrast-enhanced magnetic resonance imaging in the evaluation of early stage endometrial cancer. Zhongguo Yi Xue Ke Xue Yuan Xue Bao 2012; 34(5):486–91.
42. Andreano A, Rechichi G, Rebora P, et al. MR diffusion imaging for preoperative staging of myometrial invasion in patients with endometrial cancer: a systematic review and meta-analysis. Eur Radiol 2014; 24(6):1327–38.
43. Deng L, Wang QP, Chen X, et al. The combination of diffusion- and t2-weighted imaging in predicting deep myometrial invasion of endometrial cancer: a systematic review and meta-analysis. J Comput Assist Tomogr 2015;39(5):661–73.
44. Gallego JC, Porta A, Pardo MC, et al. Evaluation of myometrial invasion in endometrial cancer: comparison of diffusion-weighted magnetic resonance and intraoperative frozen sections. Abdom Imaging 2014;39(5):1021–6.
45. Hori M, Kim T, Onishi H, et al. Endometrial cancer: preoperative staging using three-dimensional T2-weighted turbo spin-echo and diffusion-weighted MR imaging at 3.0 T: a prospective comparative study. Eur Radiol 2013;23(8):2296–305.
46. Lin G, Ng KK, Chang CJ, et al. Myometrial invasion in endometrial cancer: diagnostic accuracy of diffusion-weighted 3.0-T MR imaging–initial experience. Radiology 2009;250(3):784–92.
47. Nougaret S, Reinhold C, Alsharif SS, et al. Endometrial cancer: combined MR volumetry and diffusion-weighted imaging for assessment of myometrial and lymphovascular invasion and tumor grade. Radiology 2015;276(3):797–808.
48. Manfredi R, Mirk P, Maresca G, et al. Local-regional staging of endometrial carcinoma: role of MR imaging in surgical planning. Radiology 2004;231(2): 372–8.
49. Seki H, Takano T, Sakai K. Value of dynamic MR imaging in assessing endometrial carcinoma involvement of the cervix. AJR Am J Roentgenol 2000; 175(1):171–6.
50. Luomaranta A, Leminen A, Loukovaara M. Magnetic resonance imaging in the assessment of high-risk features of endometrial carcinoma: a meta-analysis. Int J Gynecol Cancer 2015;25(5):837–42.
51. Lin G, Huang YT, Chao A, et al. Endometrial cancer with cervical stromal invasion: diagnostic accuracy of diffusion-weighted and dynamic contrast enhanced MR imaging at 3T. Eur Radiol 2017; 27(5):1867–76.
52. Koplay M, Dogan NU, Erdogan H, et al. Diagnostic efficacy of diffusion-weighted MRI for pre-operative assessment of myometrial and cervical invasion and pelvic lymph node metastasis in endometrial carcinoma. J Med Imaging Radiat Oncol 2014; 58(5):538–46 [quiz: 648].
53. Hendrickson M, Ross J, Eifel P, et al. Uterine papillary serous carcinoma: a highly malignant form of endometrial adenocarcinoma. Am J Surg Pathol 1982;6(2):93–108.
54. Bancher-Todesca D, Gitsch G, Williams KE, et al. p53 protein overexpression: a strong prognostic factor in uterine papillary serous carcinoma. Gynecol Oncol 1998;71(1):59–63.
55. Boruta DM 2nd, Gehrig PA, Fader AN, et al. Management of women with uterine papillary serous cancer: a Society of Gynecologic Oncology (SGO) review. Gynecol Oncol 2009;115(1):142–53.
56. Growdon WB, Rauh-Hain JJ, Cordon A, et al. Prognostic determinants in patients with stage I uterine papillary serous carcinoma: a 15-year multi-institutional review. Int J Gynecol Cancer 2012; 22(3):417–24.
57. AlHilli MM, Dowdy SC, Weaver AL, et al. Incidence and factors associated with synchronous ovarian and endometrial cancer: a population-based case-control study. Gynecol Oncol 2012;125(1):109–13.
58. Soliman PT, Slomovitz BM, Broaddus RR, et al. Synchronous primary cancers of the endometrium and ovary: a single institution review of 84 cases. Gynecol Oncol 2004;94(2):456–62.
59. Bese T, Sal V, Kahramanoglu I, et al. Synchronous Primary cancers of the endometrium and ovary

with the same histopathologic type versus endometrial cancer with ovarian metastasis: a single institution review of 72 cases. Int J Gynecol Cancer 2016; 26(2):394–406.
60. Aalders JG, Thomas G. Endometrial cancer–revisiting the importance of pelvic and para aortic lymph nodes. Gynecol Oncol 2007;104(1):222–31.
61. Muallem MZ, Sehouli J, Almuheimid J, et al. Risk factors of lymph nodes metastases by endometrial cancer: a retrospective one-center study. Anticancer Res 2016;36(8):4219–25.
62. Kim SH, Kim SC, Choi BI, et al. Uterine cervical carcinoma: evaluation of pelvic lymph node metastasis with MR imaging. Radiology 1994;190(3):807–11.
63. Yang WT, Lam WW, Yu MY, et al. Comparison of dynamic helical CT and dynamic MR imaging in the evaluation of pelvic lymph nodes in cervical carcinoma. AJR Am J Roentgenol 2000;175(3):759–66.
64. Choi HJ, Kim SH, Seo SS, et al. MRI for pretreatment lymph node staging in uterine cervical cancer. AJR Am J Roentgenol 2006;187(5):W538–43.
65. Brown G, Richards CJ, Bourne MW, et al. Morphologic predictors of lymph node status in rectal cancer with use of high-spatial-resolution MR imaging with histopathologic comparison. Radiology 2003; 227(2):371–7.
66. Shen G, Zhou H, Jia Z, et al. Diagnostic performance of diffusion-weighted MRI for detection of pelvic metastatic lymph nodes in patients with cervical cancer: a systematic review and meta-analysis. Br J Radiol 2015;88(1052):20150063.
67. Cerny M, Dunet V, Prior JO, et al. Initial staging of locally advanced rectal cancer and regional lymph nodes: comparison of diffusion-weighted MRI With 18F-FDG-PET/CT. Clin Nucl Med 2016;41(4): 289–95.
68. Eiber M, Beer AJ, Holzapfel K, et al. Preliminary results for characterization of pelvic lymph nodes in patients with prostate cancer by diffusion-weighted MR-imaging. Invest Radiol 2010;45(1): 15–23.
69. Heijnen LA, Lambregts DM, Mondal D, et al. Diffusion-weighted MR imaging in primary rectal cancer staging demonstrates but does not characterise lymph nodes. Eur Radiol 2013;23(12):3354–60.
70. Thoeny HC, Froehlich JM, Triantafyllou M, et al. Metastases in normal-sized pelvic lymph nodes: detection with diffusion-weighted MR imaging. Radiology 2014;273(1):125–35.
71. Rockall AG, Sohaib SA, Harisinghani MG, et al. Diagnostic performance of nanoparticle-enhanced magnetic resonance imaging in the diagnosis of lymph node metastases in patients with endometrial and cervical cancer. J Clin Oncol 2005;23(12): 2813–21.
72. Chang MC, Chen JH, Liang JA, et al. 18F-FDG PET or PET/CT for detection of metastatic lymph nodes in patients with endometrial cancer: a systematic review and meta-analysis. Eur J Radiol 2012;81(11): 3511–7.
73. Chung HH, Cheon GJ, Kim HS, et al. Preoperative PET/CT standardized FDG uptake values of pelvic lymph nodes as a significant prognostic factor in patients with endometrial cancer. Eur J Nucl Med Mol Imaging 2014;41(9):1793–9.
74. Fehniger J, Thomas S, Lengyel E, et al. A prospective study evaluating diffusion weighted magnetic resonance imaging (DW-MRI) in the detection of peritoneal carcinomatosis in suspected gynecologic malignancies. Gynecol Oncol 2016; 142(1):169–75.
75. Ghezzi F, Uccella S, Cromi A, et al. Lymphoceles, lymphorrhea, and lymphedema after laparoscopic and open endometrial cancer staging. Ann Surg Oncol 2012;19(1):259–67.
76. Yost KJ, Cheville AL, Al-Hilli MM, et al. Lymphedema after surgery for endometrial cancer: prevalence, risk factors, and quality of life. Obstet Gynecol 2014;124(2 Pt 1):307–15.
77. Todo Y, Kato H, Kaneuchi M, et al. Survival effect of para-aortic lymphadenectomy in endometrial cancer (SEPAL study): a retrospective cohort analysis. Lancet 2010;375(9721):1165–72.
78. Benedetti Panici P, Basile S, Maneschi F, et al. Systematic pelvic lymphadenectomy vs. no lymphadenectomy in early-stage endometrial carcinoma: randomized clinical trial. J Natl Cancer Inst 2008; 100(23):1707–16.
79. Ferraioli D, Chopin N, Beurrier F, et al. The incidence and clinical significance of the micrometastases in the sentinel lymph nodes during surgical staging for early endometrial cancer. Int J Gynecol Cancer 2015;25(4):673–80.
80. Rossi EC, Jackson A, Ivanova A, et al. Detection of sentinel nodes for endometrial cancer with robotic assisted fluorescence imaging: cervical versus hysteroscopic injection. Int J Gynecol Cancer 2013; 23(9):1704–11.
81. Holloway RW, Bravo RA, Rakowski JA, et al. Detection of sentinel lymph nodes in patients with endometrial cancer undergoing robotic-assisted staging: a comparison of colorimetric and fluorescence imaging. Gynecol Oncol 2012; 126(1):25–9.
82. Barlin JN, Khoury-Collado F, Kim CH, et al. The importance of applying a sentinel lymph node mapping algorithm in endometrial cancer staging: beyond removal of blue nodes. Gynecol Oncol 2012;125(3):531–5.
83. Khoury-Collado F, Murray MP, Hensley ML, et al. Sentinel lymph node mapping for endometrial cancer improves the detection of metastatic disease to regional lymph nodes. Gynecol Oncol 2011;122(2): 251–4.

84. Frimer M, Khoury-Collado F, Murray MP, et al. Micrometastasis of endometrial cancer to sentinel lymph nodes: is it an artifact of uterine manipulation? Gynecol Oncol 2010;119(3):496–9.
85. Koh WJ, Greer BE, Abu-Rustum NR, et al. Uterine neoplasms, version 1.2014. J Natl Compr Canc Netw 2014;12(2):248–80.
86. Imai K, Kato H, Katayama K, et al. A preoperative risk-scoring system to predict lymph node metastasis in endometrial cancer and stratify patients for lymphadenectomy. Gynecol Oncol 2016;142(2):273–7.
87. Holloway RW, Gupta S, Stavitzski NM, et al. Sentinel lymph node mapping with staging lymphadenectomy for patients with endometrial cancer increases the detection of metastasis. Gynecol Oncol 2016; 141(2):206–10.
88. Sadowski EA, Robbins JB, Guite K, et al. Preoperative pelvic MRI and serum cancer antigen-125: selecting women with grade 1 endometrial cancer for lymphadenectomy. AJR Am J Roentgenol 2015; 205(5):W556–64.
89. Todo Y, Watari H, Kang S, et al. Tailoring lymphadenectomy according to the risk of lymph node metastasis in endometrial cancer. J Obstet Gynaecol Res 2014;40(2):317–21.
90. Colombo N, Creutzberg C, Amant F, et al. ESMO-ESGO-ESTRO consensus conference on endometrial cancer: diagnosis, treatment and follow-up. Ann Oncol 2016;27(1):16–41.
91. Batista TP, Cavalcanti CL, Tejo AA, et al. Accuracy of preoperative endometrial sampling diagnosis for predicting the final pathology grading in uterine endometrioid carcinoma. Eur J Surg Oncol 2016;42(9): 1367–71.
92. Williams AR, Brechin S, Porter AJ, et al. Factors affecting adequacy of Pipelle and Tao Brush endometrial sampling. BJOG 2008;115(8):1028–36.
93. Dijkhuizen FP, Mol BW, Brolmann HA, et al. The accuracy of endometrial sampling in the diagnosis of patients with endometrial carcinoma and hyperplasia: a meta-analysis. Cancer 2000;89(8):1765–72.
94. Kishimoto K, Tajima S, Maeda I, et al. Endometrial cancer: correlation of apparent diffusion coefficient (ADC) with tumor cellularity and tumor grade. Acta Radiol 2016;57(8):1021–8.
95. Woo S, Cho JY, Kim SY, et al. Histogram analysis of apparent diffusion coefficient map of diffusion-weighted MRI in endometrial cancer: a preliminary correlation study with histological grade. Acta Radiol 2014;55(10):1270–7.
96. Takahashi M, Kozawa E, Tanisaka M, et al. Utility of histogram analysis of apparent diffusion coefficient maps obtained using 3.0T MRI for distinguishing uterine carcinosarcoma from endometrial carcinoma. J Magn Reson Imaging 2016;43(6):1301–7.
97. Mainenti PP, Pizzuti LM, Segreto S, et al. Diffusion volume (DV) measurement in endometrial and cervical cancer: a new MRI parameter in the evaluation of the tumor grading and the risk classification. Eur J Radiol 2016;85(1):113–24.
98. Inoue C, Fujii S, Kaneda S, et al. Apparent diffusion coefficient (ADC) measurement in endometrial carcinoma: effect of region of interest methods on ADC values. J Magn Reson Imaging 2014;40(1):157–61.
99. Fukunaga T, Fujii S, Inoue C, et al. Accuracy of semiquantitative dynamic contrast-enhanced MRI for differentiating type II from type I endometrial carcinoma. J Magn Reson Imaging 2015;41(6):1662–8.

MR Imaging of Cervical Cancer

Krupa Patel-Lippmann, MD[a], Jessica B. Robbins, MD[b], Lisa Barroilhet, MD[c], Bethany Anderson, MD[d], Elizabeth A. Sadowski, MD[b,c,*], James Boyum, MD[e]

KEYWORDS

• Cervical cancer • MR imaging • PET/CT • Staging • FIGO

KEY POINTS

- Cervical cancer is the second most frequent cause of cancer-related death for women worldwide.
- Cervical cancer is clinically staged using the International Federation of Gynecology and Obstetrics (FIGO) classification system, which suffers from poor accuracy in higher-stage disease.
- It is now well established that pretreatment imaging with MR imaging and PET/computed tomography (CT) improves patient outcomes.
- MR imaging is highly accurate for staging cervical cancer that is stage IB or greater, and FIGO supports the use of MR imaging in conjunction with PET/CT to increase the accuracy of staging, in areas where it is available.

INTRODUCTION

Cervical cancer is the third most common cancer in women worldwide and accounts for more than 300,000 deaths annually.[1] Eighty-five percent of cervical carcinomas are the squamous cell subtype, with adenocarcinoma, adenosquamous carcinoma, and undifferentiated carcinoma constituting the remaining 15%. Most cervical cancers are caused by the sexually transmitted human papillomavirus (HPV), with greater than 70% cancers associated with high-risk subtypes HPV-16 and HPV-18.[1] Increased compliance with screening Pap smears for the detection of precancerous lesions, as well as the recent US Food and Drug Administration approval of HPV prevention vaccines, have drastically decreased the rate of cervical cancer in the United States and other developed regions of the world.[2–4] Despite a marked decrease in the incidence of cervical cancer, those women who develop the disease have nearly a 40% chance of dying from their disease and cervical cancer remains the number 1 cause of cancer-related death in women younger than 35 years of age.[3–7] MR imaging plays a significant role in guiding the primary treatment in women diagnosed with cervical cancer and has been shown to improve patient outcomes.[5–15] In turn, radiologists may substantially contribute not only to the initial assessment of cervical cancer but also to treatment response assessment and surveillance. This article discusses the appropriate use of MR imaging in the diagnosis and treatment of cervical cancer.

Disclosure: The authors have nothing to disclose.

[a] Department of Radiology and Radiological Sciences, Vanderbilt University, Medical Center North, 1161 21st Avenue South, Nashville, TN 37232, USA; [b] Department of Radiology, University of Wisconsin Hospital and Clinics, 600 Highland Avenue, Madison, WI 53792, USA; [c] Department of Obstetrics and Gynecology, University of Wisconsin Hospital and Clinics, 600 Highland Avenue, Madison, WI 53792, USA; [d] Department of Radiation Oncology, University of Wisconsin Hospital and Clinics, 600 Highland Avenue, Madison, WI 53792, USA; [e] Department of Radiology, Mayo Clinic, 200 First Street Southwest, Rochester, MN 55902, USA
* Corresponding author.
E-mail address: esadowski@uwhealth.org

Magn Reson Imaging Clin N Am 25 (2017) 635–649
http://dx.doi.org/10.1016/j.mric.2017.03.007

mri.theclinics.com

MR IMAGING IN THE DIAGNOSIS AND TREATMENT OF CERVICAL CANCER

Cervical cancer is a clinically staged cancer based on the International Federation of Gynecology and Obstetrics (FIGO) classification system, recently revised in 2009 (**Table 1**). The initial clinical stage is assigned after gynecologic bimanual and speculum examinations, colposcopy, and cervical biopsy. In regions where MR imaging and PET/computed tomography (CT) are not available, additional invasive techniques, including an examination under anesthesia, cystoscopy, intravenous urography, and sigmoidoscopy or barium enema, can be performed when assessing for advanced disease.[4,5,8,9,16] Although clinical staging is fairly accurate in early-stage disease, approaching 85% in stage IA to IB1, accuracy in later-stage disease decreases significantly, to less than 35% in stage IIA and 21% in stage IIB[8,10] when correlated with surgical findings. MR imaging can accurately assess for important prognostic indicators such as tumor size, parametrial invasion, pelvic sidewall invasion, and lymph node metastasis, and has been shown to have accuracy up to 95% for stage IB or greater.[9–12,17–20] As such, FIGO supports the use of MR imaging in conjunction with PET/CT to increase the accuracy of staging, in areas where available.[9,10,12–15,17–24]

Treatment decisions for patients with cervical cancer are determined by the FIGO clinical stage (**Fig. 1**).[16] Patients with early-stage disease, tumor confined to the uterus, and tumors less than 4 cm (stage I–IB1), are treated with primary surgical resection and lymphadenectomy.[5,18,22,25–28] Many centers treat women with more advanced-stage disease, defined as stage IB2 or greater, using concurrent chemoradiation as definitive therapy without surgery. This approach is a recent change from previous recommendations to treat only women with stage IIB or higher with chemoradiation.[6,7,9–11,20,29–31] In addition, women with advanced-stage disease (IVB) are offered

Table 1
2009 International Federation of Gynecology and Obstetrics staging classification

Stage	Description	Subtype	Subtype Divisions
I	Confined to the uterus	IA: invasive carcinoma diagnosed only with microscopy with deepest invasion ≤5 mm and largest extension ≤7 mm	IAI: stromal invasion ≤3 mm IA2: stromal invasion >3 mm and ≤5 mm
		IB: clinically visible lesions greater than stage IA	IBI: clinically visible lesion ≤4 cm in greatest dimension IB2: clinically visible lesion >4 cm in greatest dimension
II	Carcinoma invades beyond the uterus, but not to the pelvic wall or lower one-third of the vagina	IIA: without parametrial involvement	IIA1: clinically visible lesion ≤4 cm in greatest dimension IIA2: clinically visible lesion >4 cm in greatest dimension
		IIB: obvious parametrial invasion	
III	Tumor extends to the pelvic wall, involves the lower one-third of the vagina, and/or causes hydronephrosis or a nonfunctioning kidney	IIIA: tumor involves the lower one-third of the vagina IIIB: extension to the pelvic wall, hydronephrosis, or nonfunctioning kidney	
IV	Tumor extends beyond the true pelvis or has involved the bladder or rectum	IVA: spread of growth to adjacent organs (mucosal involvement of bladder or rectum) IVB: spread to distant organs (including peritoneal, supraclavicular, mediastinal, or para-aortic lymph nodes)	

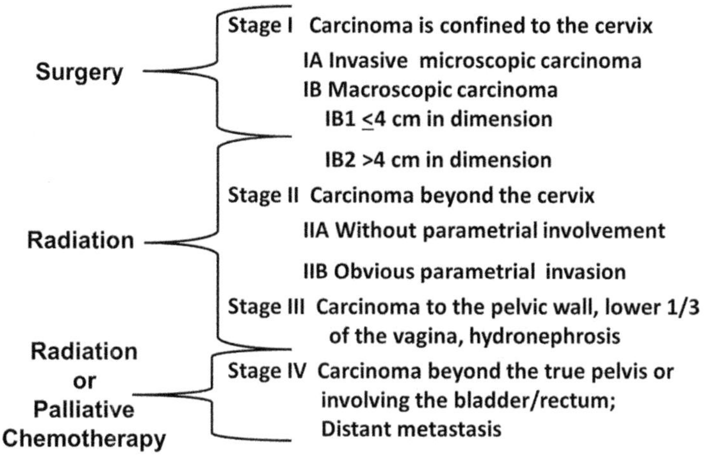

Fig. 1. Treatment of cervical cancer, based on clinical stage.

palliative chemotherapy and symptom control. MR imaging is valuable in determining size of tumor, parametrial invasion, and local metastasis, whereas PET/CT can identify local and distant metastasis and ensure that the radiation treatment volume encompasses clinically involved and high-risk areas.[25,29,30,32] The ultimate goal of advanced imaging is to appropriately stratify patients into treatment groups, to avoid the morbidity and mortality associated with unnecessary surgery, and to ensure all regions of suspected disease are included in the radiation treatment fields.

Magnetic Resonance Protocol

Patient preparation for pelvic MR imaging for cervical cancer includes steps to minimize artifacts and improve visualization of the cervix. It is recommended that patients fast for 4 to 6 hours before the examination to minimize bowel peristalsis. Some institutions choose to administer antiperistaltic medications to further minimize bowel-related motion artifacts. Having the patient void before imaging can help reduce bladder-related artifacts. In addition, vaginal gel can improve visualization of the cervix. Imaging can be performed on either 1.5-T or 3-T magnets with a dedicated pelvic, cardiac, or torso coil. A comprehensive cervical cancer protocol should include the following sequences: Coronal non-fat saturated T2-weighted single shot fast spin echo (FSE) images, axial non-fat saturated T1-weighted FSE images, Axial or axial oblique non-fat saturated T2-weighted FSE images, axial diffusion weighted images, post-contrast axial and sagittal fat saturated T1-weighted spoiled gradient echo images. An example of an MR protocol is provided in **Table 2**. Of note, many experts emphasize the importance of true short-axis views of the cervix for small-field-of-view T2-weighted images, whereas others prefer to acquire this series in the true axial plane for the sake of simplicity and reproducibility.

Interpretation

The normal anatomy of the cervix is best visualized on standard fast spin echo T2-weighted images. The normal premenopausal cervix is approximately 3 to 4 cm in length and has a trilaminar appearance: hyperintense endocervical mucosa with a band of low signal intensity representing the cervical stroma deep to the mucosal glands and intermediate-signal-intensity stroma extending to the parametrium (**Fig. 2**A). The appearance of the cervical stroma changes as the woman ages, becoming more uniformly hypointense in the postmenopausal cervix (see **Fig. 2**B).

The size, location, and extent of cervical tumors are best evaluated on standard, non-fat saturated T2-weighted and diffusion-weighted images. On T2-weighted images, the tumor shows intermediate to high signal intensity compared with the smooth muscle or myometrium of the uterus (**Fig. 3**A, B). On diffusion-weighted images, the tumor shows intermediate to high signal on $B = 0$ images with increase in signal on high B value images and corresponding low signal on apparent diffusion coefficient (ADC) images, reflecting diffusion restriction within the cellular tumor (see **Fig. 3**C). Diffusion-weighted images can increase visualization of small tumors that are difficult to delineate on T2-weighted images or in younger patients when the normal cervix is more intermediate in signal intensity, mimicking tumor signal.[33,34] On dynamic contrast-enhanced images, small

Table 2
Example MR imaging protocol parameters for imaging cervical cancer

Sequence	Coronal T2	Axial T1	Sagittal T2	Axial T2	Axial DWI	Axial T1	Sagittal T1	Axial T1
Fat Saturated	No	No	Yes	No	No	Yes	Yes	Yes
Time After Injection of Contrast (s)	—	—	—	—	—	40	90	180
Sequence	Single-shot fast spin echo	Fast spin echo	Fast recovery fast spin echo	Fast recovery fast spin echo	Echo planar	Spoiled gradient echo	Spoiled gradient echo	Spoiled gradient echo
Number of Dimensions	2	2	2	2	2	3	3	3
TE (ms)	90	9	90	86	65	1.8	1.8	1.8
TR (ms)	2400	600	3400	3400	10,000	3.8	3.8	3.8
Echo Train Length	—	4	21	21	—	InvPrep TI = 20	InvPrep TI = 20	InvPrep TI = 20
Flip Angle (degrees)	90	90	90	90	90	12	12	12
Number of Excitations	2	4	3	3	8	1	1	1
FOV (cm)	36	26	26	26	32	28	28	28
Slice Thickness/ interval (mm)	6/0	5/1.5	4/1	4/1	4/1	4.2	4.2	4.2
Matrix Size	256 × 224	256 × 224	320 × 256	320 × 256	160 × 160	256 × 192	256 × 192	256 × 192
b Value (s/mm^2)	—	—	—	—	0, 500	—	—	—
Approximate Acquisition Time (min:s)	1:15	4:36	3:30	3:30	2:50	0:27	0:27	0:27

Abbreviations: DWI, diffusion-weighted imaging; FOV, field of view; TE, echo time; TR, recovery time.

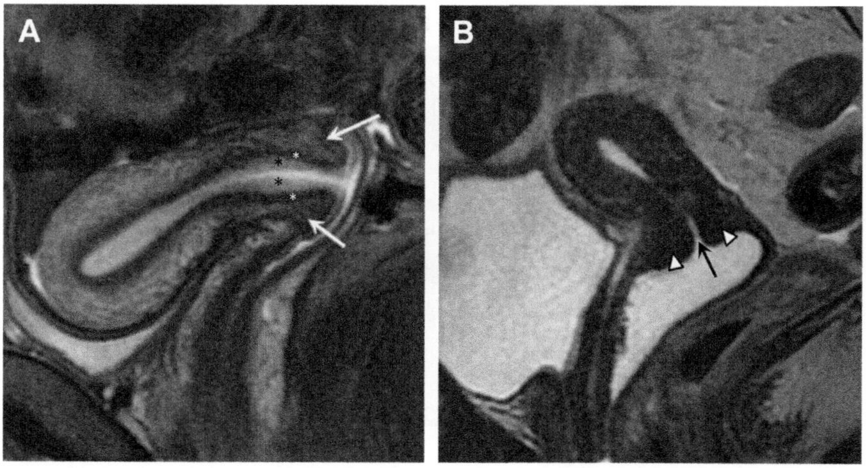

Fig. 2. Normal premenopausal and postmenopausal appearance of the cervix. (*A*) Sagittal fat-saturated T2-weighted MR image shows the normal premenopausal trilaminar appearance of the cervix, with hyperintense endocervical mucosa (*black asterisks*), band of low-signal-intensity cervical stroma deep to the glands (*white asterisks*), and intermediate-signal-intensity stroma in the remainder of the cervix (*white arrows*). (*B*) Sagittal T2-weighted MR image shows the normal postmenopausal appearance of the cervix. The endocervical mucosa remains hyperintense (*black arrow*) and the cervical stroma (*white arrowheads*) appears homogeneously hypointense.

tumors show increased early homogeneous hyperenhancement relative to the adjacent normal cervix, whereas larger tumors often show heterogeneous enhancement secondary to necrosis[17,35] (see **Fig. 3**D). Contrast-enhanced images are useful in larger tumors for delineation of tumor extent when evaluating for bladder, rectal, adnexal, or pelvic side wall invasion, or when evaluating for recurrent disease.[9,36–38]

Although nodal involvement is not part of FIGO staging, it is essential for treatment planning and is a key prognostic indicator. According to Sakuragi,[39] 5-year survival for patients with low-stage disease is 95% in the absence of lymph node metastases and decreases to less than 80% if pelvic lymph node metastases are present and less than 40% if para-aortic lymph node metastases are present. There are 3 main lymphatic drainage pathways for the cervix. After spread to the parametrial nodes, lymphatic drainage occurs anteriorly to the external iliac lymph nodes, laterally to the obturator nodes and the internal iliac lymph nodes, and posteriorly to the uterosacral ligament and sacral lymph nodes. All nodal pathways eventually drain into the common iliac and para-aortic lymph nodes.[39,40]

MR imaging is able to assess for lymph node metastasis with sensitivities up to 73% and specificities up to 96%.[14,18,26,28,41–44] Lymph nodes are optimally assessed on MR imaging using a combination of fat-saturated T2-weighted, diffusion-weighted, and T1-weighted postcontrast images. Imaging features of metastatic lymph nodes include size (>1 cm), rounded morphology, multiplicity, and central necrosis. Size, morphology, and multiplicity can be assessed on MR images. On T1-weighted and T2-weighted images, abnormal lymph nodes are often similar in signal intensity to the primary tumor with good conspicuity relative to the hyperintense surrounding fat (**Fig. 4**A, B). Postcontrast the lymph nodes are seen to enhance unless portions of the lymph node are necrotic (see **Fig. 4**C).

On diffusion-weighted images, lymph nodes are similar to the primary tumor with mild hyperintensity on B = 0 images that increases on high B value images with corresponding low ADC signal (see **Fig. 4**D). Some studies have shown that metastatic lymph nodes have a markedly decreased ADC value compared with benign lymph nodes and metastatic nodes as small as 5 mm can be detected with diffusion-weighted imaging.[33,42] Although a useful tool, there are several important caveats when evaluating lymph nodes on diffusion-weighted images. First, varying studies have noted that some metastatic lymph nodes do not restrict diffusion.[9,10,36] Second, both reactive and normal lymph nodes may appear to restrict diffusion. If a lymph node otherwise shows benign morphologic features (eg, fatty hilum and uniform cortical thickness), low signal on ADC images should be cautiously interpreted with close follow-up and/or correlation with PET/CT.

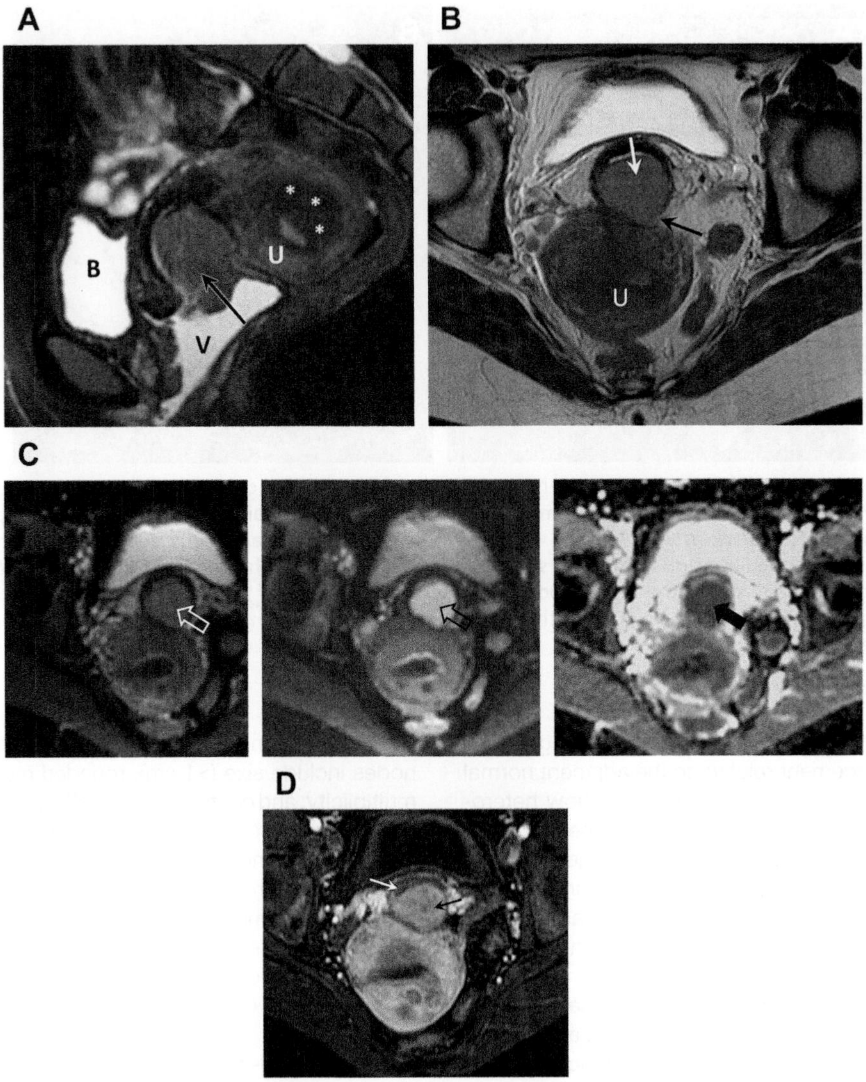

Fig. 3. A 48-year-old woman with stage IIB squamous cell carcinoma of the cervix. (*A*) Sagittal fat-saturated T2-weighted MR image shows the cervical tumor (*black arrow*) as intermediate signal intensity compared with the myometrium of the uterus (U). Adenomyosis (*white asterisks*) is seen in the anterior uterine body/fundus. (*B*) On the axial T2-weighted MR image, the intermediate signal of the cervical tumor (*white arrow*) is seen extending through the hypointense signal of the normal cervical stroma and invading the parametrium posteriorly on the left (*black arrow*). (*C*) Axial diffusion-weighted images show the tumor as isointense on the B = 0 image (*open white arrow*), hyperintense on the B = 500 image (*open black arrow*), and hypointense on the apparent diffusion coefficient (ADC) map (*solid black arrow*), signifying restricted diffusion. (*D*) Axial fat-saturated T1-weighted postcontrast image shows the increased enhancement of the cervical tumor (*black arrow*) relative to the normal adjacent cervical stroma (*white arrow*). B, bladder; V, gel in vagina.

STAGING CERVICAL CANCER ON MR IMAGING

After a new cervical cancer diagnosis, the goal of MR imaging is to assess tumor size, location, and extrauterine spread as well as detection of local metastasis. Given the limitations of clinical staging, FIGO encourages the use of MR imaging where available to help guide initial treatment decisions, as detailed earlier. Importantly, during interpretation, special attention should be paid to determining the tumor size (> or <4 cm), whether there is extension of the tumor into the lower third of the vagina, the presence of parametrial invasion or local organ invasion, and the presence of metastatic lymphadenopathy, because these findings both change the clinical stage and triage patients

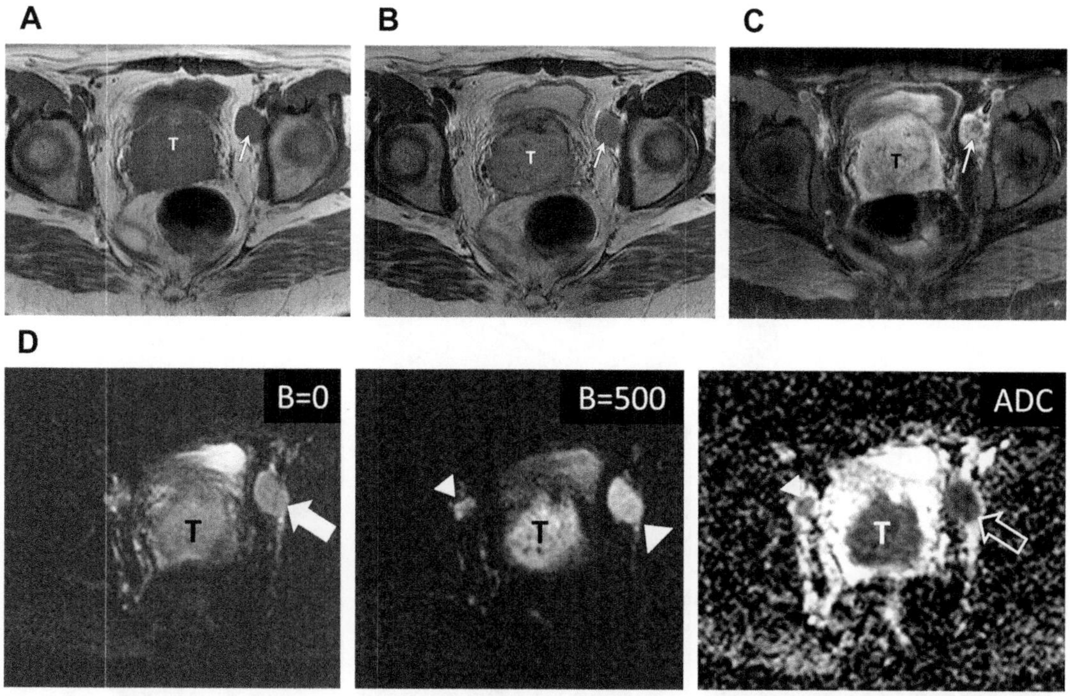

Fig. 4. A 47-year-old woman with stage IIB adenocarcinoma of the cervix. (*A*) Axial T1-weighted MR image shows an enlarged, morphologically abnormal (round) lymph node (*white arrow*) in the left pelvis, with similar signal to the primary cervical tumor (T). (*B*) Axial T2-weighted MR image shows an enlarged, morphologically abnormal (round) pelvic lymph node (*white arrow*) in the left pelvis, also with similar signal to the primary tumor (T). (*C*) Axial fat-saturated T1-weighted postcontrast image shows heterogeneous enhancement of the enlarged pelvic lymph node (*white arrow*), possibly necrosis. (*D*) Axial diffusion-weighted images show the enlarged lymph node in the left pelvis as isointense on B = 0 image (*white arrow*), hyperintense on B = 500 image (large *white arrowhead*), and hypointense on ADC map (*white open arrow*), signifying restricted diffusion. A smaller lymph node (small *white arrowheads* on B = 500 and ADC map) is noted in the right pelvis.

into different first-line treatment. In addition, MR imaging can provide valuable pretreatment planning information for intracavitary radiation therapy as well as assess response to radiation therapy. In addition, MR imaging is often used as a surveillance tool to evaluate for locally recurrent disease after surgical resection or after definitive chemoradiation.[6,17,45–49]

Stage I

Stage I disease is defined as tumor strictly confined to the cervix and is further subdivided into IA and IB. Stage IA is microinvasive tumor with further stratification based on degree of stromal invasion into IA1 (<3 mm) and IA2 (3–5 mm). The lateral extent of the tumor for both IA1 and IA2 is less than 7 mm. MR imaging cannot delineate these microinvasive tumors and thus plays no role in the evaluation of stage IA lesions. Stage IB tumors are defined as clinically visible lesions that do not meet criteria for IA lesions. These lesions are now subdivided into stage IB1, which encompasses tumors less than 4 cm in maximum dimension, and stage IB2, which are tumors greater than 4 cm in the revised FIGO staging[8] (**Figs. 5** and **6**). Correct distinction of stage IB2 tumors is of great importance because many centers treat these patients with primary chemoradiation rather than primary surgical resection.[6,9–11,20,29–31,36]

Measurement of size and location is especially important in the evaluation of younger patients who desire fertility-sparing trachelectomy, or surgical removal of the uterine cervix leaving the uterine body intact. In order to be eligible for trachelectomy, the tumor must be less than 2 cm and at least 1 cm from the internal os[17] (**Fig. 7**). In younger patients, this evaluation can be made more difficult by hormonal changes, which result in more intermediate signal of the cervix, sometimes obscuring tumor margins and location. In some cases, preoperative MR imaging is unable to determine whether a trachelectomy is possible and this decision is made in the operating room based on intraoperative frozen section at proposed margins.[50]

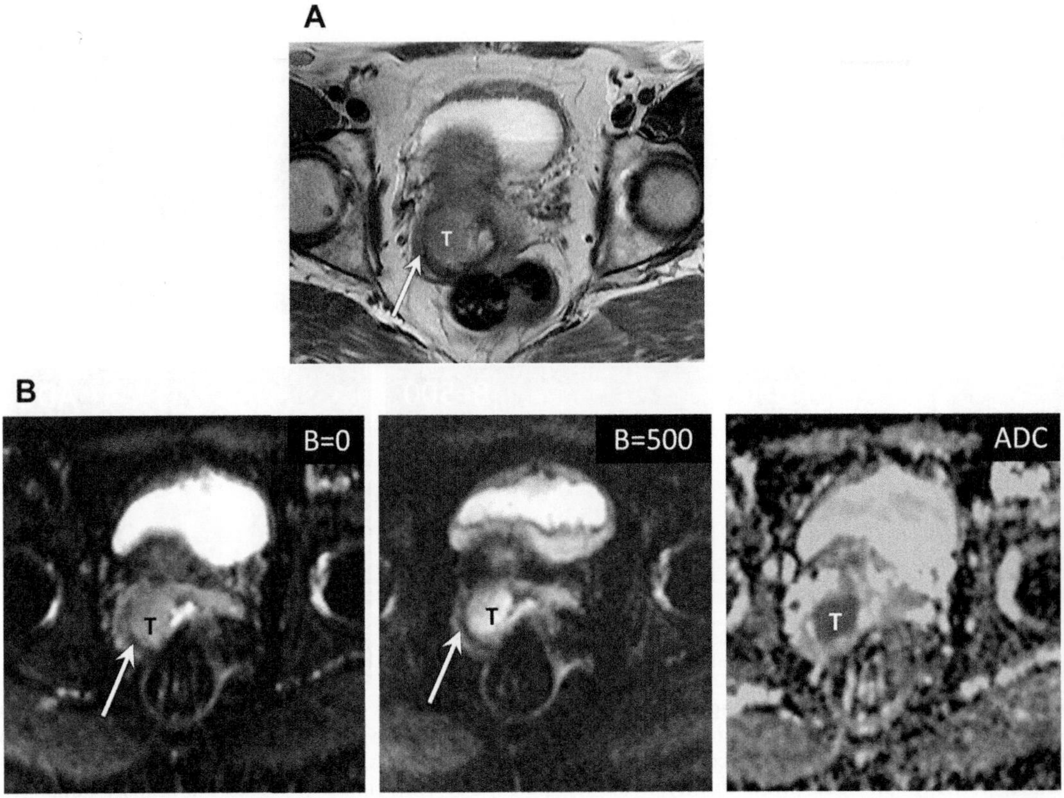

Fig. 5. A 69-year-old woman with stage IB1 squamous cell carcinoma (*A*) Axial T2-weighted MR image shows a 2.2-cm tumor (T) within the cervix that has intermediate signal. An intact hypointense stromal ring (*white arrow*) excludes parametrial invasion. (*B*) Axial diffusion-weighted MR images, B = 0 (*left*), B = 500 (*middle*), and ADC (*right*), show the 2.2-cm tumor (T) and the intact cervical stromal ring (*white arrows*).

Stage II

Stage II tumor extends outside the uterus, but not to the pelvic sidewall or lower one-third of the vagina. Stage II is further subdivided based on parametrial invasion into IIA (absent parametrial invasion) lesions and IIB (present parametrial invasion) lesions. Furthermore, stage IIA tumors are now divided into IIA1 (tumors <4 cm) and IIA2 (tumors >4 cm) based on prognostic differences seen between the two groups.[8]

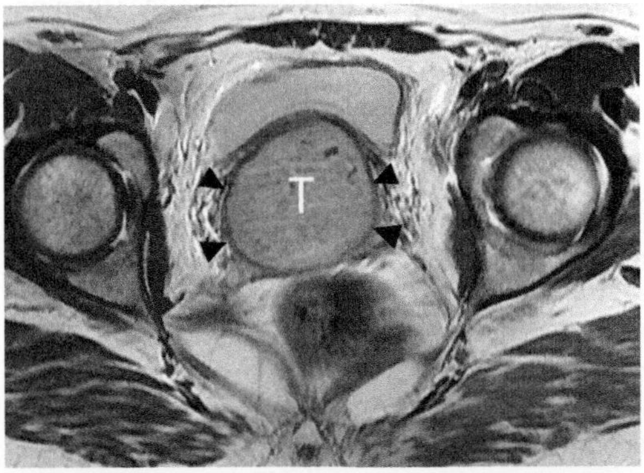

Fig. 6. A 47-year-old woman with stage IB2 squamous cell carcinoma of the cervix. Axial T2-weighted MR image shows a 5.1-cm tumor (T) confined to the cervix. The intact hypointense stromal ring (*black arrowheads*) indicates no parametrial invasion.

In addition to lesion size, tumor location, and lymph node status, parametrial invasion can influence treatment planning. Tumors that are greater than 4 cm, have parametrial invasion, or show obvious disease outside the pelvis are primarily treated with chemoradiation. The parametrium consists of the uterosacral and cardinal ligaments as well as fat, lymphatics, and vessels. Parametrial invasion is best seen on non-fat saturated T2-weighted images with full-thickness disruption of the normal cervix stroma with extension of nodular or spiculated soft tissue into the adjacent parametrium (**Fig. 8**A).[11,40] Periuterine vessel encasement in low cervical tumors and disruption of the hypointense vaginal wall in tumors with vaginal extension are both signs of parametrial invasion (see **Fig. 8**B, C).[40] The sensitivity of MR imaging for detecting parametrial invasion is

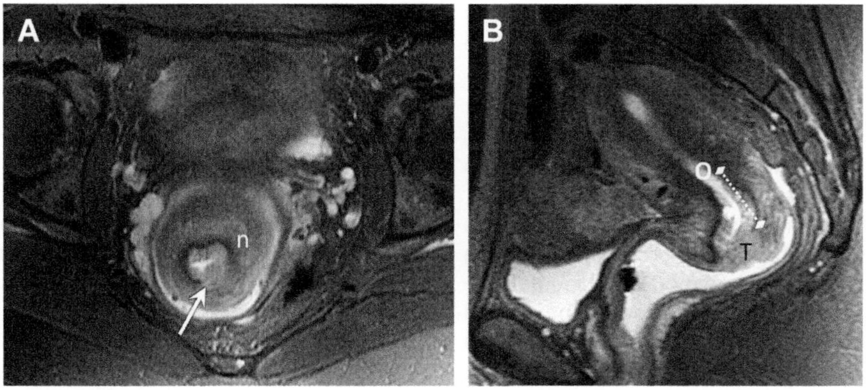

Fig. 7. A 29-year-old woman with stage IB1 cervical cancer presenting for fertility-sparing trachelectomy. (*A*) Axial fat-saturated T2-weighted MR image shows a 1.8-cm tumor contained within the cervix (*white arrow*). The tumor is isointense to the normal cervical stroma (n), but disrupts the hypointense stromal ring at the mucosal-stroma interface (*white arrow*). (*B*) Sagittal fat-saturated T2-weighted MR image shows a 1.8-cm cervical tumor (T) located near the external cervical os. The tumor was located 3.2 cm from the internal cervical os (O), depicted by the dotted line showing the distance of the most proximal edge of tumor to the internal cervical os.

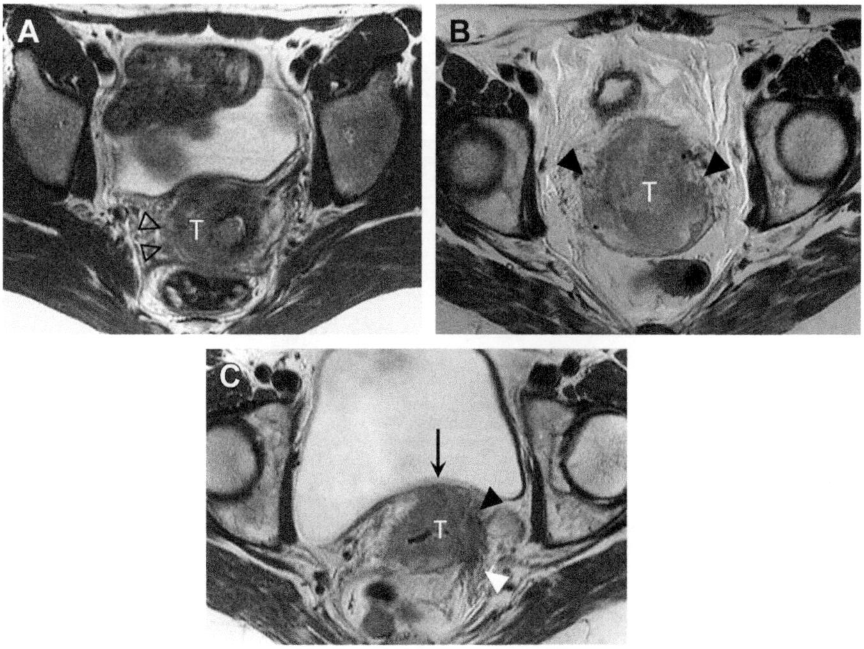

Fig. 8. Examples of stage IIB cervical cancer. (*A*) Axial T2-weighted MR image shows tumor (T) along the right side of the cervix (6 o'clock to 12 o'clock). The tumor is seen in the cervical canal and invades the full thickness of the cervix into the right parametrium (*black open arrowheads*). (*B*) Axial T2-weighted MR image shows a large cervical tumor (T) replacing the normal cervical tissue. There is bilateral parametrial invasion with spicules of tumor extending into the parametrial fat and along the parametrial vessels (*black arrowheads*). (*C*) Axial T2-weighted MR image shows tumor within the cervix (T), with spiculated parametrial tumor invasion from 12 o'clock to 5 o'clock on the left (*black arrowhead*) and tumor infiltrating along the uterosacral ligament at 5 o'clock (*white arrowhead*). There is tumor signal abutting the posterior bladder wall; however, the hypointense signal of the bladder wall was intact (*black arrow*), signifying no bladder wall invasion.

greater than 90%, with specificities greater than 80% and negative predictive values of 94% to 100%.[9,10,12,20]

Stage III

Stage III tumor is divided into stage IIIA, which is tumor involving the lower one-third of the vagina, and stage IIIB tumor, which is involvement of the pelvic sidewall with possible ureteral obstruction resulting in a hydronephrotic or atrophic nonfunctioning kidney. In stage IIIA disease, the normal hypointense T2 signal of the lower third of the vaginal vault is disrupted by hyperintense tumor. Visualization of tumor within 3 mm of the obturator internus, levator ani, piriformis muscles, or the iliac vessels is highly concerning for stage IIIB disease[20,51] (**Fig. 9**).

Stage IV

Stage IV tumor is extension of tumor beyond the true pelvis. Stage IVA is tumor extension into the mucosa of the bladder or rectum (**Fig. 10**). Although the traditional FIGO staging required invasive testing such as sigmoidoscopy and cystoscopy to assess for local invasion, the revised system now endorses the use of MR

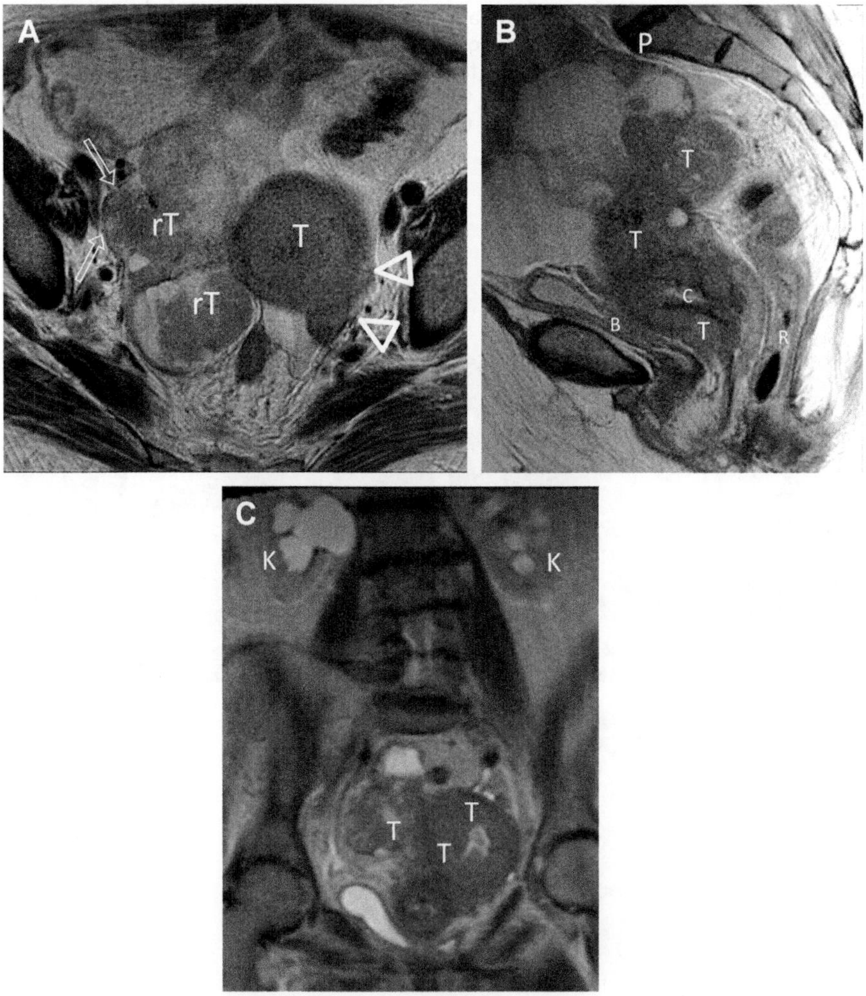

Fig. 9. A 70-year-old woman with stage IIIB clear cell carcinoma of the cervix. (*A*) Axial T2-weighted MR image shows tumor involving the uterus (T) with extension into the right adnexa (rT) and right pelvic side wall (*open white arrows*). The tumor also invades the left parametrium and appears to be within 3 mm of iliac vessels, suspicious for pelvic side wall invasion (*open white arrowheads*). (*B*) Sagittal T2-weighted MR image shows the extensive cervical tumor (T) within and outside of the uterus. The fat planes between the tumor and bladder (B)/rectum (R) appear intact, excluding invasion. The tumor appears confined to the true pelvis, because it is located below the sacral promontory (P) and no distant metastasis were noted on PET/CT. (*C*) Coronal T2-weighted MR image shows extensive tumor (T) in the pelvis, within and outside of the uterus. Bilateral hydronephrosis in the kidneys (K) is noted, which is a feature of stage IIIB disease. C, cervical canal.

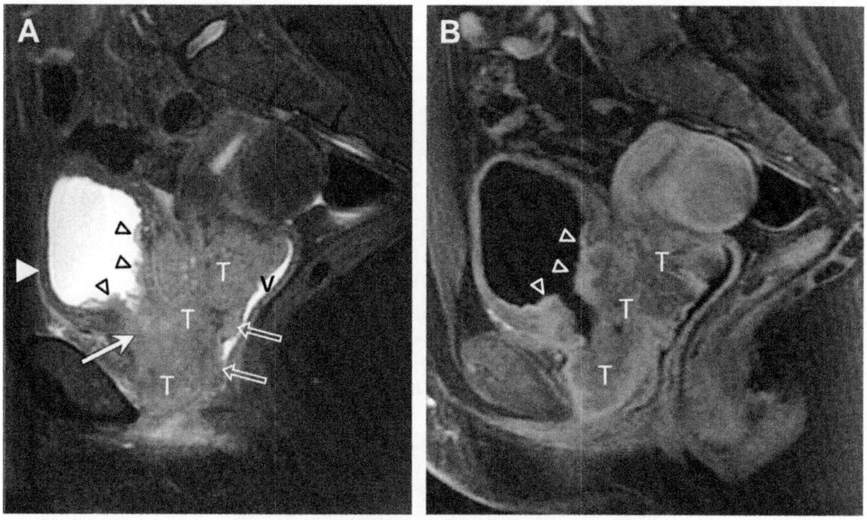

Fig. 10. A 52-year-old woman with stage IVA squamous cell carcinoma of the cervix, vagina, bladder, and urethra. (*A*) Sagittal fat-saturated T2-weighted MR image shows extensive tumor (T) in the cervix. The tumor replaces the normal cervical tissue and extends anteriorly to invade the lower posterior bladder wall, with tumor in the lumen of the bladder (*black open arrowheads*). Note the intermediate tumor signal within the posterior bladder wall compared with the normal anterior wall (*white arrowhead*). There is intermediate tumor signal involving the urethra (*white arrow*), both the upper two-thirds and lower one-third of the anterior vaginal wall (*open white arrows*). (*B*) Sagittal fat-saturated T1-weighted postcontrast MR image shows the heterogeneous enhancement of the large cervical tumor (T) invading the vagina, bladder, and urethra. The tumor invades the full thickness of the bladder wall and enhancing tumor is seen in the lumen of the bladder (*white open arrowheads*). V, gel within the vagina.

imaging to evaluate for these findings.[8] MR imaging findings of bladder or rectal invasion include focal or segmental loss of normal T2 hypointense bladder wall or loss of normal T2-hypointense muscularis propria rectal wall, with or without intraluminal soft tissue mass. A preserved fat plane between the tumor and bladder/rectum essentially excludes invasion, but the presence of uniform increased T2 signal within the luminal wall is nonspecific and can be seen in the setting of edema or inflammation. A specific pitfall in the evaluation of the bladder is bullous edema, which is a T2 hyperintense band along the interior bladder wall and can mimic tumor.[52] MR has a sensitivity of 71% to 100% for bladder and rectal invasion, with a specificity of 88% to 91% and a negative predictive value close to 100%.[17]

Stage IVB tumor is distant metastatic disease, with involvement of para-aortic or inguinal lymph nodes, liver, lung, and/or bones. PET/CT plays an important role in evaluation of metastatic lymph nodes as well as additional distant solid organ and osseous metastasis. Accurate assessment of metastatic disease is important for appropriate treatment planning and to ensure that all suspected areas of disease are included in the radiation treatment plan. A key advantage to PET/CT is its ability to detect lymph node metastasis in nodes that may not otherwise be considered abnormal on conventional MR or CT imaging based on size criteria of 1 cm and morphology. The reported PET sensitivity for lymph node detection ranges from 79% to 91% with specificity from 93% to 100%.[43,53–55]

POSTTREATMENT MONITORING

MR imaging plays an important role in evaluating treatment response as well as identifying recurrent disease. In posthysterectomy patients, typical postoperative MR appearance includes a linear configuration to the residual vaginal cuff with intact T2 hypointense vaginal wall.[47] In addition, there may be areas of fibrosis and scarring along the vaginal vault that show low signal on T2-weighted and the high b value images.[47] Findings of tumor response after radiotherapy on MR imaging includes reconstitution of the normal zonal anatomy of the cervix[56] (**Fig. 11**). Marked decrease in the size and signal intensity of the tumor in the first 2 to 3 months after initiation of treatment is highly suggestive of eventual complete tumor response.[57]

Recurrent disease is defined as local tumor regrowth in the pelvis or development of distant metastatic disease 6 months after treatment. In

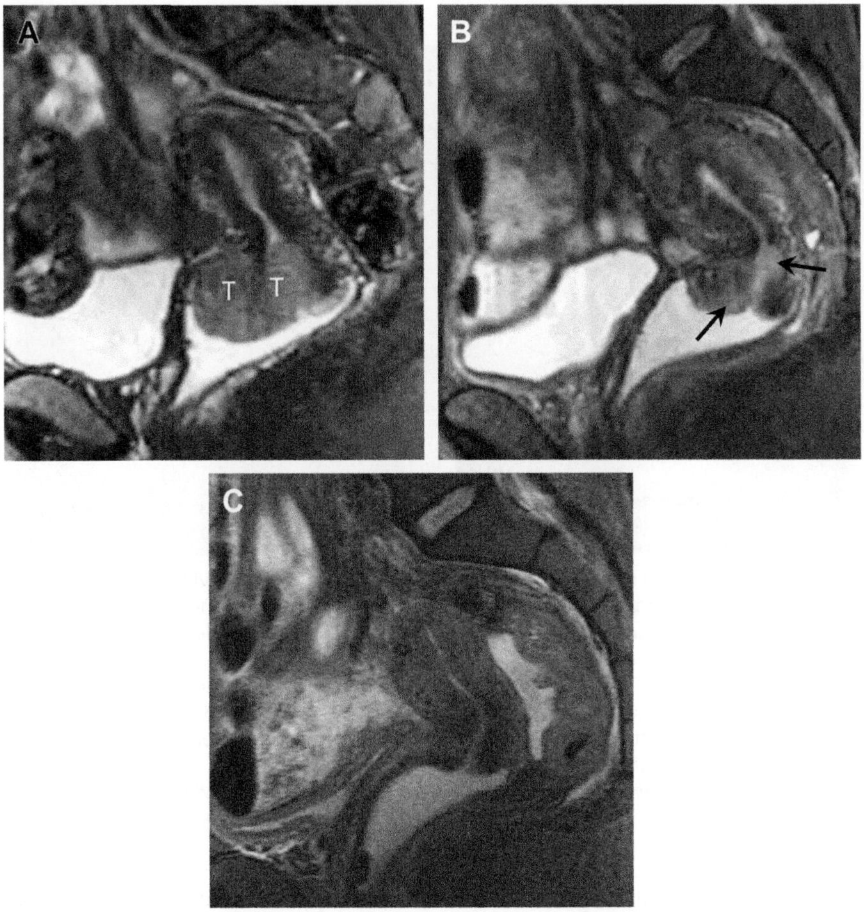

Fig. 11. A 65-year-old woman with stage IIB adenocarcinoma of the cervix treated with chemoradiation. (*A*) Sagittal fat-saturated T2-weighted MR image from the baseline MR examination shows an intermediate-signal cervical tumor (T) involving the endocervical canal and anterior lip of the cervix. (*B*) Sagittal fat-saturated T2-weighted MR image from the post–external beam radiation treatment MR examination, shows areas of intermediate T2 signal in the posterior endocervical canal and anterior cervical lip (*black arrows*), which relate to residual tumor. The patient subsequently underwent brachytherapy. (*C*) Sagittal fat-saturated T2-weighted MR image from the 3-month postbrachytherapy MR examination shows a normal-appearing cervix.

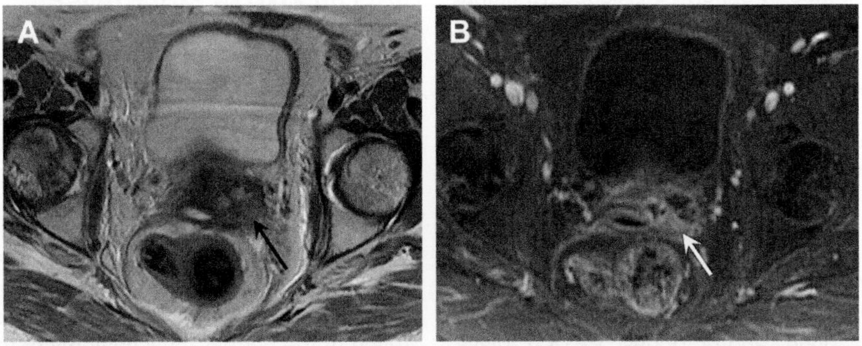

Fig. 12. A 56-year-old woman with stage IIB squamous cell carcinoma of the cervix, treated with chemoradiation. MR examination performed 12 weeks after treatment with chemoradiation. (*A*) Axial T2-weighted MR image shows an ill-defined focus of intermediate T2 signal in the left lower cervix/upper vagina concerning for residual/recurrent disease versus radiation changes (*black arrow*). (*B*) Axial fat-saturated T1-weighted postcontrast MR image shows enhancement in the ill-defined focus (*white arrow*) noted on the T2-weighted image; however, this is nonspecific and can be seen in both recurrent and treated disease. PET/CT was performed for further evaluation and was positive for hypermetabolic activity in this same location (not shown). Biopsy was subsequently obtained and was negative for malignancy. The signal abnormality decreased on a follow-up examination 6 weeks later (not shown) and therefore this was pericervical inflammatory tissue related to radiation therapy.

patients who have undergone surgical resection without radiation therapy, recurrence has a similar appearance to the primary tumor. Recurrent disease in postradiation patients is often more difficult to delineate, because posttreatment changes can have a similar appearance. In the long term, radiation-related fibrosis shows low T2 signal, enabling differentiation between posttreatment changes and intermediate-signal recurrent tumor. However, early postradiation edema, inflammatory changes, and superimposed infection can show intermediate T2 signal similar to the primary tumor (**Fig. 12**). Although studies have shown that recurrent tumor can be distinguished from postradiation changes based on postcontrast appearance, with tumor showing optimal enhancement from 45 to 90 seconds,[56] in practice these two entities can be difficult to distinguish confidently and often require further evaluation with PET/CT, serial MR examinations, and/or biopsy.

SUMMARY

Cervical cancer is a significant cause of morbidity and mortality worldwide despite advances in screening and prevention. Although cervical cancer is still clinically staged, the 2009 FIGO committee has encouraged the use of advanced imaging modalities, including MR imaging, to increase the accuracy of staging and help guide treatment, radiation treatment planning/monitoring, and detection of recurrence. Understanding the staging scheme and impact on treatment; appearance of important radiologic findings such as tumor size, parametrial invasion, and metastatic lymphadenopathy; and common pitfalls in interpretation helps radiologists render accurate and helpful reports to clinicians to optimize treatment planning in these patients.

REFERENCES

1. "Cervical Cancer" fact sheet. Available at: https://report.nih.gov/nihfactsheets/ViewFactSheet.aspx?csid=76&key=C#C. Accessed August 21, 2016.
2. "Cervical cancer incidence statistics." Available at: http://www.cancerresearchuk.org/health-professional/cancer-statistics/statistics-by-cancer-type/cervical-cancer/incidence. Accessed August 21, 2016.
3. "USA causes of death by age and gender." Available at: http://www.worldlifeexpectancy.com/usa-cause-of-death-by-age-and-gender. Accessed April 22, 2016.
4. "World Health Organization: Latest world cancer statistics." Available at: http://www.iarc.fr/en/media-centre/pr/2013/pdfs/pr223_E.pdf. Accessed April 22, 2016.
5. Lea JS, Lin KY. Cervical cancer. Obstet Gynecol Clin North Am 2012;39(2):233–53.
6. Barwick TD, Taylor A, Rockall A. Functional imaging to predict tumor response in locally advanced cervical cancer. Curr Oncol Rep 2013;15(6):549–58.
7. Green JA, Kirwan JM, Tierney JF, et al. Survival and recurrence after concomitant chemotherapy and radiotherapy for cancer of the uterine cervix: a systematic review and meta-analysis. Lancet 2001;358(9284):781–6.
8. Pecorelli S, Zigliani L, Odicino F. Revised FIGO staging for carcinoma of the cervix. Int J Gynecol Obstet 2009;105(2):107–8.
9. Kido A, Fujimoto K, Okada T, et al. Advanced MRI in malignant neoplasms of the uterus. J Magn Reson Imaging 2013;37(2):249–64.
10. Sala E, Rockall AG, Freeman SJ, et al. The added role of MR imaging in treatment stratification of patients with gynecologic malignancies: what the radiologist needs to know. Radiology 2013;266(3):717–40.
11. Freeman SJ, Aly AM, Kataoka MY, et al. The REVISED FIGO Staging System for Uterine Malignancies: implications for MR imaging. Radiographics 2012;32(6):1805–27.
12. Koyama T, Tamai K, Togashi K. Staging of carcinoma of the uterine cervix and endometrium. Eur Radiol 2007;17(8):2009–19.
13. Mitchell DG, Snyder B, Coakley F, et al. Early invasive cervical cancer: tumor delineation by magnetic resonance imaging, computed tomography, and clinical examination, verified by pathologic results, in the ACRIN 6651/GOG 183 intergroup study. J Clin Oncol 2006;24(36):5687–94.
14. Chung HH, Kang KW, Cho JY, et al. Role of magnetic resonance imaging and positron emission tomography/computed tomography in preoperative lymph node detection of uterine cervical cancer. Am J Obstet Gynecol 2010;203(2):156.e1-5.
15. Narayan K. Arguments for a magnetic resonance imaging–assisted FIGO staging system for cervical cancer. Int J Gynecol Cancer 2005;15:573–82.
16. Pecorelli S. Revised FIGO staging for carcinoma of the vulva, cervix, and endometrium. Int J Gynecol Obstet 2009;105(2):103–4.
17. Sala E, Wakely S, Senior E, et al. MRI of malignant neoplasms of the uterine corpus and cervix. Am J Roentgenol 2007;188(6):1577–87.
18. Sheu M-H, Chang C-Y, Wang J-H, et al. Preoperative staging of cervical carcinoma with MR imaging: a reappraisal of diagnostic accuracy and pitfalls. Eur Radiol 2001;11(9):1828–33.
19. Togashi K, Nishimura K, Sagoh T, et al. Carcinoma of the cervix: staging with MR imaging. Radiology 1989;171(1):245–51.
20. Zand KR, Reinhold C, Abe H, et al. Magnetic resonance imaging of the cervix. Cancer Imaging 2007;7(1):69–76.

21. Qin Y, Peng Z, Lou J, et al. Discrepancies between clinical staging and pathological findings of operable cervical carcinoma with stage IB–IIB: A retrospective analysis of 818 patients. Aust N Z J Obstet Gynaecol 2009;49(5):542–4.
22. Lai C-H, Yen T-C, Ng K-K. Surgical and radiologic staging of cervical cancer. Curr Opin Obstet Gynecol 2010;22(1):15–20.
23. Amendola MA, Hricak H, Mitchell DG, et al. Utilization of diagnostic studies in the pretreatment evaluation of invasive cervical cancer in the United States: results of intergroup protocol ACRIN 6651/GOG 183. J Clin Oncol 2005;23(30):7454–9.
24. Hricak H, Gatsonis C, Chi DS, et al. Role of imaging in pretreatment evaluation of early invasive cervical cancer: results of the Intergroup Study American College of Radiology Imaging Network 6651–Gynecologic Oncology Group 183. J Clin Oncol 2005; 23(36):9329–37.
25. Patel CN, Nazir SA, Khan Z, et al. 18F-FDG PET/CT of cervical carcinoma. Am J Roentgenol 2011; 196(5):1225–33.
26. Bellomi M, Bonomo G, Landoni F, et al. Accuracy of computed tomography and magnetic resonance imaging in the detection of lymph node involvement in cervix carcinoma. Eur Radiol 2005;15(12):2469–74.
27. Hori M, Kim T, Murakami T, et al. Uterine cervical carcinoma: preoperative staging with 3.0-T MR imaging—comparison with 1.5-T MR imaging. Radiology 2009;251(1):96–104.
28. Chung HH, Kang S-B, Cho JY, et al. Can preoperative MRI accurately evaluate nodal and parametrial invasion in early stage cervical cancer? Jpn J Clin Oncol 2007;37(5):370–5.
29. Landoni F, Maneo A, Colombo A, et al. Randomised study of radical surgery versus radiotherapy for stage Ib-IIa cervical cancer. Lancet 1997; 350(9077):535–40.
30. Peters WA, Liu PY, Barrett RJ, et al. Concurrent chemotherapy and pelvic radiation therapy compared with pelvic radiation therapy alone as adjuvant therapy after radical surgery in high-risk early-stage cancer of the cervix. J Clin Oncol 2000;18(8):1606–13.
31. Sedlis A, Bundy BN, Rotman MZ, et al. A randomized trial of pelvic radiation therapy versus no further therapy in selected patients with stage IB carcinoma of the cervix after radical hysterectomy and pelvic lymphadenectomy: a Gynecologic Oncology Group Study. Gynecol Oncol 1999;73(2):177–83.
32. Rockall AG, Cross S, Flanagan S, et al. The role of FDG-PET/CT in gynaecological cancers. Cancer Imaging 2012;12(1):49–65.
33. Punwani S. Diffusion weighted imaging of female pelvic cancers: concepts and clinical applications. Eur J Radiol 2011;78(1):21–9.
34. Dhanda S, Thakur M, Kerkar R, et al. Diffusion-weighted imaging of gynecologic tumors: diagnostic pearls and potential pitfalls. RadioGraphics 2014; 34(5):1393–416.
35. Seki H, Azumi R, Kimura M, et al. Stromal invasion by carcinoma of the cervix: assessment with dynamic MR imaging. Am J Roentgenol 1997;168(6): 1579–85.
36. Pandharipande PV, Choy G, del Carmen MG, et al. MRI and PET/CT for triaging stage IB clinically operable cervical cancer to appropriate therapy: decision analysis to assess patient outcomes. Am J Roentgenol 2009;192(3):802–14.
37. Punwani S. Contrast enhanced MR imaging of female pelvic cancers: established methods and emerging applications. Eur J Radiol 2011;78(1): 2–11.
38. Hricak H, Hamm B, Semelka RC, et al. Carcinoma of the uterus: use of gadopentetate dimeglumine in MR imaging. Radiology 1991;181(1):95–106.
39. Sakuragi N. Up-to-date management of lymph node metastasis and the role of tailored lymphadenectomy in cervical cancer. Int J Clin Oncol 2007; 12(3):165–75.
40. Kaur H, Silverman PM, Iyer RB, et al. Diagnosis, staging, and surveillance of cervical carcinoma. Am J Roentgenol 2003;180(6):1621–31.
41. Grigsby PW. The contribution of new imaging techniques in staging cervical cancer. Gynecol Oncol 2007;107(1):S10–2.
42. Lin G, Ho K-C, Wang J-J, et al. Detection of lymph node metastasis in cervical and uterine cancers by diffusion-weighted magnetic resonance imaging at 3T. J Magn Reson Imaging 2008;28(1):128–35.
43. Choi HJ, Roh JW, Seo S-S, et al. Comparison of the accuracy of magnetic resonance imaging and positron emission tomography/computed tomography in the presurgical detection of lymph node metastases in patients with uterine cervical carcinoma. Cancer 2006;106(4):914–22.
44. Park W, Park YJ, Huh SJ, et al. The usefulness of MRI and PET imaging for the detection of parametrial involvement and lymph node metastasis in patients with cervical cancer. Jpn J Clin Oncol 2005; 35(5):260–4.
45. Tanderup K, Georg D, Pötter R, et al. Adaptive management of cervical cancer radiotherapy. Semin Radiat Oncol 2010;20(2):121–9.
46. Kim HS, Kim CK, Park BK, et al. Evaluation of therapeutic response to concurrent chemoradiotherapy in patients with cervical cancer using diffusion-weighted MR imaging. J Magn Reson Imaging 2013; 37(1):187–93.
47. Jeong YY, Kang HK, Chung TW, et al. Uterine cervical carcinoma after therapy: CT and MR imaging findings. RadioGraphics 2003;23(4):969–81.
48. Levy A, Caramella C, Chargari C, et al. Accuracy of diffusion-weighted echo-planar MR imaging and ADC mapping in the evaluation of residual cervical

carcinoma after radiation therapy. Gynecol Oncol 2011;123(1):110–5.
49. Kuang F, Yan Z, Wang J, et al. The value of diffusion-weighted MRI to evaluate the response to radiochemotherapy for cervical cancer. Magn Reson Imaging 2014;32(4):342–9.
50. Chênevert J, Têtu B, Plante M, et al. Indication and method of frozen section in vaginal radical trachelectomy. Int J Gynecol Pathol 2009;28(5):480–8.
51. Hricak H, Yu KK. Radiology in invasive cervical cancer. Am J Roentgenol 1996;167(5):1101–8.
52. Scheidler J, Heuck AF. Imaging of cancer of the cervix. Radiol Clin North Am 2002;40(3):577–90.
53. Havrilesky LJ, Kulasingam SL, Matchar DB, et al. FDG-PET for management of cervical and ovarian cancer. Gynecol Oncol 2005;97(1):183–91.
54. Sironi S, Buda A, Picchio M, et al. Lymph node metastasis in patients with clinical early-stage cervical cancer: detection with integrated FDG PET/CT. Radiology 2006;238(1):272–9.
55. Reinhardt MJ, Ehritt-Braun C, Vogelgesang D, et al. Metastatic lymph nodes in patients with cervical cancer: detection with MR imaging and FDG PET. Radiology 2001;218(3):776–82.
56. Hricak H, Swift PS, Campos Z, et al. Irradiation of the cervix uteri: value of unenhanced and contrast-enhanced MR imaging. Radiology 1993;189(2):381–8.
57. Flueckiger F, Ebner F, Poschauko H, et al. Cervical cancer: serial MR imaging before and after primary radiation therapy–a 2-year follow-up study. Radiology 1992;184(1):89–93.

MR Imaging in Gynecologic Brachytherapy

Jessica B. Robbins, MD[a,*], Elizabeth A. Sadowski, MD[a,b], Shruti Jolly, MD[c], Katherine E. Maturen, MD, MS[d,e]

KEYWORDS

• Cervical cancer • Radiation therapy • Brachytherapy

KEY POINTS

- There are 2 main classes of brachytherapy applicators: intracavitary and interstitial.
- Image-guided adaptive brachytherapy (IGABT) improves local control, increases overall survival, and minimizes toxicity to the adjacent organs at risk (OARs).
- After external beam radiation, the cervical tumor often becomes much smaller, more heterogenous, and more irregular in configuration.

INTRODUCTION

Radiotherapy (RT) has long been the mainstay in the treatment of advanced cervical cancer. Primary chemoradiation, composed of a combination of external beam RT (EBRT), intracavitary brachytherapy (BT) with or without interstitial needles, and cisplatin-based chemotherapy, is currently the standard of care for treatment of locally advanced (stage IIB and greater) and bulky stage IB2 tumors.[1–3] BT is also used in the adjuvant and recurrent settings for a subset of endometrial, vaginal, and vulvar cancers. Recent implementation of 3-D IGABT[4,5] has further improved patient outcomes. Magnetic resonance (MR)-based IGABT is gaining popularity in the United States. Development and implementation of a robust MR-based IGABT program requires close collaboration between radiologists and radiation oncologists. The purpose of this article is to familiarize radiologists with IGABT by describing its history, detailing MR imaging techniques, describing treatment considerations, and reviewing image interpretation.

HISTORY OF IMAGE-GUIDED ADAPTIVE BRACHYTHERAPY

Traditionally, gynecologic BT was prescribed according the Manchester principles.[6,7] Orthogonal radiographs of the pelvis were obtained with applicators in place. A 2-D point-based technique configuring a standard dose centered on a fixed point, point A, at predetermined distance from the applicators was then used,[8,9] commonly conforming to the Manchester technique. The prevailing

The authors have nothing to disclose.
[a] Department of Radiology, University of Wisconsin School of Medicine and Public Health, E3/311 Clinical Science Center, 600 Highland Avenue, Madison, WI 53792-3525, USA; [b] Department of Obstetrics and Gynecology, University of Wisconsin School of Medicine and Public Health, E3/311 Clinical Science Center, 600 Highland Avenue, Madison, WI 53792-3525, USA; [c] Department of Radiation Oncology, University of Michigan Health System, University Hospital Floor B2 Room C490, 1500 East Medical Center Drive, Ann Arbor, MI 48109, USA; [d] Department of Radiology, University of Michigan Health System, 1500 East Medical Center Drive, B1D530H, Ann Arbor, MI 48109-5030, USA; [e] Department of Obstetrics and Gynecology, University of Michigan Health System, 1500 East Medical Center Drive, B1D530H, Ann Arbor, MI 48109-5030, USA
* Corresponding author.
E-mail address: jrobbins@uwhealth.org

Magn Reson Imaging Clin N Am 25 (2017) 651–666
http://dx.doi.org/10.1016/j.mric.2017.03.006
1064-9689/17/

assumptions for the Manchester technique are that all tumors are uniform in size and shape and that the location of OARs are the same for all individuals.[9,10] The 2-D technique does not account for the changes in tumor configuration that occur as a result of the preceding EBRT or the changes in the position of the OARs as a result in the changing tumoral topography.[4,11] Not surprisingly, cervical cancers are uniform in neither size nor shape prior to EBRT.[12] Contrary to the assumptions of the 2-D technique, cervical tumors tend to become more complex and nonconcentric over the course of RT.[12] The 2-D technique is also unable to accurately account for the OARs in individual patients. In the setting of gynecologic malignancies, the OARs include the small bowel, urinary bladder, rectosigmoid colon, and vagina.

Modern IGABT incorporates cross-sectional imaging, such as CT and MR, allowing for prescription of dose to a 3-D tumor volume while concurrently considering the anatomy of the OARs. Additionally, IGABT yields a fourth dimension, a temporal component, which can account for changes in anatomy during imaging and treatment (ie, respiratory-induced organ motion) and/or longitudinal changes of tumor shrinkage over the course of treatment.[8,13] Real-time imaging during BT is not widely used in the setting of cervical cancer. There is significant change, however, in tumoral topography and adjacent OARs over the course of treatment[2,13]; therefore, the added benefit of the longitudinal imaging capacity of IGABT is paramount. Several studies have shown improved local control, better overall survival, and reduction in toxicity to adjacent OARs in the setting of IGABT.[5,14–16] Tumors that respond poorly to initial EBRT also benefit from the IGABT technique because the dose can be more accurately tailored to the residual tumor than was previously possible in the age of the 2-D technique.[4]

CONTEMPORARY MAGNETIC RESONANCE GUIDANCE FOR BRACHYTHERAPY TREATMENT PLANNING

Imaging Technique

To optimize the utility of MR for BT treatment planning, patients should have a complete diagnostic pelvic MR imaging prior to the initiation of therapy (pre-RT MR imaging) and subsequently during BT fractions (BT MR imaging). Pre-RT MR imaging assists with disease staging of the primary malignancy[1] or delineating the extent of recurrent disease in the pelvis.[17] For gynecologic IGABT, BT MR imaging is ideally obtained while the BT applicators are in situ. Because the most substantial changes in tumor topography occur over the course of EBRT, before initiation of BT,[12,13] it is optimal to incorporate BT MR imaging for at least the first fraction,[13] even if local infrastructure may not allow for MR imaging with every BT fraction. In situations where it is not possible to obtain BT MR imaging with the applicators in situ, it is best to obtain the BT MR imaging near the conclusion of EBRT to optimize BT planning.

Although physical examination is ultimately necessary for determination for vaginal invasion, evaluation of the vagina on pre-RT MR imaging is optimized by inserting vaginal contrast, such as gel[2,18] (**Fig. 1**). Vaginal gel distends the lumen of

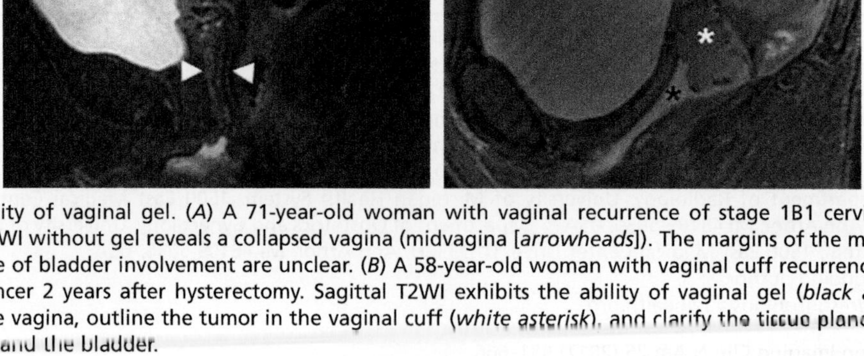

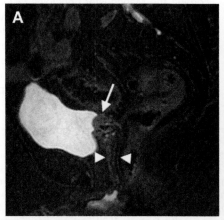

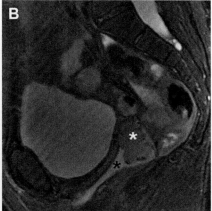

Fig. 1. Utility of vaginal gel. (*A*) A 71-year-old woman with vaginal recurrence of stage 1B1 cervical cancer. Sagittal T2WI without gel reveals a collapsed vagina (midvagina [*arrowheads*]). The margins of the mass (*arrow*) and degree of bladder involvement are unclear. (*B*) A 58-year-old woman with vaginal cuff recurrence of endometrial cancer 2 years after hysterectomy. Sagittal T2WI exhibits the ability of vaginal gel (*black asterisk*) to distend the vagina, outline the tumor in the vaginal cuff (*white asterisk*), and clarify the tissue planes between the tumor and the bladder.

the vagina and reduces redundancy in the walls. This technique allows for more accurate determination of vaginal invasion and improves the ability to determine the extent of bladder or rectal invasion, if present.[18] During BT MR imaging, the vagina is distended with packing material, instruments, and applicators; therefore, there is limited utility for vaginal gel during BT MR imaging.

A pelvic surface coil is sufficient for both pre-RT MR imaging and BT MR imaging. Intracavitary coils are not recommended because the local anatomy is altered by the presence of the coil. Because BT is rendered without the coil in place, imaging for the purposes of planning should be obtained with the pelvic organs in their native orientation.[2] Bowel preparation prior to BT fraction is optional.[2] Motion artifact from enteric peristalsis can have an impact on pelvic imaging. Some centers include an antiperistaltic agent, such as glucagon, prior to imaging.[2]

Example scan parameters for pre-RT MR imaging and BT MR imaging are provided in **Table 1** and **Table 2**. Standard diagnostic MR imaging of the pelvis (pre-RT MR imaging) includes a coronal single-shot fast spin-echo sequence to include the pelvis and kidneys (evaluating for renal collecting system obstruction), sagittal T2-weighted imaging (T2WI) fast spin-echo with or without fat-saturation, axial T2WI without fat-saturation (often oblique perpendicular to the long axis of the cervix), sagittal T1-weighted imaging (T1W1) with fat-saturation before and after gadolinium-based contrast, and axial diffusion-weighted (DW) (often oblique perpendicular to the long axis of the cervix).

The Gynaecological Groupe Européen de Curiethérapie and the European Society for Therapeutic Radiology and Oncology (GYN GEC-ESTRO) Working Group has published basic parameters for BT MR imaging.[2] GYN GEC-ESTRO requires imaging the pelvis in 3 T2WI planes—axial, coronal, and sagittal—each oblique with respect to the cervix; fat saturation is not applied to these images.[2] Optional sequences include an axial T2WI without fat saturation in the standard axial plane (ie, perpendicular to the MR gantry) and T1WI images. The cranial-caudal extent of the axial images should extend from above the uterine fundus through at least 3 cm below the caudal extent of the vaginal applicator(s) or through the entire vagina in the instance of distal vaginal tumor.[2]

Treatment Considerations

For primary treatment of locally advanced cervical cancer, the initial step of gynecologic RT is EBRT with concurrent cisplatin-based chemotherapy. The goal of EBRT is to shrink the primary tumor, treat microscopic nodal disease within the pelvis, and treat macroscopic nodal pelvic and/or para-ortic disease, if present, with an external-beam boost.[9] The goal of BT is to treat residual disease within the cervix and local surrounding tissues.[9] A combination of EBRT and BT may also be used in the adjuvant or recurrent setting for endometrial, vaginal, or vulvar cancer.[19] Recurrent tumors are often large and complex in shape, making them ideal candidates for IGABT.[19,20]

BT can be administered via low-dose rate (LDR) or high-dose rate (HDR) techniques. LDR is administered continuously for prolonged periods of time requiring an in-patient hospital stay for the duration of therapy,[21] whereas HDR can be administered over several fractions, often in an outpatient setting. In the setting of primary cervical cancer, LDR and HDR have been shown to have equivalent outcomes with respect to mortality, pelvic recurrence, and associated OARs complications.[9,21,22] Because of convenience, patient and operator preference, and decrease in radiation exposure to patient and staff, HDR is the contemporary treatment of choice in the setting of primary cervical cancer.

The choice between LDR and HDR for vaginal masses (either recurrent endometrial or cervical cancer or advanced primary vulvar or vaginal cancer) is less clear; specifically, a single continuous LDR prescription and up to twice-daily fractions of HDR are acceptable options.[19,23,24] For vaginal tumors less than or equal to 0.5 cm in thickness, intracavitary BT (using a vaginal cylinder, paired colpostats and ovoids, or a ring device) alone is sufficient.[19] For larger vaginal masses (>0.5 cm), however, the high dose needed for tumor coverage has unacceptable vaginal epithelial dose from an intracavitary approach and interstitial implants are usually needed (discussed in more detail later).[19]

For each HDR fraction, patients are generally anesthetized with either general or spinal techniques for the duration of instrumentation, imaging, treatment planning, and treatment phases.[9,19] Patients undergoing LDR BT generally have spinal anesthesia with an epidural catheter.[19] Therefore, it is imperative that all members of the care team are aware of MR safety considerations.[25] In the setting of spinal anesthesia, care must be taken to implant an MR-compatible spinal catheter. In the setting of general anesthesia, the team must be prepared to transport and care for patients within zone IV, the room in which the MR scanner is located.[25]

The physical layout of each local institution determines which transportation factors must be

Table 1
Example magnetic resonance parameters for preradiotherapy MR imaging

Sequence	Orientation	Coverage	Parameters: Fat Saturation	Repetition Time (ms)	Echo Time (ms)	Echo Train Length	Maximum Field of View (cm)	Matrix (Frequency × Phase)	Number of Excitations	Slice Thickness (mm)/ Interval (mm)	Comments
T2 SSFSE	Coronal	Kidneys through pelvis	No	Minimum	90		36–40	256 × 256	2	6/1	Evaluate for renal collecting system dilation
T2 FRFSE	Sagittal	Acetabulum to acetabulum	Yes	3400	90	21	26	320 × 256	3	5/1.5	
T2 FRFSE	Axial	L4-L5 interspace through perineum; may oblique perpendicular to long axis of cervix	No	3400	86	21	26	320 × 256	3	5/1.5	
T1 FSE without contrast	Axial	L4-L5 interspace through perineum	Yes	600	9	4	26	256 × 224	4	5/1.5	
T1 FSE with contrast	Axial	L4-L5 interspace through perineum	Yes	600	9	4	28	256 × 192	1	4.6/1	40 s after contrast
T1 FSE with contrast	Sagittal	Acetabulum to acetabulum	Yes	600	9	4	28	256 × 192	1	4.6/1	90 s after contrast
T1 FSE with contrast	Axial	Level of the left renal vein through perineum	Yes	600	9	4	32	256 × 192	2	6/1	180 s after contrast
DW	Axial	L4-L5 interspace through perineum; may oblique perpendicular to long axis of cervix	No	10,000	65		32	160 × 160		3/0.5	b values (s/mm^2): 0, 500

Vaginal gel is instilled prior to imaging. Glucagon may be considered.
Abbreviations: FRFSE, fast-recovery fast spin-echo; FSE, fast spin-echo; SSFSE, single-shot fast spin-echo.

Table 2
Example magnetic resonance parameters for brachytherapy MR imaging

			Parameters								
Sequence	**Orientation**	**Coverage**	**Fat Saturation**	**Repetition Time (ms)**	**Echo Time (ms)**	**Echo Train Length**	**Maximum Field of View (cm)**	**Matrix (Frequency × Phase)**	**Number of Excitations**	**Slice Thickness (mm)/ Interval (mm)**	**Comments**
Optional T2 FRFSE	Sagittal	Acetabulum to acetabulum	Yes	3000	90	21	26	320 × 256	2	5/1.5	First opportunity to ensure adequate position of applicators. Use to prescribe subsequent sequences.
T2 FRFSE	Axial oblique, perpendicular to long axis of tandem/cervix	1 cm above uterine fundus to 3 cm below caudal margin of vaginal applicators	No	3000	90	21	26	320 × 256	3	5/1	
T2 FRFSE	Sagittal oblique, parallel to long axis of tandem/ cervix	Acetabulum to acetabulum	No	3000	90	21	26	320 × 256	3	5/1	
T2 FRFSE	Coronal oblique, parallel to long axis of tandem/ cervix	Body of uterus and entire tumor	No	3000	90	21	26	320 × 256	3	5/1	

(*continued on next page*)

Table 2
(*continued*)

			Parameters							
Sequence	Orientation	Coverage	Fat Saturation	Repetition Time (ms)	Echo Time (ms)	Echo Train Length	Maximum Field of View (cm)	Matrix (Frequency × Phase)	Number of Excitations	Slice Thickness (mm)/ Interval (mm)	Comments
Optional T2 FRFSE	Axial, perpendicular to the MR gantry	1 cm above uterine fundus to 3 cm below caudal margin of vaginal applicators	No	3000	90	21	26	320 × 256	3	5/1	
Optional high-resolution T2 FRFSE	Axial oblique, perpendicular to long axis of tandem/cervix	1 cm above uterine fundus to 3 cm below caudal margin of vaginal applicators	No	3000	90	21	26	320 × 256	3	2/interleaved	This could replace the axial oblique T2 FSE. With near isotropic voxels, this can be reconstructed in multiple planes by some planning software.
Optional axial T1 FSE	Axial, perpendicular to the MR gantry	1 cm above uterine fundus to 3 cm below caudal margin of vaginal applicators	No	625	9	4	26	256 × 192	2	5/1	

MR compatible applicators are placed prior to imaging.
Abbreviations: FRFSE, fast-recovery fast spin-echo; FSE, fast spin-echo.

considered. In some institutions, the MR scanner is located within the radiation oncology department itself, in which case the transportation demands are minimal. In other institutions, the MR scanner is distant from the radiation oncology department, requiring substantial transportation to and from the scanner. The greater the transportation distance, the more time the care team has to monitor patients in transport. Regardless of the geographic separation between the radiation oncology department and MR scanner, great care needs to be taken to ensure that the applicators are not disturbed during patient transfer to and from the MR gantry and during transportation.

Brachytherapy Applicators and Instruments

It is important to understand the BT applicators and instruments that are used in conjunction with IGABT. There are 2 broad classes of applicators: intracavitary and interstitial. Intracavitary applicators are seated within the uterus or vagina and do not penetrate anatomic tissue planes. Interstitial applicators are placed directly into the soft tissues of the pelvis (often the parametria) or into recurrent tumors in the vaginal cuff, pelvis, and/or perineum.

Patients with an in situ uterus have a tandem advanced through the cervix into the endometrial canal. The tandem is a hollow catheter with gentle angulation to mimic the version of the uterus. The radiation source, mounted on a flexible insertion device usually advanced by an afterloader machine, is routed through the central channel of the tandem. Optimally, the tandem is situated such that the tip abuts the fundal endometrium but does not penetrate into or through the myometrium (**Fig. 2**). Transabdominal ultrasound may be used during instrumentation to ensure appropriate positioning and prevent uterine perforation.[26] Some practitioners place an indwelling intrauterine tube (Smit sleeve) into the cervical os concurrent with the initial tandem placement; the Smit sleeve remains in place over the course of several BT fractions easing the task of cervical dilation and tandem placement.[27,28] The Smit sleeve should align with the axis of the endocervical canal and should not extend beyond the cervix, and the caudal margin should be flush with the ectocervix (**Fig. 3**).

The 2 most common vaginal applicators are paired colpostats and ovoids (see **Fig. 2**) or a ring device (**Fig. 4**). Both types of applicators sit flush with the cervix or in the vaginal fornices and may contain fine perforations to optionally guide interstitial needles into the parametria.[4,29] Both the ovoids and the ring serve to displace the vaginal mucosa from the epicenter of the radiation field. Each ovoid is situated in one of the lateral vaginal fornices whereas the ring encircles the cervix at the vaginal apex. The colpostat is a linear device, which is angulated approximately 30° at the cephalad end; the ovoid is threaded on the angulated portion of the colpostat (see **Fig. 2**C). Like the tandem, both the colpostat and ring applicator are hollow; the radiation source courses through the central source channel. In the setting of paired ovoids and colpostats, a flange is placed on the tandem, advanced until it sits flush with the inferior margin of the cervix, and holds the paired ovoids snug with the tandem (see **Fig. 2**A, B). In the setting of a ring device, the tandem courses through the center of the ring (see **Fig. 4**).

The vagina is packed with gauze to secure the instruments in place and to additionally displace the vaginal walls from the radiation source[2] (see **Fig. 2**D). The gauze should remain inferior to the caudal margin of the vaginal applicators and should not be interposed between the cervix and the applicators. A rectal retractor is situated in the posterior vagina to posteriorly displace the rectum from the radiation source (see **Figs. 2**B and **4**B).

In other settings, direct placement of BT applicators into tumor is needed. Interstitial needles allow a radiation oncologist to achieve adequate tumor coverage in locally advanced disease, especially in the lateral extent of the tumor and in the setting of bulky (>0.5 cm) vaginal recurrence or advanced vaginal cancer.[19,20,23,29] The needles alter the configuration of the radiation field such that it extends further into the parametrial space(s), fully encompassing the target while minimizing dose to the OARs.[29] Like the other applicators, the interstitial needles are hollow to accommodate the temporary insertion of the radiation source. Interstitial needles should follow a relatively straight course. They should be positioned within the parametria and/or measurable residual tumor.[19] Care must be taken to avoid placement of interstitial needles into adjacent bladder, rectum, and/or small bowel.[19] When used in conjunction with vaginal intracavitary applicators, interstitial needles are passed through the perforations in either the ovoids or ring into either one or bilateral parametrial regions (**Fig. 5**).

When intracavitary applicators are not indicated, interstitial needles can be passed through the perineum in a free-hand technique or through

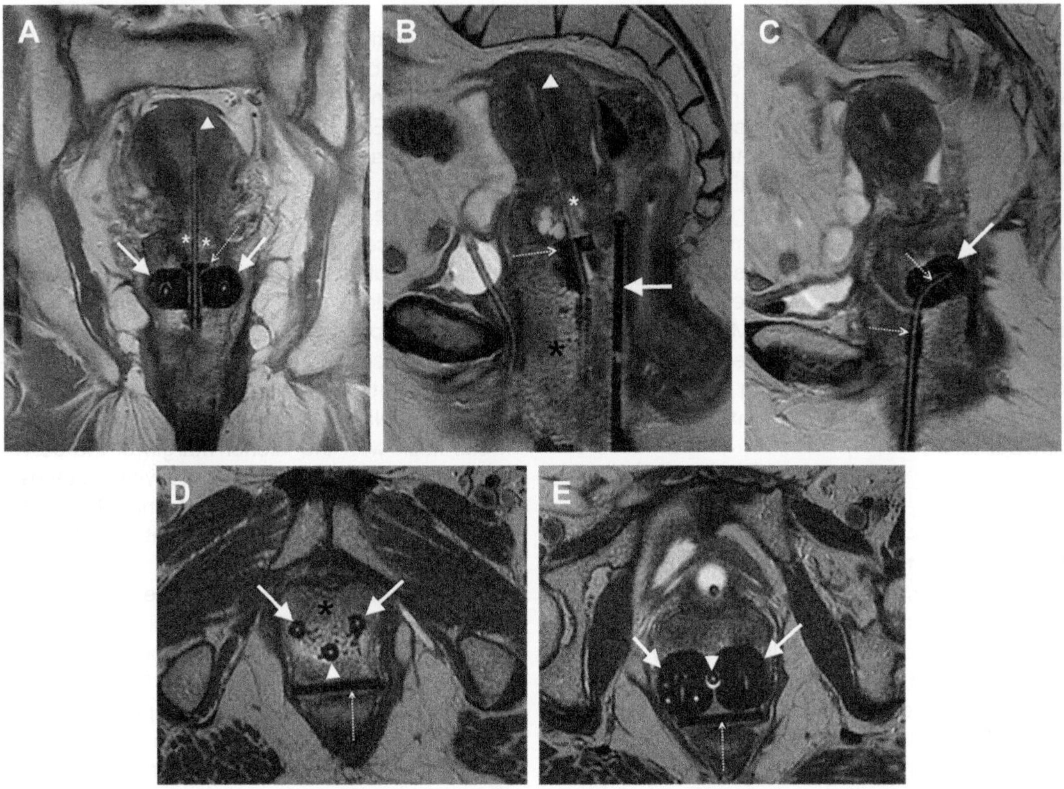

Fig. 2. Applicator anatomy. A 44-year-old woman with stage IIB cervical cancer and BT applicators in place. (*A*) Coronal T2WI without fat saturation. Minimal residual infiltrative tumor (*white asterisks*) remains within the cervix. Tandem (*arrowhead*) is situated centrally within the endometrial canal and is fully inserted. Paired ovoids (*solid white arrows*) lie within the vaginal fornices. Flange (*dashed white arrow*) is flush with cervix. (*B*) Sagittal T2WI in midline illustrates residual infiltrative tumor (*white asterisk*), with flange (*dashed white arrow*) flush with the cervix in midline. Vagina is packed with gauze (*black asterisk*) and the rectal retractor (*white arrow*) is situated in posterior vagina. Tandem (*arrowhead*) is fully inserted within the endometrial canal. (*C*) Right paramidline sagittal T2WI demonstrates one of the colpostats (*white dashed arrows*); the ovoid (*solid white arrow*) is seated on the angulated end of the colpostat. (*D*) Axial T2WI in low pelvis shows gauze packing (*black asterisk*) and rectal retractor (*dashed white arrow*). Paired colpostats (*white arrows*) and tandem (*arrowhead*) are seen in cross-section. (*E*) Axial T2WI in midpelvis shows paired ovoids (*solid white arrows*) in fornices. Tandem (*arrowhead*) and rectal retractor (*dashed white arrow*) are seen in cross-section.

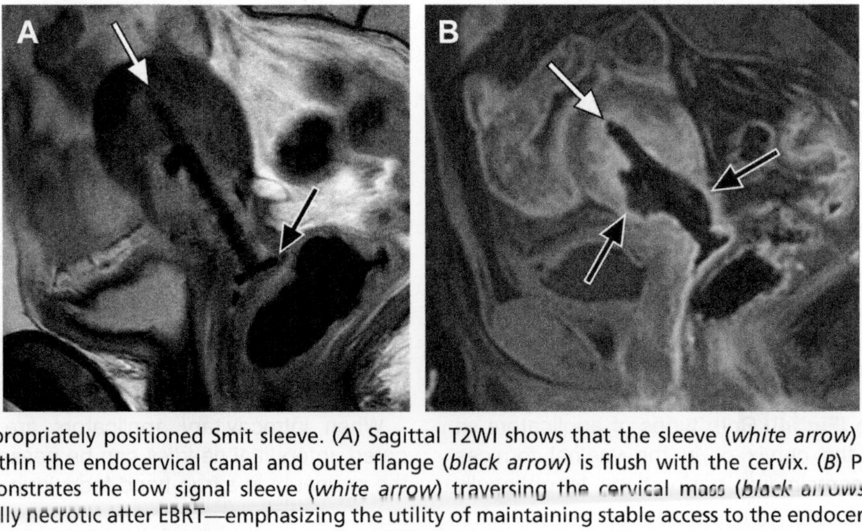

Fig. 3. Appropriately positioned Smit sleeve. (*A*) Sagittal T2WI shows that the sleeve (*white arrow*) is centrally aligned within the endocervical canal and outer flange (*black arrow*) is flush with the cervix. (*B*) Postcontrast T1WI demonstrates the low signal sleeve (*white arrow*) traversing the cervical mass (*black arrows*), which is now partially necrotic after EBRT—emphasizing the utility of maintaining stable access to the endocervical canal.

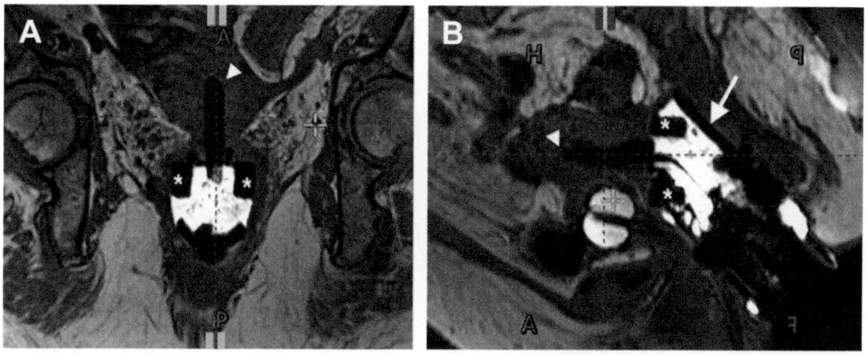

Fig. 4. Ring and tandem applicator on coronal (*A*) and sagittal (*B*) PDWI. The tip of the tandem (*arrowhead*) is situated within the endometrial canal. The ring (*asterisks*), seen in cross-section in both images, sits flush with the cervix. The rectal retractor (*arrow*) is positioned posteriorly within the vagina.

a perineal template.[19] In some cases of recurrent cancer, interstitial needles may be placed in conjunction with gynecologic surgeons performing laparoscopy; the radiation oncologist advances the interstitial needles through the perineum while the surgeon laparoscopically guides the needle within the pelvis, assuring adequate placement.[19] If a perineal template is used, it is secured to the perineum for the duration of treatment (**Fig. 6**). The perforations in a perineal template are evenly spaced, allowing for uniform interstitial needle distribution. Whether the interstitial needles are placed free-hand or are guided through a perineal template or vaginal applicator, less than or equal to 1 cm spacing between the needles is the goal; ideally, the target tissue is encompassed with a 1-cm margin[19] (see **Fig. 6**).

For apical or upper vaginal tumors, a vaginal obturator (also referred to as a vaginal cylinder) is added to the perineal template.[19] The obturator is a cylindrical applicator and is advanced through the center of the perineal template into the vaginal cuff. Small grooves, coursing around the periphery of the obturator and running the length of the cylinder, guide the interstitial needles in a tight circumference around the periphery of the obturator.

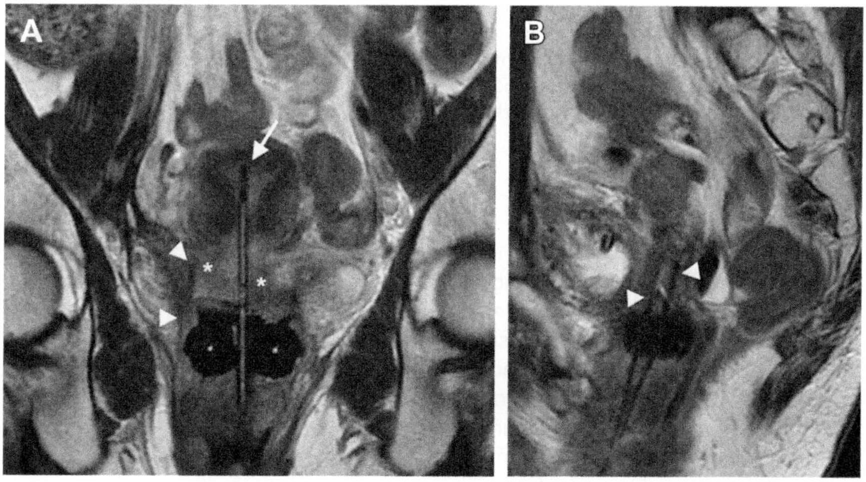

Fig. 5. Ring and tandem applicator with interstitial needles in a 44-year-old woman with stage 4 cervical cancer. (*A*) Coronal T2WI shows asymmetric residual tumor extending into the right parametrium (*white asterisks*), with lateral extension beyond optimal coverage with tandem geometry. Intracavitary applicators, including the tandem (*white arrow*) and ovoids, are appropriately positioned. Interstitital needles (*arrowheads*) have been advanced through perforations in the right ovoid into right parametrium. (*B*) Sagittal T2WI shows 2 of the right interstitial needles longitudinally (*arrowheads*).

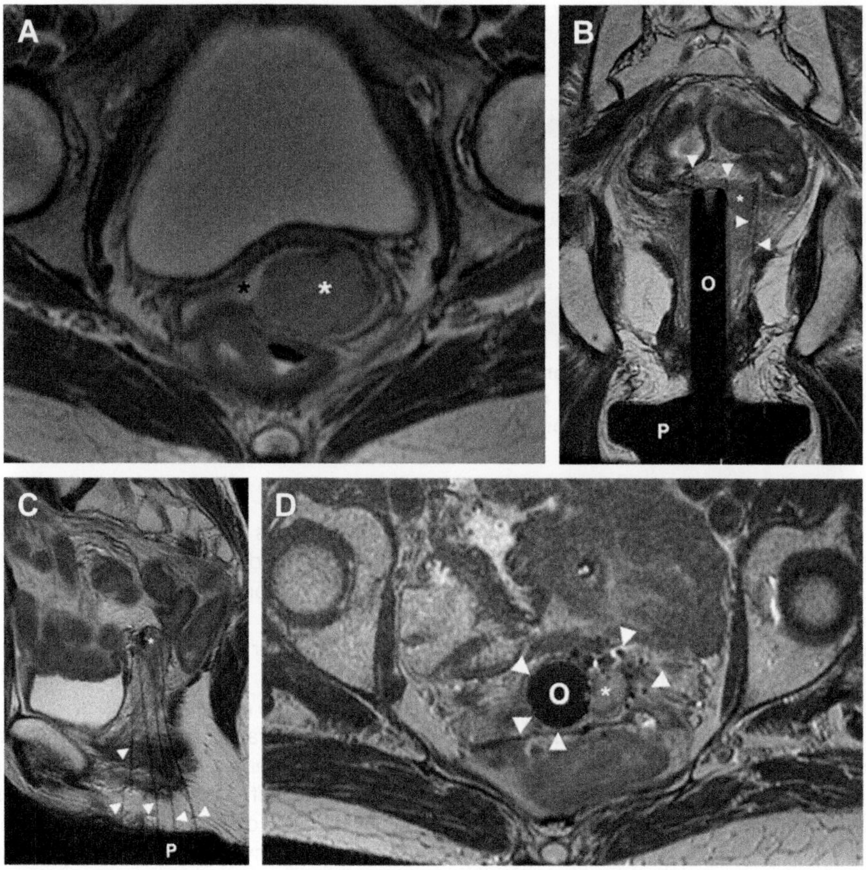

Fig. 6. Vaginal obturator with interstitial needles. A 58-year-old woman with vaginal cuff recurrence of endometrial cancer, too bulky to be treated with vaginal cylinder alone. (*A*) Axial T2WI shows the large soft tissue mass in the left vaginal cuff (*white asterisk*), outlined by vaginal gel (*black asterisk*). After EBRT, BT was administered via vaginal obturator, perineal template, and interstitial needles. (*B*) Coronal T2WI shows small residual tumor (*asterisk*) in the left vaginal cuff. Perineal template (P) is sutured to perineum and the cylindrical vaginal obturator (O) is advanced through the center of the template into the vaginal cuff, whereas interstitial needles (*arrowheads*) are advanced through the template according to the distribution of tumor. (*C*) Left paramidline sagittal T2WI shows perineal template (P) and interstitial needles (*arrowheads*) directed at the residual tumor (*asterisk*). (*D*) Axial T2WI at the cephalad aspect of the obturator (O) shows more than 20 interstitial needles (*arrowheads*) visible as punctate signal voids around the residual tumor (*asterisk*).

IMAGE INTERPRETATION

Techniques for primary diagnosis and staging of cervical cancer on MR are described in detail elsewhere.[1,18,30] Pre-RT MR imaging assists with pelvic staging and helps radiation oncologists forecast the type of BT needed for individual patients. The configuration of the primary tumor before EBRT may inform the configuration of IGABT that is used. Uniformly circumferential tumors likely are treated with a standard intracavitary tandem and ovoid or ring and tandem set up (see **Figs. 2** and **4**), both of which result in a pear-shaped radiation field; the target includes residual disease, the entire uterus, and immediate parametria.[4,9] Interstitial needles guided through the vaginal applicators may be placed directly into tumors with extensive or asymmetric parametrial invasion and/or unfavorable response after EBRT[29] (see **Fig. 5**). In the setting of vaginal recurrence or advanced primary vulvar cancer, the combination of intracavitary and interstitial applicators depends on the tumor configuration[19] (see **Fig. 6**). Interstitial needles allow a radiation oncologist to alter the configuration of the radiation field such that it extends further into the parametrial space(s), fully encompassing the target, while minimizing dose to the OARs.[29]

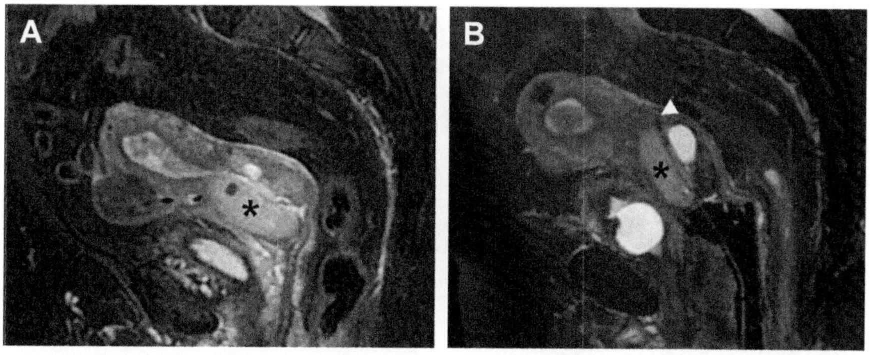

Fig. 7. Large residual tumor after EBRT. An 81-year-old woman with stage 1B2 cervical cancer. (*A*) Sagittal T2WI at diagnosis shows a large mass centered within the anterior lip of the cervix (*asterisk*). The tumor is confined to the cervix, but due to the patient's age and medical comorbidities, she was treated with primary chemoradiation rather than surgery. (*B*) Sagittal T2WI after EBRT shows residual tumor (*asterisk*). Additionally, the tandem was malpositioned (*arrowhead*); the tip of the tandem is situated at the level of the internal cervical os.

Prior to the initiation of RT, patients may also be imaged with standard CT of the abdomen and pelvis or PET/CT to identify factors that may affect the EBRT field, such as pelvic or paraaortic lymph nodes, which are treated with an EBRT boost.[9] Alternatively, if distant metastatic disease is identified, RT may not be indicated.

After EBRT, the tumor may be much smaller, more heterogenous, and more irregular in configuration in response to EBRT but usually remains intermediate to high signal intensity on T2WI.[1,12,18] Therefore, radiation oncologists can contour the margins of the target volume (the tissue to be treated), based on the oblique T2WI obtained at BT MR imaging[2,31] (**Table 2**). It is important to describe large volume and/or asymmetric residual tumor (see **Figs. 5**A; **Fig. 7**A) and its distribution on BT MR imaging because it may alter the IGABT approach. Similarly, enlarging pelvic lymph nodes should be noted because this could be a sign of disease that is either unresponsive to EBRT or excluded from the EBRT field. After EBRT, some metastatic lymph nodes may undergo cystic necrosis; their numerous locules may have the appearance of ovaries with multiple follicles (**Fig. 8**). The ovaries become atrophic, however, and decrease in signal intensity after EBRT[32]; therefore, they are small and dark on T2WI and contain few, if any, follicles. Alternatively, other metastatic lymph nodes are necrotic prior to the initiation of RT; these may involute over the course of therapy (**Fig. 9**).

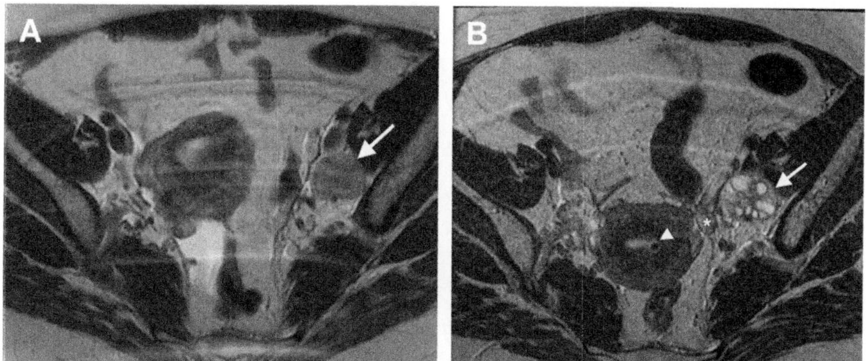

Fig. 8. Cystic necrosis of pelvic lymph nodes in a 44-year-old woman with stage 2B cervical cancer after EBRT. (*A*) At diagnosis, there were several bulky pelvic nodes, including a 2.5-cm solid left external iliac lymph node (*arrow*). (*B*) After EBRT, the left external iliac lymph node had undergone cystic necrosis (*arrow*). The multiple loculations could be mistaken for ovarian follicles; however, the normal but atrophic left ovary is situated along the medial margin of the lymph node (*asterisk*). The tandem is appropriately positioned within the endometrial canal (*arrowhead*).

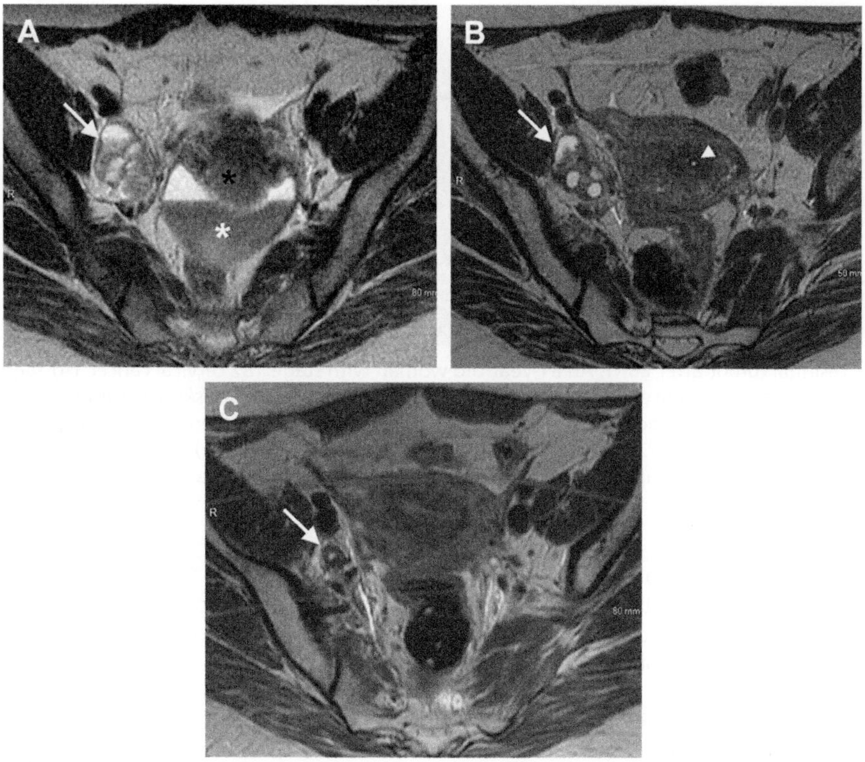

Fig. 9. Cystic necrosis of pelvic lymph nodes at diagnosis in a 37-year-old woman with stage 4 cervical cancer invading bladder. (*A*) The patient presented to the emergency department with heavy vaginal bleeding and a large amount of hematocolpos (*white asterisk*). The caudal aspect of the cervical tumor is included in this image (*black asterisk*). At presentation, the external iliac lymph nodes were enlarged and demonstrated cystic necrosis (*arrow*). (*B*) At BT MR imaging, the right external iliac lymph node has diminished in size (*arrow*). The tandem (*arrowhead*) is appropriately positioned within the endometrial cavity. (*C*) Four months after completion of chemoradiation, the right external iliac lymph node has nearly completely involuted (*arrow*).

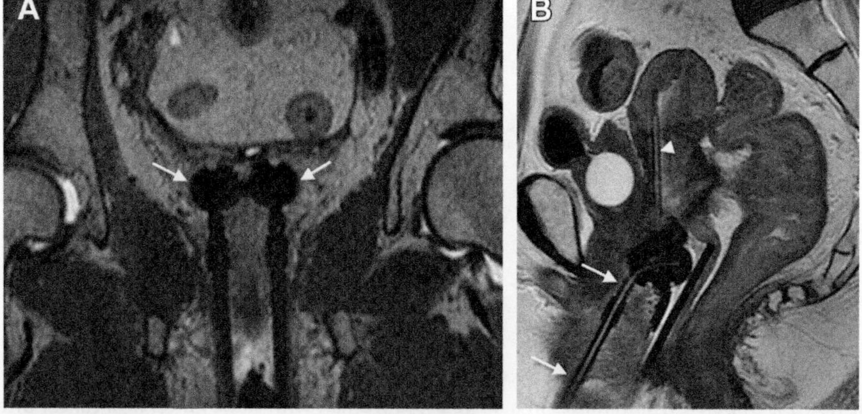

Fig. 10. Highlighting source channel with gadolinium-filled catheter. (*A*) A 32-year-old woman with recurrent cervical cancer after hysterectomy, treated with paired ovoids (*arrows*) and colpostats. The low-signal, empty central source channels of the paired colpostats are difficult to discern on this coronal T2WI. (*B*) Compare with this sagittal T2WI of a 61-year-old woman with stage IIB cervical cancer. Gadolinium-filled catheters are present within the source channels of the colpostat (*arrow*) and tandem (*arrowhead*).

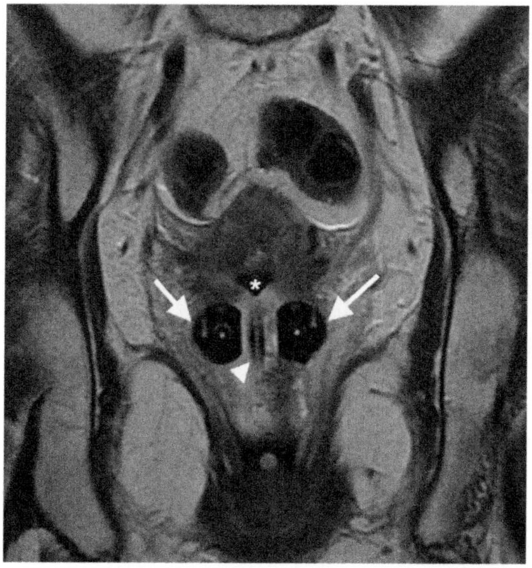

Fig. 11. Migration of vaginal applicators in a 35-year-old woman with stage 2B cervical cancer. Coronal T2WI without fat saturation shows that the flange (*asterisk*) is flush with the cervix but no longer in contact with the ovoids (*arrows*). Each of the paired ovoids is inferiorly and laterally displaced and is not in contact with the tandem (*arrowhead*).

All the gynecologic BT applicators are dark on T1WI and T2WI. At baseline, the source channel of the applicators is filled with air also resulting in dark T2WI signal. As a result, it can be nearly impossible to identify the location of the source channel (**Fig. 10**A), which is important for radiation dosimetry. To increase the conspicuity of the source channel on the T2WI planning sequences, a fine-caliber catheter filled with oil, copper sulfate,[4,33] or gadolinium can be advanced into the lumen of the tandem, colpostats, or ring applicator prior to BT MR imaging (see **Fig. 10**B); the catheter is removed prior to BT. Because the caliber of the interstitial needles is too small to accommodate an insert, the source channel cannot be similarly accentuated (see **Figs. 5**B and **6**B–D).

Routinely, the position of the applicators on BT MR imaging should be described. **Figs. 2–6** illustrate the expected appearance and location of the applicators. The tip of the tandem should be situated within the endometrial canal near the fundus. The vaginal applicator(s) should abut the inferior margin of the cervix. If interstitial needles are present, they should be situated within the parametrium and/or residual tumor. Unexpected positioning of the applicators on BT MR imaging should be described. Although transabdominal ultrasound may be used during initial positioning,[26] the tandem may migrate during patient transportation and/or transfer to the MR gantry (see **Fig. 7**A). Similarly, the vaginal or interstitial applicators may migrate (**Fig. 11**); the interstitial needles may pierce adjacent structures, such as the bladder, rectum, sigmoid, or small bowel (**Fig. 12**); or the Smit sleeve may have been malpositioned (**Fig. 13**). It is even possible for the tandem to perforate through the fundal myometrium or friable cervical tumor (**Fig. 14**) or for the vaginal obturator to perforate through the vaginal cuff (**Fig. 15**). Finally, all devices and applicators are removed from patients at the completion of treatment (unlike LDR approaches, such as prostate BT with

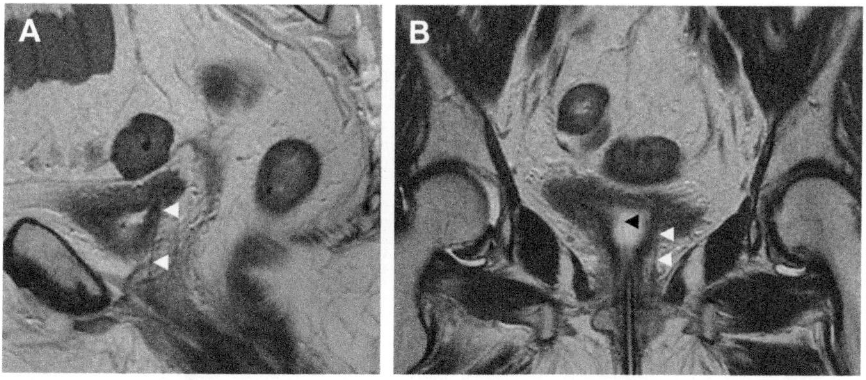

Fig. 12. Malpositioned interstitial needles in a 56-year-old woman with vaginal squamous cell carcinoma. This patient was not a surgical candidate and was, therefore, treated with BT administered via interstitial needles. (*A*) Sagittal and (*B*) coronal T2WI illustrate interstitial needles piercing the posterior wall of the bladder (*white arrowheads*) and within the bladder lumen (*black arrowhead*).

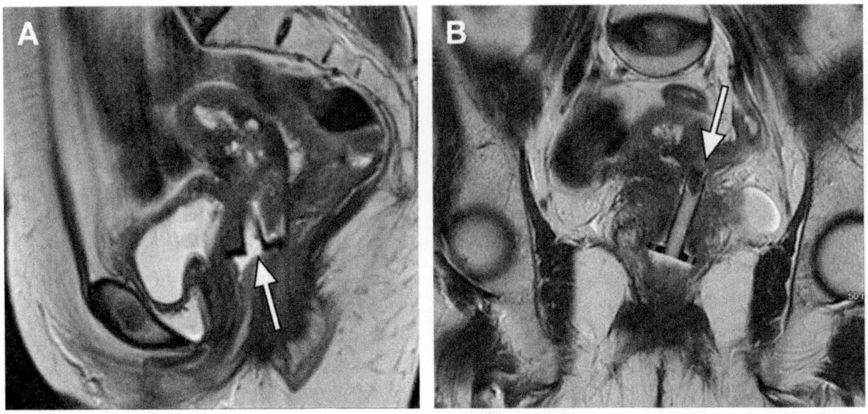

Fig. 13. Malpositioned Smit sleeve (*arrows*) on sagittal (*A*) and coronal (*B*) T2WI. Although the external flange is flush with the cervix, the sleeve is not centered within the canal, instead angling to the left and perforating tumor in the lower uterine segment.

permanent radioactive seeds), so there should not be any metallic devices or fragments in the pelvis on post-therapeutic imaging.

FUTURE DIRECTIONS

Functional imaging exploits the physiologic properties of tissue rather than relying solely on tissue composition. Current functional techniques include PET/CT for metabolic information; DW MR, which infers information about cellular density and integrity of cell membranes; and dynamic contrast-enhanced MR to evaluate microvascularity and perfusion of the tumor.[34–37] Although a detailed discussion of the breadth and capacity of functional imaging of the female pelvis is beyond the scope of this article, it may become increasingly important in the setting of personalized RT. For instance, regional alterations in DW signal or dynamic contrast-enhanced pattern within a tumor after EBRT may inform dose prescription for subsequent BT.[34,36] Hypoxic cervical cancers tend to respond poorly to RT; therefore, a functional MR sequence, such as blood oxygen level dependent, which predicts tissue oxygenation may hold promise in predicting response and/or guiding personalized RT prescriptions.[38,39]

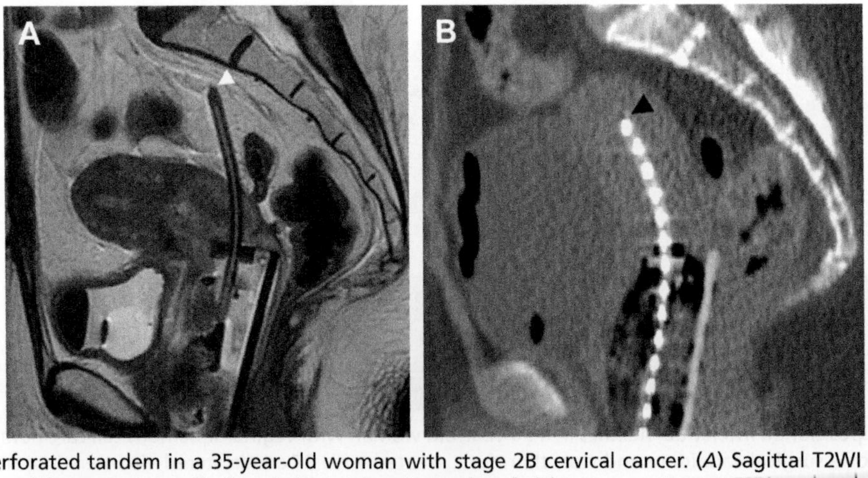

Fig. 14. Perforated tandem in a 35-year-old woman with stage 2B cervical cancer. (*A*) Sagittal T2WI documents perforation of the posterior wall of cervix by tandem (*arrowhead*). (*B*) Instruments were replaced and subsequent CT confirms appropriate position of the tandem within the endometrial canal (*arrowhead*).

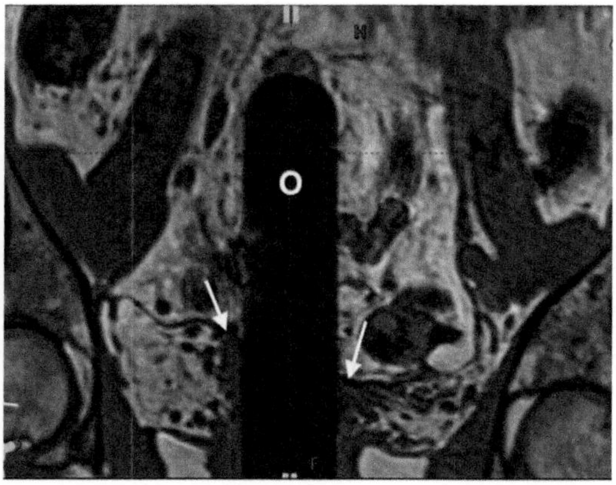

Fig. 15. Vaginal obturator (O) extends into the peritoneal space due to vaginal cuff (*arrows*) dehiscence, as seen on this sagittal proton-density weighted image from treatment planning software.

SUMMARY

The transition from historical BT planning methods to contemporary IGABT has improved local control, increased overall survival, and reduced toxicity to adjacent OARs in the setting of gynecologic malignancies. MR imaging is critical to the success of IGABT. Knowledge of applicator selection, expected applicator configuration, and projected natural history of gynecologic malignancies treated with RT will improve the interpretive ability of radiologists.

REFERENCES

1. Freeman SJ, Aly AM, Kataoka MY, et al. The revised FIGO staging system for uterine malignancies: implications for MR imaging. Radiographics 2012;32(6):1805–27.
2. Dimopoulos JC, Petrow P, Tanderup K, et al. Recommendations from Gynaecological (GYN) GEC-ESTRO Working Group (IV): Basic principles and parameters for MR imaging within the frame of image based adaptive cervix cancer brachytherapy. Radiother Oncol 2012;103(1):113–22.
3. Vale C, Tierney JF, Stewart LA, et al. Reducing uncertainties about the effects of chemoradiotherapy for cervical cancer: a systematic review and meta-analysis of individual patient data from 18 randomized trials. J Clin Oncol 2008;26(35):5802–12.
4. Tanderup K, Nielsen SK, Nyvang GB, et al. From point A to the sculpted pear: MR image guidance significantly improves tumour dose and sparing of organs at risk in brachytherapy of cervical cancer. Radiother Oncol 2010;94(2):173–80.
5. Rijkmans EC, Nout RA, Rutten IH, et al. Improved survival of patients with cervical cancer treated with image-guided brachytherapy compared with conventional brachytherapy. Gynecol Oncol 2014;135(2):231–8.
6. Nag S, Yacoub S, Copeland LJ, et al. Interstitial brachytherapy for salvage treatment of vaginal recurrences in previously unirradiated endometrial cancer patients. Int J Radiat Oncol Phys 2002;54(4):1153–9.
7. Nag S, Erickson B, Parikh S, et al. The American brachytherapy society recommendations for high-dose-rate brachytherapy for carcinoma of the endometrium. Int J Radiat Oncol Phys 2000;48(3):779–90.
8. Barkati M, Van Dyk S, Foroudi F, et al. The use of magnetic resonance imaging for image-guided brachytherapy. J Med Imaging Radiat Oncol 2010;54(2):137–41.
9. Narayan K, Barkati M, van Dyk S, et al. Image-guided brachytherapy for cervix cancer: from Manchester to Melbourne. Expert Rev Anticancer Ther 2010;10(1):41–6.
10. Sadozye AH, Reed N. A review of recent developments in image-guided radiation therapy in cervix cancer. Curr Oncol Rep 2012;14(6):519–26.
11. Tanderup K, Georg D, Potter R, et al. Adaptive management of cervical cancer radiotherapy. Semin Radiat Oncol 2010;20(2):121–9.
12. Mayr NA, Yuh WT, Taoka T, et al. Serial therapy-induced changes in tumor shape in cervical cancer and their impact on assessing tumor volume and treatment response. AJR Am J Roentgenol 2006;187(1):65–72.
13. Dimopoulos JC, Schirl G, Baldinger A, et al. MRI assessment of cervical cancer for adaptive radiotherapy. Strahlenther Onkol 2009;185(5):282–7.
14. Lindegaard JC, Fokdal LU, Nielsen SK, et al. MRI-guided adaptive radiotherapy in locally advanced cervical cancer from a Nordic perspective. Acta Oncol 2013;52(7):1510–9.
15. Potter R, Dimopoulos J, Georg P, et al. Clinical impact of MRI assisted dose volume adaptation and dose escalation in brachytherapy of locally advanced cervix cancer. Radiother Oncol 2007;83(2):148–55.
16. Narayan K, van Dyk S, Bernshaw D, et al. Comparative study of LDR (Manchester system) and HDR image-guided conformal brachytherapy of cervical cancer: patterns of failure, late complications, and survival. Int J Radiat Oncol Biol Phys 2009;74(5):1529–35.
17. Nishie A, Stolpen AH, Obuchi M, et al. Evaluation of locally recurrent pelvic malignancy: performance of T2- and diffusion-weighted MRI with image fusion. J Magn Reson Imaging 2008;28(3):705–13.
18. Robbins J, Kusmirek J, Barroilhet L, et al. Pitfalls in imaging of cervical cancer. Semin Roentgenol 2016;51(1):17–31.

19. Beriwal S, Demanes DJ, Erickson B, et al. American Brachytherapy Society consensus guidelines for interstitial brachytherapy for vaginal cancer. Brachytherapy 2012;11(1):68–75.
20. Yoshida K, Yamazaki H, Kotsuma T, et al. Treatment results of image-guided high-dose-rate interstitial brachytherapy for pelvic recurrence of uterine cancer. Brachytherapy 2015;14(4):440–8.
21. Viani GA, Manta GB, Stefano EJ, et al. Brachytherapy for cervix cancer: low-dose rate or high-dose rate brachytherapy - a meta-analysis of clinical trials. J Exp Clin Cancer Res 2009;28:47.
22. Hareyama M, Sakata K, Oouchi A, et al. High-dose-rate versus low-dose-rate intracavitary therapy for carcinoma of the uterine cervix: a randomized trial. Cancer 2002;94(1):117–24.
23. De Ieso PB, Mullassery V, Shrimali R, et al. Image-guided vulvovaginal interstitial brachytherapy in the treatment of primary and recurrent gynecological malignancies. Brachytherapy 2012;11(4):306–10.
24. Mahantshetty U, Kalyani N, Engineer R, et al. Reirradiation using high-dose-rate brachytherapy in recurrent carcinoma of uterine cervix. Brachytherapy 2014;13(6):548–53.
25. Expert Panel on MRS, Kanal E, Barkovich AJ, et al. ACR guidance document on MR safe practices: 2013. J Magn Reson Imaging 2013;37(3):501–30.
26. van Dyk S, Bernshaw D. Ultrasound-based conformal planning for gynaecological brachytherapy. J Med Imaging Radiat Oncol 2008;52(1):77–84.
27. Smit BJ, van Wijk AL. An improved, disposable indwelling intrauterine tube ("smit sleeve") not requiring retaining stitches for brachy-radiotherapy for carcinoma of the cervix. Eur J Gynaecol Oncol 2013;34(4):289–90.
28. Smit BJ, du Toit JP, Groenewald WA. An indwelling intrauterine tube to facilitate intracavitary radiotherapy of carcinoma of the cervix. Br J Radiol 1989;62(733):68–9.
29. Dimopoulos JC, Kirisits C, Petric P, et al. The Vienna applicator for combined intracavitary and interstitial brachytherapy of cervical cancer: clinical feasibility and preliminary results. Int J Radiat Oncol Biol Phys 2006;66(1):83–90.
30. Sala E, Wakely S, Senior E, et al. MRI of malignant neoplasms of the uterine corpus and cervix. AJR Am J Roentgenol 2007;188(6):1577–87.
31. Haie-Meder C, Potter R, Van Limbergen E, et al. Recommendations from Gynaecological (GYN) GEC-ESTRO Working Group (I): concepts and terms in 3D image based 3D treatment planning in cervix cancer brachytherapy with emphasis on MRI assessment of GTV and CTV. Radiother Oncol 2005;74(3):235–45.
32. Addley HC, Vargas HA, Moyle PL, et al. Pelvic imaging following chemotherapy and radiation therapy for gynecologic malignancies. Radiographics 2010;30(7):1843–56.
33. Haack S, Nielsen SK, Lindegaard JC, et al. Applicator reconstruction in MRI 3D image-based dose planning of brachytherapy for cervical cancer. Radiother Oncol 2009;91(2):187–93.
34. Barwick TD, Taylor A, Rockall A. Functional imaging to predict tumor response in locally advanced cervical cancer. Curr Oncol Rep 2013;15(6):549–58.
35. Kido A, Fujimoto K, Okada T, et al. Advanced MRI in malignant neoplasms of the uterus. J Magn Reson Imaging 2013;37(2):249–64.
36. Mayr NA, Huang Z, Wang JZ, et al. Characterizing tumor heterogeneity with functional imaging and quantifying high-risk tumor volume for early prediction of treatment outcome: cervical cancer as a model. Int J Radiat Oncol Biol Phys 2012;83(3): 972–9.
37. Sala E, Rockall A, Rangarajan D, et al. The role of dynamic contrast-enhanced and diffusion weighted magnetic resonance imaging in the female pelvis. Eur J Radiol 2010;76(3):367–85.
38. Kim CK, Park SY, Park BK, et al. Blood oxygenation level-dependent MR imaging as a predictor of therapeutic response to concurrent chemoradiotherapy in cervical cancer: a preliminary experience. Eur Radiol 2014;24(7):1514–20.
39. Hallac RR, Ding Y, Yuan Q, et al. Oxygenation in cervical cancer and normal uterine cervix assessed using blood oxygenation level-dependent (BOLD) MRI at 3T. NMR Biomed 2012;25(12): 1321–30.

PET/MR Imaging in Gynecologic Oncology

Michael A. Ohliger, MD, PhD[a,b,*], Thomas A. Hope, MD[a,c], Jocelyn S. Chapman, MD[d,1], Lee-may Chen, MD[d,2], Spencer C. Behr, MD[a,3], Liina Poder, MD[a,4]

KEYWORDS

• PET/MR imaging • PET • MR imaging • Ovarian cancer • Cervical cancer • Endometrial cancer • Gynecology

KEY POINTS

- MR imaging and PET individually play important and complementary roles in assessing gynecologic malignancy.
- MR imaging is the modality of choice for assessing local extension of tumors, whereas PET adds value for detection of distant metastases.
- Simultaneous PET/MR imaging systems combine these advantages while reducing radiation dose compared with PET/CT.
- Novel MR imaging and PET tracers promise to extend the applications of PET/MR imaging.

INTRODUCTION

MR imaging and PET play vital roles in evaluating patients with gynecologic malignancies. MR images of the pelvis provide excellent spatial resolution and soft tissue contrast to precisely define the local extent of pelvic tumors. Diffusion-weighted imaging (DWI) and dynamic contrast enhancement (DCE) provide additional information about tissue properties.[1] PET, which is usually performed using the glucose analog 2-Deoxy-2-[^{18}F]fluoroglucose (FDG), is valuable for detecting distant metastases. Gynecologic malignancies are, therefore, natural applications for simultaneous PET/MR imaging acquisitions, which combine the advantages of both modalities into a single scan.

The goal of this article is to review the ways that PET/MR imaging acquisitions can be applied to the evaluation of gynecologic malignancies. The technical challenges of performing a PET/MR imaging scan are reviewed focusing on how these challenges have an impact on the evaluation of gynecologic malignancies. The role of PET and MR imaging alone in the evaluation of cervical cancer, endometrial cancer, and ovarian cancer is discussed. Current efforts to combine the information between two scans, including exciting initial results using dedicated PET/MR imaging systems,

Dr T.A. Hope has received a research grant and is on the speakers' bureau for GE Healthcare. Dr S.C. Behr has received a research grant from GE Healthcare. Drs M.A. Ohliger, J.C. Chapman, L. Chen, and L. Poder have nothing to disclose.

[a] Department of Radiology and Biomedical Imaging, University of California, San Francisco, 505 Parnassus Avenue, M-391, San Francisco, CA 94143-0628, USA; [b] Department of Radiology, Zuckerberg San Francisco General Hospital, 1001 Potrero Avenue, San Francisco, CA 94110, USA; [c] Department of Radiology, San Francisco Veterans Affairs Hospital, Box VAMC, 4150 Clement Street, 2D007, San Francisco, CA 94121, USA; [d] Department of Obstetrics, Gynecology and Reproductive Sciences, University of California, San Francisco, 1825 Fourth Street, Third Floor, San Francisco, CA 94158, USA
[1] Box 1702, 550 16th Street, 7442, San Francisco, CA 94158.
[2] Box 1702, 550 16th Street, 7434, San Francisco, CA 94158.
[3] Box 0628, 505 Parnassus Avenue, 332A, San Francisco, CA 94117.
[4] Box 0336, 350 Parnassus, 307F, San Francisco, CA 94117.
* Corresponding author. Box 0628, 1001 Potrero Avenue, 1X60, San Francisco, CA 94110.
E-mail address: Michael.ohliger@ucsf.edu

Magn Reson Imaging Clin N Am 25 (2017) 667–684
http://dx.doi.org/10.1016/j.mric.2017.03.012

are discussed. Finally, future directions for this rapidly developing technology, including its use with novel emerging MR imaging and PET contrast agents, are discussed.

TECHNICAL FACTORS

Technical Challenges of the PET/MR Imaging Acquisition

Detection

Combining PET and MR imaging into a single acquisition is technically challenging. PET agents, such as FDG, emit positrons, which interact with nearby electrons and emit pairs of high-energy photons. Traditionally, the photons emitted during a PET scan have been detected using photomultiplier tubes, which are sensitive to large magnetic fields and, therefore, are inappropriate for an MR imaging environment. This problem has been solved by the development of solid state PET detectors, including avalanche photodiodes, which are not as sensitive to the presence of magnetic fields.[2]

Attenuation correction

High-energy photons that are produced within the body during PET scans are attenuated by overlying soft tissue, causing structures deep within the body to have lower signal intensities than structures closer to the surface. PET images require attenuation correction to adjust the signal intensity to account for differing amounts of attenuation. In integrated PET/CT scans, the CT acquisition serves as a direct reference for the amount of x-ray attenuation.[3] Because MR imaging acquisitions are not x-ray based, they do not provide a direct attenuation reference.[4] Therefore, alternative approaches must be used.

One of the most popular methods for MR imaging–based attenuation correction relies on a Dixon-based technique,[5] where two images are acquired, one with fat and water signals in phase and one with fat and water signal out of phase. Linear combinations of these two images generate maps of the fat and water content of the body. Segmenting the body into fat, soft tissue, and lungs allows an attenuation map to be generated.[6,7]

Accounting for the attenuation of cortical bone remains a challenge for MR imaging–based attenuation correction methods. Cortical bone produces significant x-ray attenuation but has very low signal on MR imaging scans. This potentially leads to error in quantification of standardized uptake values (SUVs), potentially leading to a 10% to 18% underestimation of SUVs.[8–10] This is expected to be particularly problematic within the pelvis, which is surrounded by bone.[10]

Accounting for cortical bone during attenuation correction is an evolving area of research. One approach uses predetermined atlases to correct for how much cortical bone is expected in each patient. Another approach relies on acquisition of a specialized MR imaging pulse sequence with either ultrashort or zero echo time. In these sequences, cortical bone signal can be measured and, therefore, accounted for in attenuation correction maps.[11,12]

Lung nodules

Lung imaging using MR imaging is challenging. Because air within the lung creates numerous areas of varying magnetic susceptibility, lung tissue has a very short T_2* and, therefore, low signal on most MR imaging pulse sequences. In addition, the spatial resolution of MR imaging acquisitions tends to be much lower than CT acquisitions. Both of these facts cause MR imaging to be less sensitive to small lung nodules compared with CT.[13] Ultrashort-echo and zero-echo time pulse potentially could be used to detect smaller nodules,[14] but this reduced sensitivity to small lung nodules remains a limitation of PET/MR imaging compared with PET/CT. The clinical importance of reduced sensitivity to small lung nodules has yet to be determined and likely varies with primary cancer type.

Respiratory and bowel motion

Respiratory and bowel motion occur continuously during the PET/MR imaging acquisition and are particularly significant when acquiring the abdomen and upper pelvis. Because the MR imaging acquisition is significantly longer than the CT acquisition, this can potentially have an impact on the anatomic localization of small peritoneal implants. Because MR imaging data are being acquired throughout the acquisition, the MR imaging data potentially serve as a reference for correcting for motion in the PET acquisition,[15–17] leading to improved image quality.[18]

Bladder filling

The urinary bladder filling over the course of an PET/MR imaging acquisition may cause changes in position of the uterus between the beginning and end of the acquisition.[19] Therefore, it is especially important that the PET and MR imaging acquisitions occur simultaneously. Otherwise, significant errors could occur in the localization of uterine tumors in particular.

MR Imaging Sequences for Gynecologic Malignancies

MR imaging of gynecologic malignancies is based on high-resolution imaging of the local extent of tumor, together with characterization of the chemical composition of tumor using fat-sensitive sequences. Further characterization of the tissue properties of tumors can be obtained using DWI and DCE (described later).

High-resolution T_2-weighted imaging

The most important pulse sequences for imaging the female pelvis are high-resolution T_2-weighted fast spin-echo (FSE) pulse sequences performed without fat saturation. The use of non–fat-saturated sequences allows for precise definition of tissue planes and serosal margins. T_2-weighted imaging also permits identification of fluid collections and ascites. For patients with cervical and endometrial malignancies, it can be useful to choose image planes that are perpendicular to the axis of the tumor to better assess parametrial or endometrial invasion.[20] There is currently interest in replacing traditional 2-D FSE pulse sequences with novel 3-D T_2-weighted FSE sequences (CUBE [GE Healthcare, Waukesha, WI] and T_2 SPACE [Siemens Medical Systems, Erlangen, Germany]).[21] Because 3-D FSE sequences obtain volumetric data they can, in principle, be reformatted into multiple image planes. Further research is required to determine if these reconstructed sequences have the same image contrast properties and diagnostic utility as their primarily acquired 2-D T_2 counterparts.

T_1-weighted gradient-echo sequences

Multiecho T_1 gradient-echo sequences acquired without fat saturation are obtained with a field of view that encompasses the entire pelvis. Microscopic fat within lesions can be detected by measuring signal loss that occurs when fat and water are acquired with their signals out of phase.[22] Macroscopic fat can be detected by looking for "India ink" artifact that occurs at lesion boundaries or by comparing T_1-weighted images acquired with and without fat saturation. Because blood products have intrinsically high signals on T_1-weighted sequences, these pulse sequences can aid in the diagnosis of endometriomas (**Fig. 1**A–C). The presence of macroscopic fat permits the diagnosis of definitively benign lesions, such as dermoid cysts (**Fig. 1**D–F).[22]

Contrast-enhanced spoiled gradient echo

T_1-weighted spoiled gradient-echo (SPGR) images with fat saturation can be obtained in a high-resolution volumetric acquisition and are

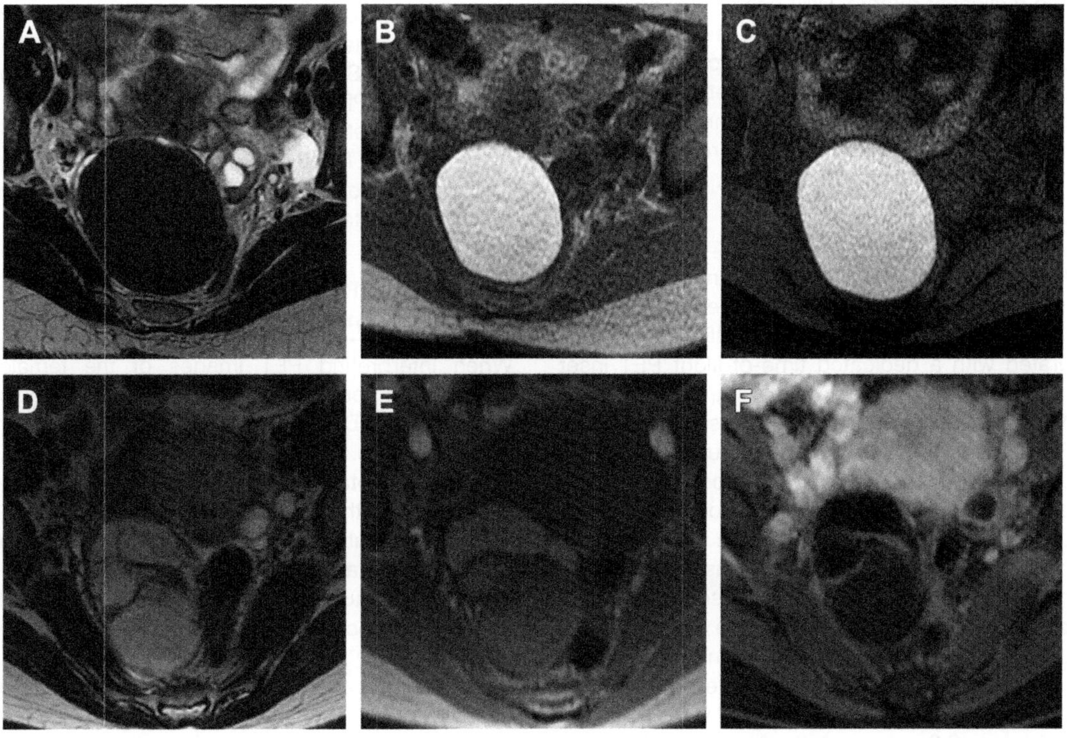

Fig. 1. Use of MR imaging to diagnose definitively benign processes. (*A–C*) Cystic mass that is hypointense on (*A*) T_2-weighted images and hyperintense on T_1-weighted images (*B*) with and (*C*) without fat saturation, characteristic of an endometrioma. (*D–F*) Complex mass that is hyperintense on (*D*) T_2-weighted images but follows fat signal on T_1-weighted images (*E*) with and (*F*) without fat saturation, diagnostic of a dermoid.

typically acquired before and after administration of gadolinium contrast. Among many other uses, gadolinium enhancement can enhance the conspicuity of endometrial masses relative to the myometrium[20,23] and identify solid enhancing nodules within adnexal masses. Contrast-enhanced images are generally acquired in multiple contrast phases, which can vary in terms of tumor conspicuity.

Diffusion-weighted imaging

DWI has gained increasing attention in characterizing gynecologic malignancies. In DWI, image contrast is related to how freely water molecules can diffuse within tissues. Molecules that are in a more restrictive environment have higher signal on DWI and molecules that can move more freely have lower signal on DWI. The diffusion properties of tissues are quantified by computing the apparent diffusion coefficient (ADC), which is the rate that signal decays across multiple DWIs. Because the ADC is, in principle, an intrinsic property of the material being studied, there is great interest in using ADC as a quantitative biomarker of disease. Many small studies have suggested that low ADC may be related to tumor aggressiveness and used to predict malignancy.[1,24–27] There is still considerable overlap, however, between benign and malignant tumors. DWI has also been shown to make peritoneal metastases more conspicuous.[28] Because DWI and PET probe different properties of tissues, namely metabolic activity and cell density, it is hoped that through PET/MR imaging examinations they may provide complementary information about tumors.

PET/MR Imaging Protocol

At the authors' institution, simultaneous PET/MR imaging examinations are performed using a system based on a 3T wide-bore MR imager integrated with a dedicated time-of-flight PET inset (Signa, GE Healthcare, Waukesha, WI). PET and MR imaging data are acquired simultaneously. For gynecologic malignancy evaluation, the authors use a combined whole-body acquisition and a dedicated pelvis bed position (**Fig. 2**). The dedicated pelvis acquisition uses the pulse sequences described in the previous section, with high-resolution T_2-weighted FSE sequences in 3 planes, obliqued with respect to the cervix or uterus, depending on the location of the tumor (see **Fig. 2**B). High-resolution T_2-weighted images are obtained with 4-mm slices and voxels that are 0.6 mm to 0.9 mm on a side. A small field-of-view diffusion-weighted acquisition is acquired, covering the primary tumor only (slice thickness 5 mm and voxel size 1.5 mm × 1.5 mm; see **Fig. 2**C). Subsequently, a time-resolved 3-D gradient-echo T_1-weighted image SPGR acquisition is acquired for evaluation of DCE[29] (see **Fig. 2**D). For ovarian masses, a 2-D dual-echo gradient echo is added to evaluate for fat.

For the whole-body PET and MR imaging portion of the examination (see **Fig. 2**E–F), each bed position is imaged for 3 minutes, and simultaneously a postgadolinium T_1-weighted SPGR image is acquired in the axial plane as well as single-shot FSE (SSFSE) acquisitions in the axial and coronal plane. T_1-weighted SPGR images are acquired using a dual-echo Dixon-based approach that can then be used to produce fat and soft tissue maps that are used for attenuation correction.

The dedicated pelvis acquisition takes approximately 20 minutes in total to acquire, and the whole-body acquisition requires an additional 20 minutes. Patient set up (coil placement, localizer acquisition, and plane placement) takes between 10 minutes and 15 minutes, resulting in a total acquisition time of approximately 60 minutes.

One subtle but important detail of the PET/MR imaging acquisition is that the isocenter of the MR image acquisition must be the same as the center of the bed position of the PET acquisition. For optimal image quality, however, the isocenter is ideally placed at the location of the tumor. For this reason, the authors also acquire a sagittal T_2-weighted SSFSE image of the pelvis prior to beginning the PET acquisition to identify the tumor location and determine the best location selection of the pelvis PET bed position (see **Fig. 2**A). During the remainder of the study, PET and MR data are acquired simultaneously.

IMAGE INTERPRETATION

Physiologic Uptake

When interpreting PET images of the female pelvis, it is important to understand the physiologic variations in FDG uptake that may occasionally mimic disease.[30,31] In premenopausal patients, endometrial uptake varies cyclically with the menstrual cycle, with increased SUVs seen in menstruating and ovulating patients and lower SUVs seen in proliferative and secretory phases.[32] The presence of an intrauterine device has also been noted to cause increased FDG uptake in the endometrium.[33]

Abnormal ovarian uptake can be seen during ovulation, which can be potentially avoided by scheduling PET examinations just after menstruation.[34,35] In premenopausal women, corpus luteum cysts avidly take up FDG and can mimic a metastatic lymph nodes, particularly on

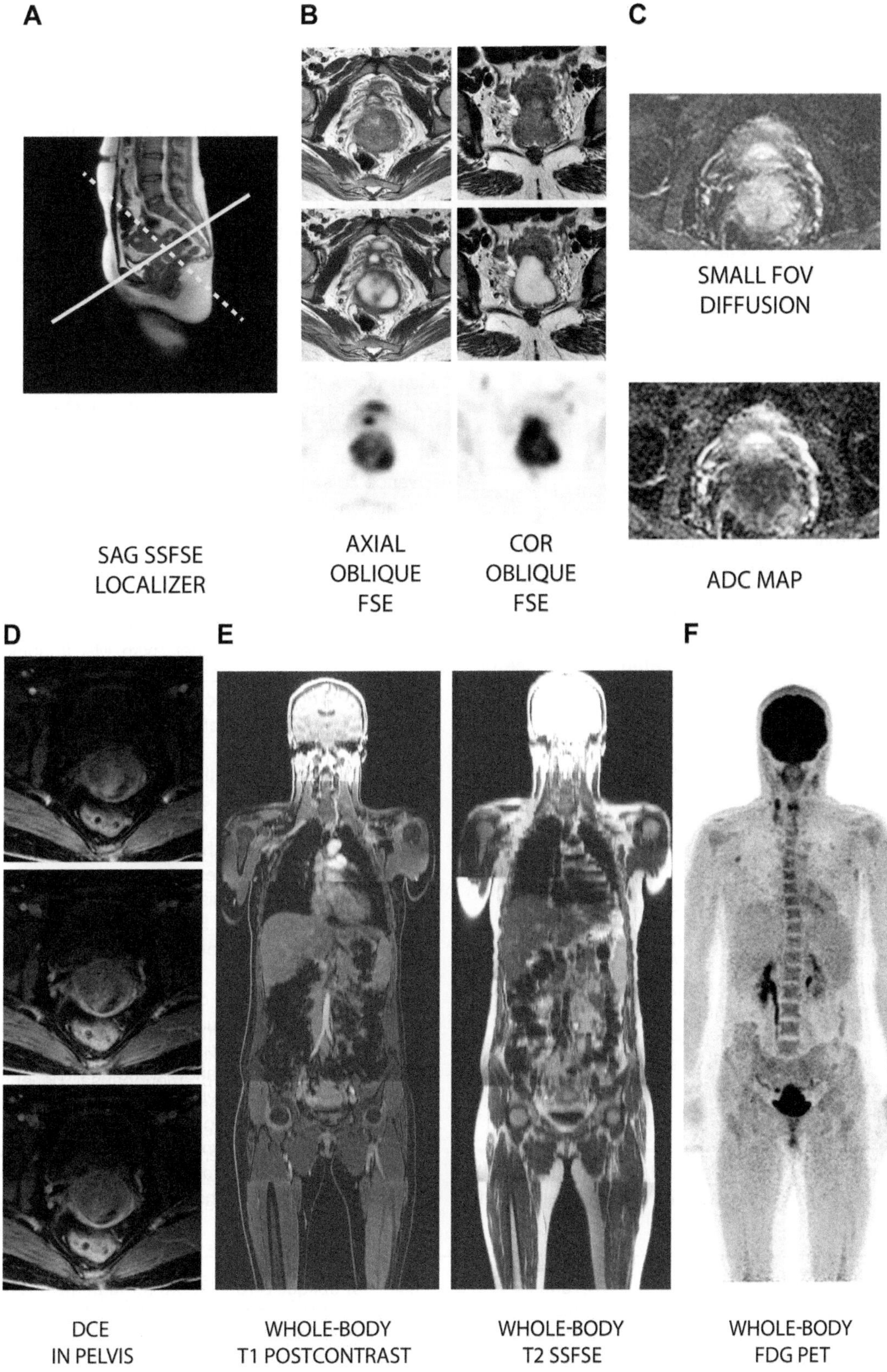

Fig. 2. PET/MR imaging protocol used at the authors' institution, shown in a patient with a cervical mass. (*A*) Large field-of-view sagittal (SAG) T_2-weighted image for localization of tumor and choice of oblique image

PET/CT examinations that are performed without CT contrast. Ovarian hyperstimulation in the setting of oocyte retrieval has been noted to cause increased FDG uptake and should not be confused with malignancy.[36] In contrast, increased ovarian uptake in postmenopausal women should be taken as a sign of malignancy.[32]

In addition to the ovaries and endometrium, fallopian tubes demonstrate increased FDG uptake in the midportion of the menstrual cycle.[37] Inflammatory processes in the fallopian tubes, such as salpingitis, can also cause increased FDG uptake[38] (**Fig. 3**). Physiologic uptake in the fallopian tubes can be particularly problematic in light of emerging evidence that the fallopian tubes may represent the site of origin for serous ovarian cancers.[39]

Combined PET and MR Imaging in Gynecologic Malignancies

These sections review the current literature regarding the use of combined PET and MR imaging in cervical, endometrial, and ovarian cancer. The discussion focuses mainly on studies that directly compare MR imaging and PET/CT and numerous emerging reports describing simultaneous PET/MR imaging acquisition. For each malignancy, discussion is separated into the use of these imaging modalities in the initial diagnosis, detection of recurrence, and treatment response. Because experience with this emerging modality is in the early stages, it is difficult to draw general conclusions, especially because MR imaging and PET/CT are not monolithic entities, and the performance of each depends on the protocol chosen. In particular, the CT portion of the PET/CT examination can be performed with or without contrast,[40,41] and that choice affects the comparison with MR imaging for anatomic localization.[42,43] Often, when PET/CT is compared with MR imaging for characterization of lymph node metastasis, MR imaging characterization relies on morphologic criteria (size >1 cm) and not other functional parameters (DWI and DCE) often used in clinical practice.

Cervical Cancer

Worldwide, cervical cancer is the fourth most common cancer in women, with a large majority of cases and deaths occurring in developing countries (2014 World Health Organization Cancer fact sheet). Most cervical cancers are associated with the human papilloma virus and approximately 12,990 cases of cervical cancer are expected in the United States in 2016.[44] Tumors that are confined to the cervix and less than 4 cm (International Federation of Gynecology and Obstetrics [FIGO] stage IB1 or less) are generally treated with surgery, whereas those with locally advanced disease (parametrial or organ invasion) are generally treated with primary chemoradiotherapy.[45] Tumors confined to the cervix but greater than 4 cm (stage IB2) may be treated with either surgery or chemoradiotherapy, depending on clinical characteristics, such as depth of cervical stromal invasion and concern for nodal involvement. National Comprehensive Cancer Network (NCCN) guidelines in 2016 advocate whole-body PET/CT for locally advanced disease (FIGO stage II or above) and for patients where cervical cancer is found incidentally after hysterectomy.[46] MR imaging is considered optional for assessment of local extent of disease.

Initial staging

MR imaging and PET are complementary in the evaluation of cervical cancer, with MR imaging more sensitive for local disease and PET/CT better for evaluation of metastatic disease.[47,48] MR imaging has been shown in a large multicenter study to be more accurate than CT in detecting cervical tumors[49] and has a negative predictive value of approximately 100% in excluding bladder and rectal involvement.[50] In a large meta-analysis, PET was found to have a higher pooled sensitivity for metastatic lymph nodes than either MR imaging or CT.[51] In this analysis, the pooled sensitivity for PET was still low (0.58), indicating there is extensive disease that potentially remains occult on any imaging modality.

Where the combination of PET and MR imaging has been specifically evaluated, it has been shown valuable in staging of cervical cancer. In a study of 27 patients with cervical cancer using an integrated PET/MR imaging system, PET/MR imaging had high sensitivity and specificity for vaginal invasion, parametrial extension, and lymph node involvement. Both ADC and maximum SUV were correlated with tumor size and pathologic grade. A similar

planes. Solid line is plane for oblique axial and dashed line is plane for oblique coronal (COR) through the cervix. (*B*) High-resolution T_2-weighted FSE acquired in the oblique axial (*left column*) and oblique coronal (*planes*). Also shown are overlays of the PET data reformatted into the oblique planes. (*C*) Small field-of-view (FOV) DWI and ADC map, with low ADC tumor clearly seen. (*D*) Multiphase dynamic contrast-enhanced (DCE) T_1-weighted SPGR. (*E*) Whole-body imaging with T_1-weighted SPGR and T_2-weighted SSFSE. (*F*) Maximum intensity projection of whole-body PET acquisition.

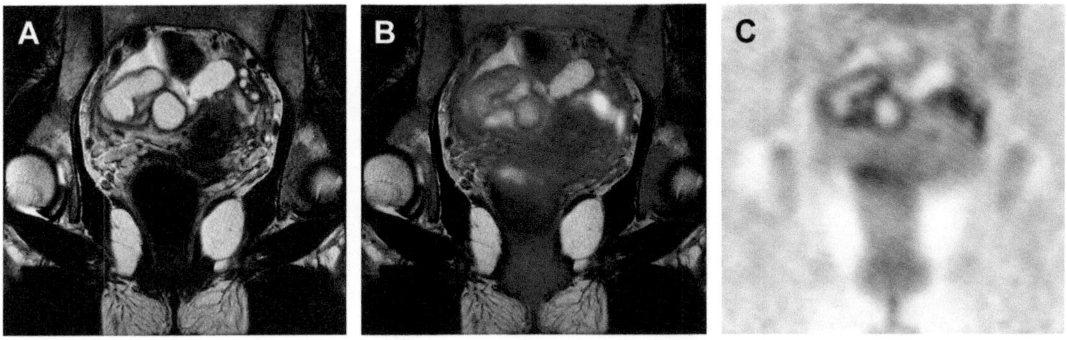

Fig. 3. Tubal uptake in a patient with chronic salpingitis. Fluid-filled tubular structure is seen on (*A*) T_2-weighted imaging with uniform FDG uptake seen on (*B*) overlays and (*C*) PET images. Patient was brought to surgery based on elevated carcinoembryonic antigen, with no evidence of malignancy and chronic salpingitis confirmed by pathology.

correlation of ADC and maximum SUV was found in a study of separately acquired PET and MR imaging scans of patients with cervical cancer.[52] In locally advanced cervical cancer (FIGO stages IB–IVA), fused PET and MR imaging allows the detection of more lymph node groups than PET alone.[53]

Fig. 4 shows examples of a primary cervical cancer lesion too small to reliably identify on T_2-weighted imaging but visible using the PET overlay. **Fig. 5** shows FDG uptake in a small anterior cervical mass without parametrial extension.

Prognosis

Both FDG PET and MR imaging have been shown to have value in predicting the prognosis of patients diagnosed with cervical cancer. The volume of tumor burden determined by FDG PET is correlated with overall survival after radiation therapy.[54]

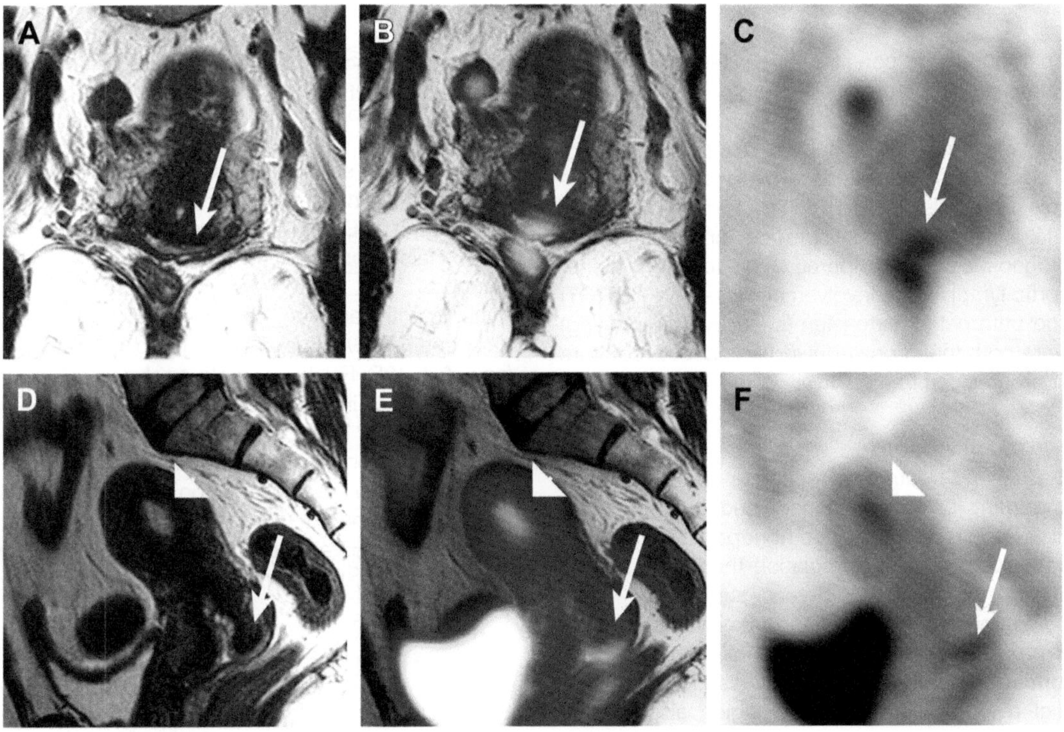

Fig. 4. FDG uptake in a small cervical mass not visible on T_2-weighted imaging (*long arrow*). (*A*) Axial and (*D*) sagittal T_2-weighted FSE demonstrates mild asymmetric soft tissue along the posterior cervix, with a clear hypermetabolic focus on (*B, E*) overlayed and (*C, F*) reformatted PET images. Arrowhead shows normal physiologic FDG uptake in the endometrium.

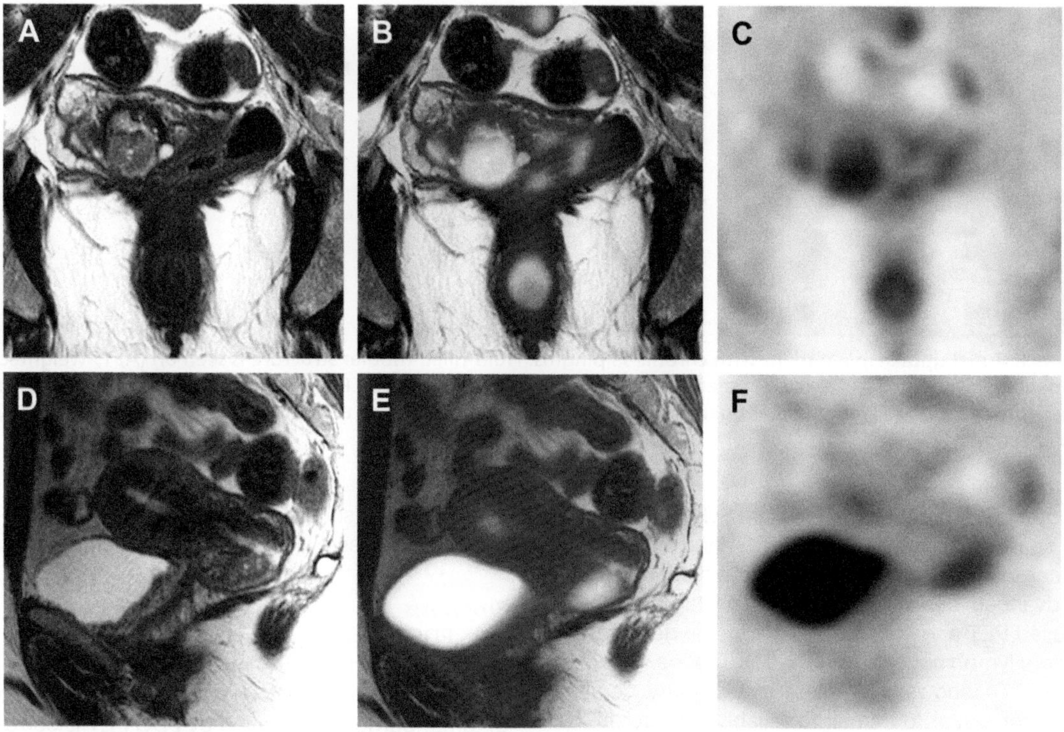

Fig. 5. Cervical mass without parametrial extension. (*A, D*) Axial-oblique and sagittal T_2-weighted FSE images show a T_2 hypointense mass arising from the anterior cervix without extension into the parametrium. FDG avidity is demonstrated by (*B, E*) overlayed and (*C, F*) reformatted PET images.

A nomogram has been created based on PET characteristics to predict overall survival and progression-free survival.[55] In a meta-analysis, high maximum SUV in both the primary tumor and metastasis has been shown to predict unfavorable prognosis.[56] Combining PET and MR imaging into a single prognostic model provides further prognostic value compared with each study alone; aortic lymph node involvement (seen by PET/CT) and parametrial extension (seen by MR imaging) were both found powerful independent predictors of progression free survival.[57]

Treatment response

Evaluating treatment response is particularly important for cervical cancer because advanced disease is typically treated nonoperatively. Residual FDG uptake after radiation therapy has been shown to predict a 5-year survival of 32%, compared with 80% if no uptake was seen.[58] In a prospective study, FDG uptake on PET performed 3 months after therapy was found to predict overall survival.[59] MR imaging also has an important role in treatment planning for brachytherapy and monitoring response.[60] In examining the prediction of treatment response, both the change in maximum SUV and change in ADC have been found predictive of disease progression after radiation therapy.[61]

Surveillance

PET imaging is sensitive and specific for detection of recurrent cervical cancer,[62] with correlative imaging, such as CT or MR imaging, helping to elucidate false-positive or false-negative PET findings.[63] **Fig. 6** shows examples of 2 different patients with recurrent cervical tumors in the vagina (see **Fig. 6**A–C) and along the pelvic sidewall (see **Fig. 6**D–F). In a meta-analyses of prior studies, other investigators have questioned the added value of PET/CT compared with MR imaging or CT alone,[64] including its cost-effectiveness.[65] The decreased radiation dose of PET/MR imaging compared with PET/CT is a major strength for surveillance imaging, particularly in young women, where multiple serial scans may be required.

Endometrial Cancer

Endometrial cancer is the most common gynecologic malignancy and tenth most common malignancy in women in the United States.[44] Approximately 60,050 cases are expected in the United States during 2016. Approximately

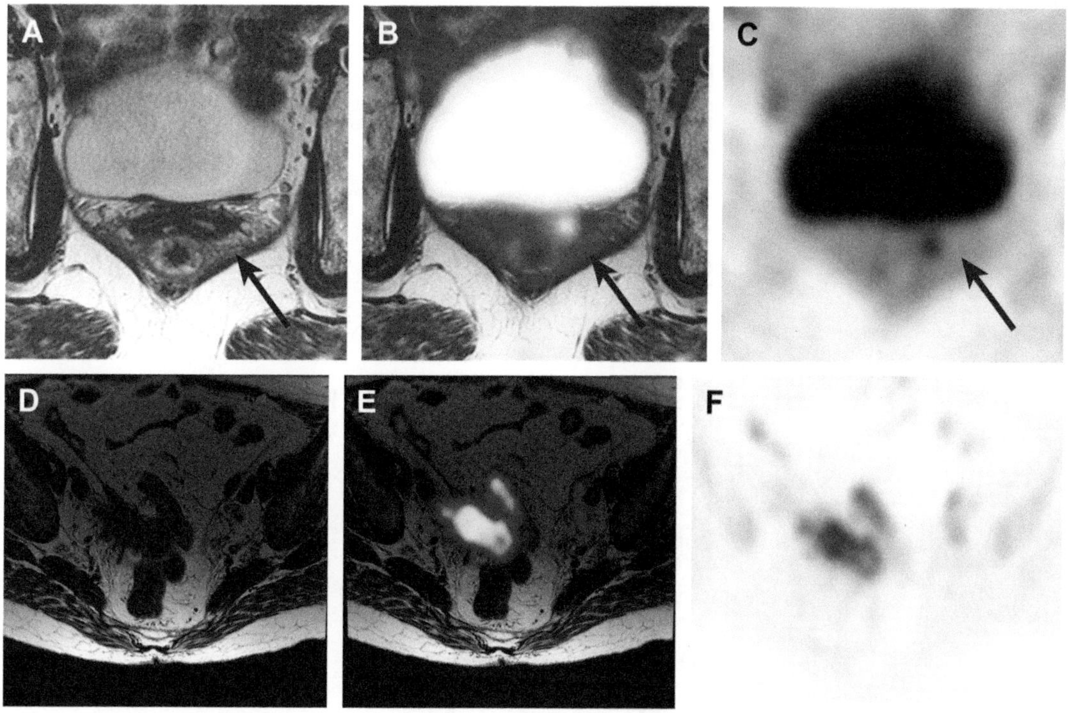

Fig. 6. Cervical cancer recurrence seen in 2 different patients. (*A–C*) Focus of uptake (*arrow*) is seen in the vaginal cuff on (*B*) overlayed and (*C*) reformatted PET images, although no discrete mass is seen on (*A*) T_2-weighted images. (*D–F*) Cervical cancer recurrence seen as a hypermetabolic infiltrative pelvic sidewall mass visible on (*D*) T_2-weighted images, (*E*) PET overlay, and (*F*) reformatted PET image.

two-thirds of endometrial cancers are diagnosed at an early stage after women present with postmenopausal bleeding. At presentation, a vast majority of patients have disease confined to the uterus.[66] Staging is typically performed surgically and based on 2010 FIGO criteria. The 2016 NCCN guidelines suggest imaging with MR imaging, CT, or PET as clinically indicated when there is suspected extrauterine disease or for patients with serous, clear cell, or carcinosarcoma found on biopsy.[67] Primary treatment of locally confined disease is surgical resection with postoperative radiation therapy or systemic chemotherapy depending on the presence of high-risk pathologic features.

Initial staging

As with cervical cancer, MR imaging and PET are complementary in the initial staging of endometrial cancer because MR imaging is more accurate for local extension and PET is more accurate for distant metastases. Although MR imaging is not part of the official FIGO staging for endometrial cancer, MR imaging can be useful for preoperative planning in determining cervical involvement, parametrial extension, and depth of myometrial invasion, which in turn informs hysterectomy type as well as the likelihood of nodal metastasis.[45,68] In a direct comparison of fused PET/MR imaging, MR imaging, and PET/CT data, PET/MR imaging and MR imaging alone were both more accurate for local staging of endometrial cancer (T-stage accuracy 80% for PET/MR imaging or MR imaging alone vs 60% for PET/CT).[69] An example of combined PET/MR imaging in a patient with endometrial cancer confined to the uterus is shown in **Fig. 7**. The sensitivity of MR imaging for endometrial invasion may also help select patients with low-grade tumors who may undergo fertility-sparing surgery.[70]

PET/CT is more sensitive than MR imaging for distant metastatic disease. Two meta-analyses have shown that PET/CT is highly sensitive and specific for distant nodal metastasis.[71,72] Although the sensitivity for lymph node metastases is higher for PET/CT than for other modalities, the pooled sensitivity of 72% found by Bollineni and colleagues[72] was still low in an absolute sense, reinforcing that a significant percentage of lymph nodes still go undetected by PET/CT. In a direct comparison of MR imaging and PET/CT for initial staging using retrospectively fused data, PET/CT was found superior for detection of metastatic lymph nodes (sensitivity 70% for PET/CT vs 34% for MR imaging).[73]

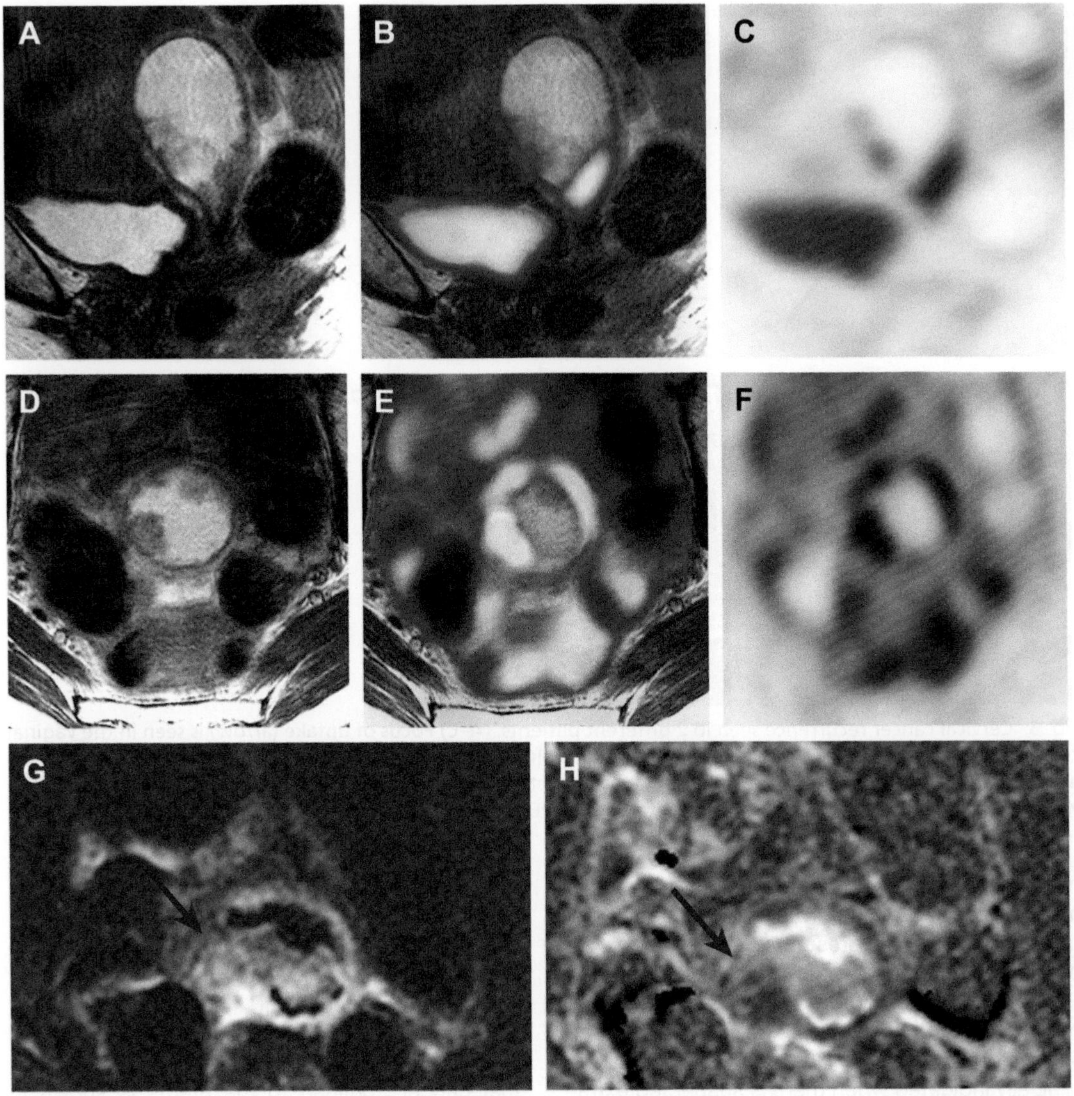

Fig. 7. Primary endometrial cancer. (*A, D*) High-resolution T_2-weighted images demonstrate frondlike soft tissue within the lower uterine segment. The endometrial cavity is also filled with fluid. Endometrial soft tissue is seen to take up FDG on both (*B, E*) overlayed and (*C, F*) reformatted PET images. The endometrial mass (*arrow*) also exhibits (*G*) increased signal on axial DWI and (*H*) decreased ADC.

Prognosis

Both PET and MR imaging features of endometrial cancer have been associated with prognosis after therapy. The preoperative maximum SUV has been correlated with the presence of high-risk or low-risk disease after surgical staging.[74] A similar result has been found using an integrated PET/MR imaging system, where tumors with high-risk features, such as deep myometrial invasion, cervical invasion, lymphovascular space involvement, and lymph node metastases, were found to have elevated maximum SUV and decreased minimum ADC on preoperative imaging.[75] The ratio of maximum SUV to minimum ADC was also correlated with higher risk or higher stage tumors. It is uncertain whether this result indicates that the ratio has independent meaning or whether they are both correlated to the same underlying abnormality.

Surveillance

In terms of recurrent disease, FDG PET has been shown highly accurate in the diagnosis of recurrent disease, with a meta-analysis showing a pooled sensitivity of 96% and specificity of 93%.[76] A patient with recurrent endometrial cancer along the vaginal cuff clearly seen on the PET overlay is shown in **Fig. 8**.

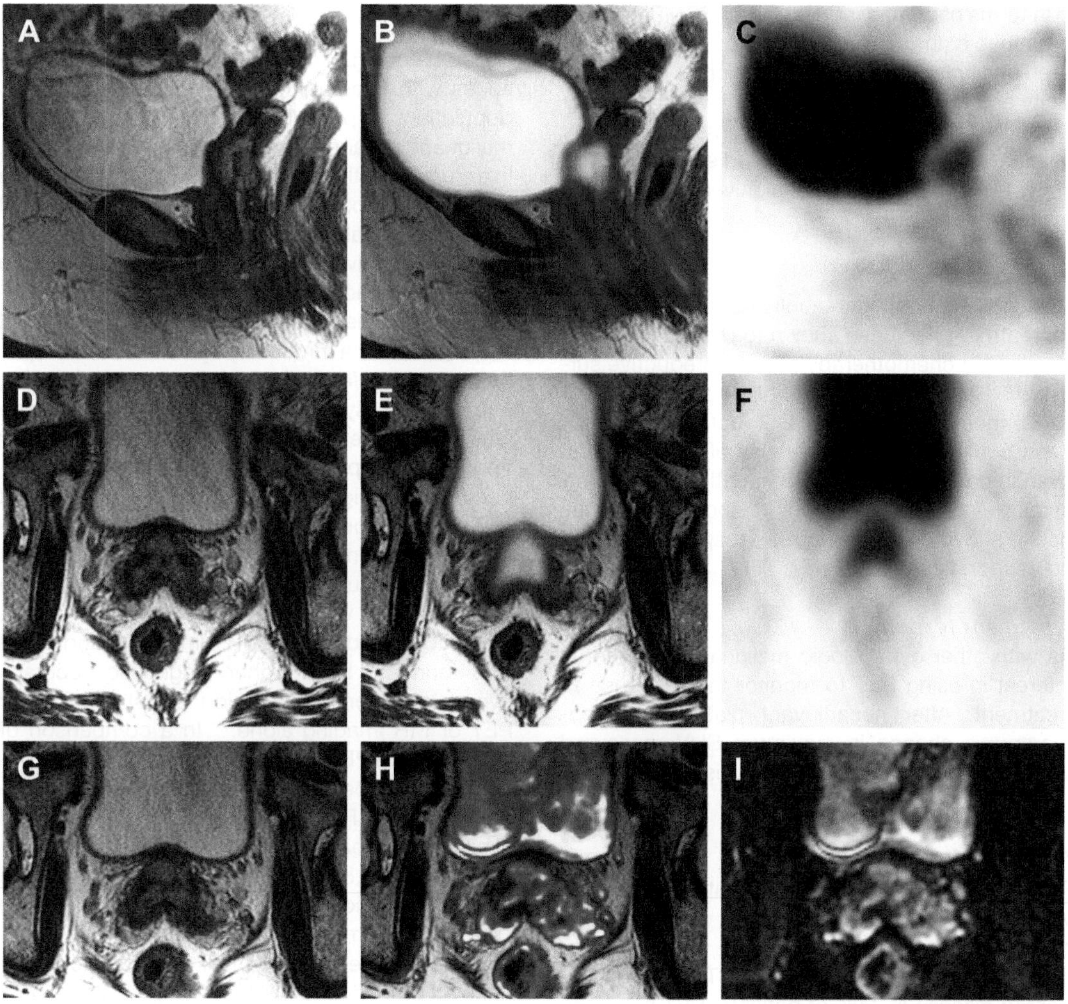

Fig. 8. Recurrent endometrial cancer occurring within the vagina. On (*A*) sagittal and (*D*) axial oblique T_2-weighted images, a mass is seen in the upper vagina, invading through the wall, clearly separate from the bladder. Hypermetabolism is seen on both (*B, E*) PET overlays and (*C, F*) reformatted primary PET data. (*G–I*) increased (*I*) DWI signal can also be seen within the mass (*H*) overlayed onto the T_2-weighted image.

Ovarian Cancer

Ovarian cancer is the second most common gynecologic malignancy but has the highest mortality, mostly because ovarian cancers are usually diagnosed at a late stage. Formal staging is entirely based on surgical findings. In the initial assessment, NCCN guidelines support chest radiograph, chest CT, and abdominal/pelvic CT, as clinically indicated.[77] PET/CT or MR imaging are suggested for indeterminate adnexal masses. For surveillance of tumor recurrence, NCCN guidelines support the use of CT, MR imaging, PET/CT, or PET for surveillance.

Initial staging

As with other types of gynecologic malignancies, PET/CT is superior to CT alone for detecting metastatic lymph nodes.[78] A recent study found better diagnostic performance for contrast-enhanced CT compared with PET/CT in evaluating patients with suspected carcinomatosis.[79] In this study, the CT portion of the PET/CT was performed without contrast, and the poor performance for PET/CT compared with contrast CT alone reflects the value of intravenous contrast when searching for metastatic peritoneal disease. The staging accuracy of MR imaging alone in assessing peritoneal disease is difficult to determine. A prospective study showed high sensitivity for pelvic sites but low sensitivity for abdominal sites.[80] In a large comparative study by the Radiological Diagnostic Oncology Group, however, CT and MR imaging were believed equally accurate.[81]

In terms of primary adnexal lesions, MR imaging is valuable in evaluating indeterminate lesions seen on ultrasound, mainly based on its high specificity and ability to delineate definitively benign lesions.[82] PET/CT is rarely used to assess primary ovarian tumors but in small studies it has been shown able to distinguish benign versus malignant masses.[83,84]

Prognosis

Using PET, the total metabolic tumor volume prior to treatment has been shown to predict response to adjuvant chemotherapy after cytoreductive surgery.[85] Beyond total metabolic volume, intratumoral heterogeneity of FDG uptake has also been correlated with higher risk of recurrence in ovarian cancer.[86] Using DWI in patients with metastatic ovarian cancer, early change in ADC has been shown to distinguish responders from nonresponders.[87]

Treatment response

As with other gynecologic malignancies, there is interest in using PET to monitor the response to treatment. After neoadjuvant platinum chemotherapy, a change in maximum SUV measured within the omentum predicted histologic tumor response.[88]

Surveillance

PET/CT has been found useful in staging patients with suspected recurrent ovarian cancer (based on elevated CA-125, clinical suspicion, or abnormal imaging study).[89] PET/CT found unsuspected disease in 44% of patients. PET has been shown to have high sensitivity in detecting recurrence on a per-patient basis but lower sensitivity on a per-lesion basis.[90] In a study of 268 ovarian cancer malignancy patients who had surveillance PET/CT, a change in management occurred in 11% of cases.[91] PET combined with contrast-enhanced CT was found statistically more sensitive, specific, and accurate compared with contrast-enhanced CT alone.[92]

Few data are available directly comparing MR imaging and PET/CT for detecting local recurrence of ovarian cancers. A small study of 36 patients found MR imaging more sensitive than PET/CT for detecting local recurrence and peritoneal lesions.[93] In this study, PET/CT was performed without contrast, which may explain why more lesions were detected using MR imaging. These results indicate that having metabolic information as well as anatomic information provided by contrast-enhanced studies should be useful and complementary, suggesting that combined PET/MR imaging should prove valuable.

Studies Involving Mixed Tumor Populations

Several recent publications describe initial experiences with integrated PET/MR imaging in mixed populations of patients with different gynecologic malignancies, and those are discussed separately. In a study directly comparing PET/MR imaging with PET/CT in a mixed set of patients with a variety of gynecologic malignancies (ovarian, cervical, endometrial, and vulvar), PET/MR imaging was found to have superior accuracy for depiction of primary tumors.[94] In this study, images were obtained sequentially on a trimodality system where the patient was transferred from dedicated MR imaging and PET/CT systems. No significant difference was found in detection of regional lymph nodes or abdominal lymph nodes. In terms of recurrent gynecologic malignancies, PET/MR imaging and PET/CT were found to have equal diagnostic accuracy in identifying distant metastatic disease.[95]

In another study examining retrospective fusion of 27 patients with cervical and ovarian cancer, PET combined with MR imaging and DWI was found to have higher diagnostic accuracy (when taken on a per-lesion basis) than either PET or MR imaging alone.[96] In a comparison of simultaneous PET/MR imaging with PET/CT in patients with suspected recurrent gynecologic malignancy, PET/MR imaging and PET/CT showed similar lesion-based sensitivity and specificity.[97] However, that PET/MR imaging had a much smaller radiation dose. Retrospectively fused PET and MR imaging data showed higher sensitivity for local recurrence of all gynecologic malignancy than PET/CT.[98]

FUTURE DIRECTIONS

PET/MR imaging technology is currently entering an exciting period. Numerous commercially available systems now exist and, as discussed previously, these systems can successfully combine the superior ability of MR imaging to assess local tumor extension with the ability of PET to assess for metastatic disease. This combination produces several potential advantages compared with conventional approaches. First, combining two examinations into a single study is tremendously more convenient for patients compared with separate PET/CT and MR imaging acquisitions. Second, there is a significant reduction in radiation exposure. The exact radiation dose savings depends on the specific CT protocol that is used, but dose reductions have been reported as high as 50%.[99] Radiation dose reduction is particularly important for gynecologic cancers that may affect young women.

Although the improvement in convenience and radiation dose savings are significant advantages to PET/MR imaging, the true power of this technology will lie in exploiting the complementary information provided by both modalities. Although this is a topic of continuing research, several potential areas where the combination of PET and MR imaging might be particularly powerful are discussed.

Multiparametric Evaluation of Tumors

DCE, DWI, and FDG uptake represent measurements of three fundamentally different tissue properties that are all altered in malignancies compared with normal tissues.[25] DCE uptake kinetics measure tissue permeability, DWI measures the dense packing of cells, and FDG measures glucose uptake and trapping, which is related to glycolysis. One area of current research is to determine whether these 3 techniques produce additive or duplicative information.

There is evidence that DWI and FDG uptake may be somewhat duplicative. In a study of 48 patients with gynecologic malignancy on an integrated whole-body PET/MR imaging system, the addition of whole-body DWI was found to have no incremental benefit over PET in terms of lesion detection.[100] Another study found similar results looking at all malignancies (not just gynecologic malignancy), where lower lesion-to-background contrast was seen for whole body diffusion compared with PET.[101]

Although these studies seem to suggest that DWI may be duplicative in terms of lesion conspicuity, they do not address any additional biological information that may be obtained from ADC measurements. As described previously, minimum ADC and maximum SUV tend to be correlated, so it remains to be determined whether these measurements provide unique information when assessing tumors. If DWI is shown to provide similar information to FDG uptake, it leaves open the possibility of other novel PET tracers in place of FDG, as described later.

Novel PET Tracers

Numerous novel PET tracers have been introduced for the evaluation of the biological activity of tumors. One such agent is [^{18}F]fluoromisonidazole (FMISO). FMISO is a PET agent that is sensitive to hypoxia. A fused multiparametric approach has been used to combine MR imaging data with PET CT data obtained using both FDG and FMISO.[102] PET and MR imaging parameters demonstrated some statistically significant correlation, but the degrees of correlation were modest, suggesting they potentially provide independent information. Two other PET markers for hypoxia, [^{18}F]fluoroazomycin arabinoside and ^{64}Cu-diacetyl-bis(N^{4}-methylthiosemicarbazone), have been tested in the context of radiotherapy for cervical cancer.[103,104]

Recently, it has been noted that the vasculature of ovarian tumors demonstrate up-regulation of prostate-specific membrane antigen (PSMA),[105] which opens a potential role for the numerous PSMA-targeting imaging agents that have been recently developed to image prostate cancer.

Novel MR Imaging Tracers

Just as alternative PET tracers can be used to replace FDG in a PET/MR imaging acquisition, novel MR imaging tracers with altered molecular specificity are under development. One novel class of tracers is composed of superparamagnetic iron oxide particles, which are taken up in metastatic lymph nodes.[106] One such agent, ferumoxytol, is Food and Drug Administration approved as an iron supplement but has been used off label to assess lymph nodes in prostate cancer.[107] Normal lymph nodes take up ferumoxytol and, therefore, have signal loss on T_2-weighted sequences (which are sensitive to iron). In lymph nodes that contain metastatic tumor, ferumoxytol is excluded, preserving the T_2 signal.

Another emerging molecular imaging tracer in MR imaging are hyperpolarized compounds containing ^{13}C. Hyperpolarized ^{13}C MR imaging is a new field in which compounds enriched with the NMR-active nucleus ^{13}C are polarized outside of the scanner and injected, allowing real-time measurements of tissue metabolism. Tumors demonstrate increased production [^{13}C]lactate from [^{13}C]pyruvate, which in preclinical studies has been correlated to tumor grade.[108,109] A clinical ^{13}C polarizer is now available, and a phase 1 clinical trial using hyperpolarized ^{13}C in pyruvate in patients in prostate cancer has been published,[110] with more studies ongoing. This novel metabolic imaging technique could be combined in a PET/MR imaging examination to obtain complementary metabolic information about tumors.

Radiation Planning and Monitoring Treatment Response

PET/MR imaging has a particularly potentially powerful role in the planning of radiation therapy. High-resolution delineation of the tumor permits precise delineation of the radiation field.[60] Metabolic information provided by FDG uptake may provide information about treatment response prior to regression on anatomic imaging, permitting radiation doses to be tailored accordingly.[111] Furthermore, as discussed previously, the use of agents, such as FMISO, to measure hypoxia may aid in determining which tissues are most susceptible to radiation, again permitting the adjustment of radiation doses.

Additive Image Information

In both PET and MR imaging acquisitions, there is interest in finding ways to generate images using as few data as possible, thus speeding up acquisition time. Currently, the MR imaging and PET acquisitions are treated separately. It could be speculated, however, that in an integrated image acquisition, spatial information provided by the PET acquisition may be used in combination with the acquired MR imaging data in a single integrated reconstruction. One application of this approach is to use a constrained joint reconstruction of PET and MR imaging data to increase the spatial resolution of PET images.[112]

SUMMARY

Both MR imaging and PET currently have important roles in diagnosis and surveillance of gynecologic malignancies, providing complementary information about local tumor staging and distant metastases, respectively. Integrating these 2 modalities into a single examination currently has clear advantages both in terms of patient convenience as well as radiation dose savings. The further integration of novel PET and MR imaging probes; expansion to new applications, such as radiation planning; and the development of advanced reconstruction techniques promise to further expand the promise of this new clinical imaging tool.

REFERENCES

1. Hameeduddin A, Sahdev A. Diffusion-weighted imaging and dynamic contrast-enhanced MRI in assessing response and recurrent disease in gynaecological malignancies. Cancer Imaging 2015;15(1):3.
2. Delso G. Ziegler S PET/MR system design. PET/MRI. Berlin; Heidelberg (Germany): Springer Berlin Heidelberg; 2013. p. 1–19.
3. Kinahan PE, Townsend DW, Beyer T, et al. Attenuation correction for a combined 3D PET/CT scanner. Med Phys 1998;25(10):2046–53.
4. Wagenknecht G, Kaiser H-J, Mottaghy FM, et al. MRI for attenuation correction in PET: methods and challenges. Magma 2012;26(1):99–113.
5. Ma J. Dixon techniques for water and fat imaging. J Magn Reson Imaging 2008;28(3):543–58.
6. Fowler KJ, McConathy J, Narra VR. Whole-body simultaneous positron emission tomography (PET)-MR: Optimization and adaptation of MRI sequences. J Magn Reson Imaging 2013;39(2): 259–68.
7. Ouyang J, Chun SY, Petibon Y, et al. Bias atlases for segmentation-based PET attenuation correction using PET-CT and MR. IEEE Trans Nucl Sci 2013; 60(5):3373–82.
8. Martinez-Möller A, Souvatzoglou M, Delso G, et al. Tissue classification as a potential approach for attenuation correction in whole-body PET/MRI: evaluation with PET/CT data. J Nucl Med 2009; 50(4):520–6.
9. Aznar MC, Sersar R, Saabye J, et al. Whole-body PET/MRI: The effect of bone attenuation during MR-based attenuation correction in oncology imaging. Eur J Radiol 2014;83(7):1177–83.
10. Schramm G, Maus J, Hofheinz F, et al. Correction of quantification errors in pelvic and spinal lesions caused by ignoring higher photon attenuation of bone in [18F]NaF PET/MR. Med Phys 2015; 42(11):6468–76.
11. Berker Y, Franke J, Salomon A, et al. MRI-based attenuation correction for hybrid PET/MRI systems: a 4-class tissue segmentation technique using a combined ultrashort-echo-time/Dixon MRI sequence. J Nucl Med 2012;53(5):796–804.
12. Leynes AP, Yang J, Shanbhag DD, et al. Hybrid ZTE/Dixon MR-based attenuation correction for quantitative uptake estimation of pelvic lesions in PET/MRI. Med Phys 2017;44(3):902–13.
13. Chandarana H, Heacock L, Rakheja R, et al. Pulmonary Nodules in Patients with Primary Malignancy: Comparison of Hybrid PET/MR and PET/CT Imaging. Radiology 2013;268(3):874–81.
14. Burris NS, Johnson KM, Larson PEZ, et al. Detection of small pulmonary nodules with ultrashort echo time sequences in oncology patients by using a PET/MR system. Radiology 2015;278: 239–46.
15. Fürst S, Grimm R, Hong I, et al. Motion correction strategies for integrated PET/MR. J Nucl Med 2015;56(2):261–9.
16. Fayad H, Lamare F, Merlin T, et al. Motion correction using anatomical information in PET/CT and PET/MR hybrid imaging. Q J Nucl Med Mol Imaging 2016;60(1):12–24.
17. Balfour DR, Marsden PK, Polycarpou I, et al. Respiratory motion correction of PET using MR-constrained PET-PET registration. Biomed Eng Online 2015;14(1):85.
18. Hope TA, Verdin EF, Bergsland EK, et al. Correcting for respiratory motion in liver PET/MRI: preliminary evaluation of the utility of bellows and navigated

hepatobiliary phase imaging. EJNMMI Phys 2015;2(1):21.
19. Heiba SI, Raphael B, Castellon I, et al. PET/CT image fusion error due to urinary bladder filling changes: consequence and correction. Ann Nucl Med 2009;23(8):739–44.
20. Rauch GM, Kaur H, Choi H, et al. Optimization of MR Imaging for Pretreatment Evaluation of Patients with Endometrial and Cervical Cancer. RadioGraphics 2014;34(4):1082–98.
21. Hecht EM, Yitta S, Lim RP, et al. Preliminary clinical experience at 3 T With a 3D T2-weighted sequence compared with multiplanar 2D for evaluation of the female pelvis. Am J Roentgenol 2011;197(2):W346–52.
22. Pereira JM, Sirlin CB, Pinto PS, et al. CT and MR imaging of extrahepatic fatty masses of the abdomen and pelvis: techniques, diagnosis, differential diagnosis, and pitfalls. RadioGraphics 2005;25(1):69–85.
23. Wu L-M, Xu J-R, Gu H-Y, et al. Predictive value of T2-weighted imaging and contrast-enhanced MR imaging in assessing myometrial invasion in endometrial cancer: a pooled analysis of prospective studies. Eur Radiol 2012;23(2):435–49.
24. Dhanda S, Thakur M, Kerkar R, et al. Diffusion-weighted imaging of gynecologic tumors: diagnostic pearls and potential pitfalls. RadioGraphics 2014;34(5):1393–416.
25. Sala E, Rockall A, Rangarajan D, et al. The role of dynamic contrast-enhanced and diffusion weighted magnetic resonance imaging in the female pelvis. Eur J Radiol 2010;76(3):367–85.
26. Namimoto T, Awai K, Nakaura T, et al. Role of diffusion-weighted imaging in the diagnosis of gynecological diseases. Eur Radiol 2009;19(3):745–60.
27. Lin G, Ho K-C, Wang J-J, et al. Detection of lymph node metastasis in cervical and uterine cancers by diffusion-weighted magnetic resonance imaging at 3T. J Magn Reson Imaging 2008;28(1):128–35.
28. Fujii S, Matsusue E, Kanasaki Y, et al. Detection of peritoneal dissemination in gynecological malignancy: evaluation by diffusion-weighted MR imaging. Eur Radiol 2007;18(1):18–23.
29. Hope TA, Petkovska I, Saranathan M, et al. Combined parenchymal and vascular imaging: High spatiotemporal resolution arterial evaluation of hepatocellular carcinoma. J Magn Reson Imaging 2015;43(4):859–65.
30. Liu Y. Benign ovarian and endometrial uptake on FDG PET-CT: patterns and pitfalls. Ann Nucl Med 2009;23(2):107–12.
31. Gorospe L, Jover-Díaz R, Vicente-Bártulos A. Spectrum of PET–CT pelvic pitfalls in patients with gynecologic malignancies. Abdom Imaging 2012;37(6):1041–65.
32. Lerman H, Metser U, Grisaru D, et al. Normal and abnormal 18F-FDG endometrial and ovarian uptake in pre- and postmenopausal patients: assessment by PET/CT. J Nucl Med 2004;45(2):266–71.
33. Julian A, Payoux P, Rimailho J, et al. Uterine uptake of F-18 FDG on positron emission tomography induced by an intrauterine device: Unusual pitfall. Clin Nucl Med 2007;32(2):128–9.
34. Kim S-K, Kang KW, Roh JW, et al. Incidental ovarian 18F-FDG accumulation on PET: correlation with the menstrual cycle. Eur J Nucl Med Mol Imaging 2005;32(7):757–63.
35. Nishizawa S, Inubushi M, Okada H. Physiological 18F-FDG uptake in the ovaries and uterus of healthy female volunteers. Eur J Nucl Med Mol Imaging 2004;32(5):549–56.
36. Bacanovic S, Stiller R, Pircher M, et al. Ovarian hyperstimulation and oocyte harvesting prior to systemic chemotherapy-a possible pitfall in 18F-FDG PET/CT staging of oncologic patients. Clin Nucl Med 2016;41(8):e394–6.
37. Yun M, Cho A, Lee JH, et al. Physiologic 18F-FDG Uptake in the Fallopian Tubes at Mid Cycle on PET/CT. J Nucl Med 2010;51(5):682–5.
38. Yildirim-Poyraz N, Kandemir Z, Ozdemir E, et al. Incidental FDG uptake in bilateral salpingitis due to Morgagni cyst hydatids on PET/CT scan in a patient with solitary pulmonary nodule. Rev Esp Med Nucl Imagen Mol 2014;33(6):394–6.
39. Erickson BK, Conner MG, Landen CN Jr. The role of the fallopian tube in the origin of ovarian cancer. Am J Obstet Gynecol 2013;209(5):409–14.
40. Berthelsen AK, Holm S, Loft A, et al. PET/CT with intravenous contrast can be used for PET attenuation correction in cancer patients. Eur J Nucl Med Mol Imaging 2005;32(10):1167–75.
41. Mawlawi O, Erasmus JJ, Munden RF, et al. Quantifying the effect of IV contrast media on integrated PET/CT: clinical evaluation. Am J Roentgenol 2006;186(2):308–19.
42. Kitajima K, Murakami K, Yamasaki E, et al. Performance of integrated FDG–PET/contrast-enhanced CT in the diagnosis of recurrent ovarian cancer: comparison with integrated FDG–PET/non-contrast-enhanced CT and enhanced CT. Eur J Nucl Med Mol Imaging 2008;35(8):1439–48.
43. Kitajima K, Suzuki K, Senda M, et al. Preoperative nodal staging of uterine cancer: is contrast-enhanced PET/CT more accurate than non-enhanced PET/CT or enhanced CT alone? Ann Nucl Med 2011;25(7):511–9.
44. American Cancer Society. Cancer Facts & Figures 2016. Atlanta: American Cancer Society; 2016.
45. Sala E, Rockall AG, Freeman SJ, et al. The added role of MR imaging in treatment stratification of patients with gynecologic malignancies: what the

radiologist needs to know. Radiology 2013;266(3): 717–40.
46. Koh W-J, Greer BE, Abu-Rustum NR, et al. Cervical Cancer NCCN Guideline, Version 2. 2017.
47. Kusmirek J, Robbins J, Allen H, et al. PET/CT and MRI in the imaging assessment of cervical cancer. Abdom Imaging 2015;40(7):2486–511.
48. Reinhardt MJ, Ehritt-Braun C, Vogelgesang D, et al. Metastatic Lymph Nodes in Patients with Cervical Cancer: Detection with MR Imaging and FDG PET. Radiology 2001;218(3):776–82.
49. Hricak H, Gatsonis C, Chi DS, et al. Role of Imaging in Pretreatment Evaluation of Early Invasive Cervical Cancer: Results of the Intergroup Study American College of Radiology Imaging Network 6651–Gynecologic Oncology Group 183. J Clin Oncol 2005;23(36):9329–37.
50. Rockall AG, Ghosh S, Alexander-Sefre F, et al. Can MRI rule out bladder and rectal invasion in cervical cancer to help select patients for limited EUA? Gynecol Oncol 2006;101(2):244–9.
51. Wu C, Lu L, Liu Y, et al. Evaluating MRI, CT, PET/CT in detection of lymph node status in cervical cancer: a meta-analysis. Int J Clin Exp Med 2016; 9(6):9917–31.
52. Ho K-C, Lin G, Wang J-J, et al. Correlation of apparent diffusion coefficients measured by 3T diffusion-weighted MRI and SUV from FDG PET/ CT in primary cervical cancer. Eur J Nucl Med Mol Imaging 2009;36(2):200–8.
53. Kim S-K, Choi HJ, Park S-Y, et al. Additional value of MR/PET fusion compared with PET/CT in the detection of lymph node metastases in cervical cancer patients. Eur J Cancer 2009;45(12):2103–9.
54. Miller TR, Grigsby PW. Measurement of tumor volume by PET to evaluate prognosis in patients with advanced cervical cancer treated by radiation therapy. Int J Radiat Oncol Biol Phys 2002;53(2):353–9.
55. Kidd EA, Naqa El I, Siegel BA, et al. FDG-PET-based prognostic nomograms for locally advanced cervical cancer. Gynecol Oncol 2012;127(1):136–40.
56. Sarker A, Im H-J, Cheon GJ, et al. Prognostic implications of the SUVmax of primary tumors and metastatic lymph node measured by 18F-FDG PET in patients with uterine cervical cancer: a meta-analysis. Clin Nucl Med 2016;41(1):34–40.
57. Sala E, Micco M, Burger IA, et al. Complementary prognostic value of pelvic magnetic resonance imaging and whole-body fluorodeoxyglucose Positron Emission Tomography/Computed Tomography in the pretreatment assessment of patients with cervical cancer. Int J Gynecol Cancer 2015;25(8):1461–7.
58. Grigsby PW, Siegel BA, Dehdashti F, et al. Posttherapy [18F] fluorodeoxyglucose positron emission tomography in carcinoma of the cervix: response and outcome. J Clin Oncol 2004;22(11):2167–71.
59. Schwarz JK, Siegel BA, Dehdashti F, et al. Association of posttherapy positron emission tomography with tumor response and survival in cervical carcinoma. JAMA 2007;298(19):2289–95.
60. Beddy P, Rangarajan RD. Sala E Role of MRI in intracavitary brachytherapy for cervical cancer: what the radiologist needs to know. AJR Am J Roentgenol 2011;196(3):W341–7.
61. Park JJ, Kim CK, Park BK. Prognostic value of diffusion-weighted magnetic resonance imaging and (18)F-fluorodeoxyglucose-positron emission tomography/computed tomography after concurrent chemoradiotherapy in uterine cervical cancer. Radiother Oncol 2016;120(3):507–11.
62. Havrilesky LJ, Kulasingam SL, Matchar DB, et al. FDG-PET for management of cervical and ovarian cancer. Gynecol Oncol 2005;97(1):183–91.
63. Sakurai H, Suzuki Y, Nonaka T, et al. FDG-PET in the detection of recurrence of uterine cervical carcinoma following radiation therapy—tumor volume and FDG uptake value. Gynecol Oncol 2006; 100(3):601–7.
64. Meads C, Davenport C, Małysiak S, et al. Evaluating PET-CT in the detection and management of recurrent cervical cancer: systematic reviews of diagnostic accuracy and subjective elicitation. BJOG 2013;121(4):398–407.
65. Auguste P, Barton P, Meads C, et al. Evaluating PET-CT in routine surveillance and follow-up after treatment for cervical cancer: a cost-effectiveness analysis. BJOG 2013;121(4):464–76.
66. Chan JK, Cheung MK, Huh WK, et al. Therapeutic role of lymph node resection in endometrioid corpus cancer. Cancer 2006;107(8):1823–30.
67. National Comprehensive Cancer Network. NCCN clinical practice guidelines in oncology (NCCN guidelines): uterine neoplasms. Version 2. 2016. 2016.
68. Rockall AG, Meroni R, Sohaib SA, et al. Evaluation of endometrial carcinoma on magnetic resonance imaging. Int J Gynecol Cancer 2007;17(1):188–96.
69. Kitajima K, Suenaga Y, Ueno Y, et al. Value of fusion of PET and MRI for staging of endometrial cancer: Comparison with 18F-FDG contrast-enhanced PET/CT and dynamic contrast-enhanced pelvic MRI. Eur J Radiol 2013;82(10):1672–6.
70. Erkanli S, Ayhan A. Fertility-sparing therapy in young women with endometrial cancer: 2010 update. Int J Gynecol Cancer 2010;20(7):1170–87.
71. Kakhki VRD, Shahriari S, Treglia G, et al. Diagnostic performance of fluorine 18 fluorodeoxyglucose positron emission tomography imaging for detection of primary lesion and staging of endometrial cancer patients: systematic review and meta-analysis of the literature. Int J Gynecol Cancer 2013;23(9):1536.
72. Bollineni VR, Ytre-Hauge S, Bollineni-Balabay O, et al. High diagnostic value of 18F-FDG PET/CT

in endometrial cancer: systematic review and meta-analysis of the literature. J Nucl Med 2016; 57(6):879–85.
73. Kim HJ, Cho A, Yun M, et al. Comparison of FDG PET/CT and MRI in lymph node staging of endometrial cancer. Ann Nucl Med 2016;30(2):104–13.
74. Ghooshkhanei H, Treglia G, Sabouri G, et al. Risk stratification and prognosis determination using 18F-FDG PET imaging in endometrial cancer patients: A systematic review and meta-analysis. Gynecol Oncol 2014;132(3):669–76.
75. Shih IL, Yen RF, Chen CA, et al. Standardized uptake value and apparent diffusion coefficient of endometrial cancer evaluated with integrated whole-body PET/MR: Correlation with pathological prognostic factors. J Magn Reson Imaging 2015; 42(6):1723–32.
76. Kadkhodayan S, Shahriari S, Treglia G, et al. Accuracy of 18-F-FDG PET imaging in the follow up of endometrial cancer patients: systematic review and meta-analysis of the literature. Gynecol Oncol 2013;128(2):397–404.
77. Morgan RJ, Armstrong DK, Alvarez RD, et al. Ovarian cancer, Version 1.2016, NCCN clinical practice guidelines in oncology. J Natl Compr Canc Netw 2016;14(9):1134–63.
78. Castellucci P, Perrone AM, Picchio M, et al. Diagnostic accuracy of 18F-FDG PET/CT in characterizing ovarian lesions and staging ovarian cancer: Correlation with transvaginal ultrasonography, computed tomography, and histology. Nucl Med Commun 2007;28(8):589–95.
79. Lopez-Lopez V, Cascales-Campos PA, Gil J, et al. Use of (18)F-FDG PET/CT in the preoperative evaluation of patients diagnosed with peritoneal carcinomatosis of ovarian origin, candidates to cytoreduction and hipec. A pending issue. Eur J Radiol 2016;85(10):1824–8.
80. Ricke J, Sehouli J, Hach C, et al. Prospective evaluation of contrast-enhanced MRI in the depiction of peritoneal spread in primary or recurrent ovarian cancer. Eur Radiol 2003;13(5):943–9.
81. Tempany CM, Zou KH, Silverman SG, et al. Staging of advanced ovarian cancer: comparison of imaging modalities–report from the Radiological Diagnostic Oncology Group. Radiology 2000;215(3):761–7.
82. Kinkel K, Lu Y, Mehdizade A, et al. Indeterminate ovarian mass at US: incremental value of second imaging test for characterization—meta-analysis and bayesian analysis. Radiology 2005;236(1): 85–94.
83. Risum S, Høgdall C, Loft A, et al. The diagnostic value of PET/CT for primary ovarian cancer—A prospective study. Gynecol Oncol 2007;105(1):145–9.
84. Park T, Lee S, Park S, et al. Value of 18F-FDG PET/CT in the detection of ovarian malignancy. Nucl Med Mol Imaging 2014;49(1):42–51.
85. Yamamoto M, Tsujikawa T, Fujita Y, et al. Metabolic tumor burden predicts prognosis of ovarian cancer patients who receive platinum-based adjuvant chemotherapy. Cancer Sci 2016;107(4): 478–85.
86. Lee M, Lee H, Cheon GJ, et al. Prognostic value of preoperative intratumoral FDG uptake heterogeneity in patients with epithelial ovarian cancer. Eur Radiol 2016;27:1–8.
87. Kyriazi S, Collins DJ, Messiou C, et al. Metastatic ovarian and primary peritoneal cancer: assessing chemotherapy response with diffusion-weighted MR imaging—value of histogram analysis of apparent diffusion coefficients. Radiology 2011; 261(1):182–92.
88. Vallius T, Peter A, Auranen A, et al. 18F-FDG-PET/CT can identify histopathological non-responders to platinum-based neoadjuvant chemotherapy in advanced epithelial ovarian cancer. Gynecol Oncol 2016;140(1):29–35.
89. Dragosavac S. Staging recurrent ovarian cancer with 18FDG PET/CT. Oncol Lett 2012;5(2):593–7.
90. Khan N, Oriuchi N, Yosmzaki A, et al. Diagnostic accuracy of FDG PET imaging for the detection of recurrent or metastatic gynecologic cancer. Ann Nucl Med 2005;19(2):137–45.
91. Han EJ, Park HL, Lee YS, et al. Clinical usefulness of post-treatment FDG PET/CT in patients with ovarian malignancy. Ann Nucl Med 2016;30:600–7.
92. Tawakol A, Abdelhafez YG, Osama A, et al. Diagnostic performance of 18F-FDG PET/contrast-enhanced CT versus contrast-enhanced CT alone for post-treatment detection of ovarian malignancy. Nucl Med Commun 2016;37(5):453–60.
93. Kim CK, Park BK, Choi JY, et al. Detection of recurrent ovarian cancer at mri: comparison with integrated PET/CT. J Comput Assist Tomogr 2007; 31(6):868–75.
94. Queiroz MA, Kubik-Huch RA, Hauser N, et al. PET/MRI and PET/CT in advanced gynaecological tumours: initial experience and comparison. Eur Radiol 2015;25(8):2222–30.
95. Beiderwellen K, Grueneisen J, Ruhlmann V, et al. [18F]FDG PET/MRI vs. PET/CT for whole-body staging in patients with recurrent malignancies of the female pelvis: initial results. Eur J Nucl Med Mol Imaging 2014;42(1):56–65.
96. Stecco A, Buemi F, Cassarà A, et al. Comparison of retrospective PET and MRI-DWI (PET/MRI-DWI) image fusion with PET/CT and MRI-DWI in detection of cervical and endometrial cancer lymph node metastases. Radiol Med 2016;121(7):537–45.
97. Grueneisen J, Schaarschmidt BM, Heubner M, et al. Implementation of FAST-PET/MRI for whole-body staging of female patients with recurrent pelvic malignancies: A comparison to PET/CT. Eur J Radiol 2015;84(11):2097–102.

98. Kitajima K, Suenaga Y, Ueno Y, et al. Value of fusion of PET and MRI in the detection of intra-pelvic recurrence of gynecological tumor: comparison with 18F-FDG contrast-enhanced PET/CT and pelvic MRI. Ann Nucl Med 2014;28(1):25–32.
99. Melsaether AN, Raad RA, Pujara AC, et al. Comparison of Whole-Body 18F FDG PET/MR Imaging and Whole-Body 18F FDG PET/CT in Terms of Lesion Detection and Radiation Dose in Patients with Breast Cancer. Radiology 2016;281(1):193–202.
100. Grueneisen J, Schaarschmidt BM, Beiderwellen K, et al. Diagnostic value of diffusion-weighted imaging in simultaneous 18F-FDG PET/MR imaging for whole-body staging of women with pelvic malignancies. J Nucl Med 2014;55(12):1930–5.
101. Buchbender C, Hartung-Knemeyer V, Beiderwellen K, et al. Diffusion-weighted imaging as part of hybrid PET/MRI protocols for whole-body cancer staging: Does it benefit lesion detection? Eur J Radiol 2013;82(5):877–82.
102. Pinker K, Andrzejewski P, Baltzer P, et al. Multiparametric [18F]Fluorodeoxyglucose/[18F]Fluoromisonidazole Positron Emission Tomography/Magnetic Resonance imaging of locally advanced cervical cancer for the non-invasive detection of tumor heterogeneity: a pilot study. PLoS One 2016;11(5):e0155333.
103. Schuetz M, Schmid MP, Pötter R, et al. Evaluating repetitive 18F-fluoroazomycin-arabinoside (18FAZA) PET in the setting of MRI guided adaptive radiotherapy in cervical cancer. Acta Oncol 2010;49(7):941–7.
104. Lewis JS, Laforest R, Dehdashti F, et al. An imaging comparison of 64Cu-ATSM and 60Cu-ATSM in cancer of the uterine cervix. J Nucl Med 2008;49(7):1177–82.
105. Wernicke AG, Kim S, Liu H, et al. Prostate-specific Membrane Antigen (PSMA) Expression in the Neovasculature of Gynecologic Malignancies: Implications for PSMA-targeted Therapy. Appl Immunohistochem Mol Morphol 2016;1. http://dx.doi.org/10.1097/PAI.0000000000000297.
106. Harisinghani MG, Dixon WT, Saksena MA, et al. MR Lymphangiography: Imaging Strategies to Optimize the Imaging of Lymph Nodes with Ferumoxtran-10. RadioGraphics 2004;24(3):867–78.
107. Turkbey B, Agarwal HK, Shih J, et al. A phase I dosing study of ferumoxytol for MR lymphography at 3 T in patients with prostate cancer. Am J Roentgenol 2015;205(1):64–9.
108. Witney TH, Brindle KM. Imaging tumour cell metabolism using hyperpolarized 13C magnetic resonance spectroscopy. Biochem Soc Trans 2010;38(5):1220–4.
109. Zhang H. The potential of hyperpolarized 13C MRI in assessing signaling pathways in cancer. Acad Radiol 2014;21(2):215–22.
110. Nelson SJ, Kurhanewicz J, Vigneron DB, et al. Metabolic imaging of patients with prostate cancer using hyperpolarized [1-13C]Pyruvate. Sci Transl Med 2013;5(198):198ra108.
111. Han K, Croke J, Foltz W, et al. A prospective study of DWI, DCE-MRI and FDG PET imaging for target delineation in brachytherapy for cervical cancer. Radiother Oncol 2016;120(3):519–25.
112. Knoll F, Koesters T, Otazo R, et al. Joint reconstruction of simultaneously acquired MR-PET data with multi sensor compressed sensing based on a joint sparsity constraint. EJNMMI Phys 2014;1(1):A26.

Printed and bound by CPI Group (UK) Ltd, Croydon, CR0 4YY
08/05/2025
01864701-0006